DATE DUE

Demco, Inc. 38-293

Magnetic Resonance in the Diagnosis of C.N.S. Disorders

Vaso Antunović, M.D., Ph.D.
Professor of Neurosurgery
Institute for Neurosurgery
Clinical Center of Serbia
School of Medicine
University of Belgrade
Belgrade, Yugoslavia

Gradimir Dragutinović, M.D., Ph.D.
Assistant Professor of Radiology
Institute for Radiology
Clinical Center of Serbia
School of Medicine
University of Belgrade
Belgrade, Yugoslavia

Zvonimir Lević, M.D., Ph.D.
Professor of Neurology
Institute for Neurology
Clinical Center of Serbia
School of Medicine
University of Belgrade
Belgrade, Yugoslavia

Miroslav Samardzić, M.D., Ph.D.
Professor of Neurosurgery
Institute for Neurosurgery
Clinical Center of Serbia
School of Medicine
University of Belgrade
Belgrade, Yugoslavia

330 illustrations

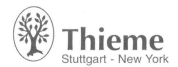 Thieme
Stuttgart - New York

 CIC Edizioni Internazionali - *Rome, 2001*

Important note:
Medicine is an ever-changing science undergoing continual development. Research and clinical experience are continually expanding our knowledge, in particular our knowledge of proper treatment and drug therapy. Insofar as this book mentions any dosage or application, readers may rest assured that the authors, editors and publishers have made every effort to ensure that such references are in accordance with the state of knowledge at the time of production of the book.

Nevertheless this does not involve, imply, or express any guarantee or responsibility on the part of the publishers in respect of any dosage instructions and forms of application stated in the book. Every user is requested to examine carefully the manufacturers' leaflets accompanying each drug and to check, if necessary in consultation with a physician or specialist, whether the dosage schedules mentioned therein or the contraindications stated by the manufacturers differ from the statements made in the present book. Such examination is particularly important with drugs that are either rarely used or have been newly released on the market. Every dosage schedule or every form of application used is entirely at the user's own risk and responsibility. The authors and publishers request every user to report to the publishers any discrepancies or inaccurancies noticed.

© Copyright 2001

 CIC Edizioni Internazionali

Corso Trieste, 42 - 00198 Rome, Italy
www.gruppocic.it

ISBN 88-7141-444-6

Distribution rights outside of Italy
Georg Thieme Verlag
Stuttgart, New York

ISBN 3-13-129781-6   (GTV)
ISBN 1-58890-073-8   (TNY)

CONTENTS

VIII. TUMORS OF THE CRANIOCERVICAL JUNCTION 171
Gradimir Dragutinović, Miodrag Rakić, Ljiljana Djordjić

IX. EXTRACRANIAL TUMORS WITH INTRACRANIAL PROPAGATION 177
Vaso Antunović, Gradimir Dragutinović, Ivan Piščević

X. TUMORS OF THE HYPOPHYSIS 183
Gradimir Dragutinović, Vaso Antunović, Miroslav Samardzić

XI. TEMPORAL LOBE EPILEPSY 197
Zvonimir Lević, Gradimir Dragutinović, Lukas Rasulić

EDITORS AND CONTRIBUTORS

Vaso Antunović, M.D., Ph.D.
Professor of Neurosurgery
Institute for Neurosurgery
Clinical Center of Serbia
School of Medicine
University of Belgrade
Belgrade, Yugoslavia

Ljiljana Djordjić, M.D., M.Sc.
Assistant in Neurosurgery
Institute for Neurosurgery
Clinical Center of Serbia
School of Medicine
University of Belgrade
Belgrade, Yugoslavia

Gradimir Dragutinović, M.D., Ph.D.
Assistant Professor of Radiology
Institute for Radiology
Clinical Center of Serbia
School of Medicine
University of Belgrade
Belgrade, Yugoslavia

Zvonimir Lević, M.D., Ph.D.
Professor of Neurology
Institute for Neurology
Clinical Center of Serbia
School of Medicine
University of Belgrade
Belgrade, Yugoslavia

Branislav Nestorović, M.D., Ph.D.
Associate Professor of Neurosurgery
Institute for Neurosurgery
Clinical Center of Serbia
School of Medicine
University of Belgrade
Belgrade, Yugoslavia

Ivan Piščević, M.D.
Assistant in Neurosurgery
Institute for Neurosurgery
Clinical Center of Serbia
School of Medicine
University of Belgrade
Belgrade, Yugoslavia

Miodrag Rakić, M.D., Ph.D.
Assistant Professor of Neurosurgery
Institute for Neurosurgery
Clinical Center of Serbia
School of Medicine
University of Belgrade
Belgrade, Yugoslavia

Lukas Rasulić, M.D., Ph.D.
Assistant in Neurosurgery
Institute for Neurosurgery
Clinical Center of Serbia
School of Medicine
University of Belgrade
Belgrade, Yugoslavia

Miroslav Samardzić, M.D., Ph.D.
Professor of Neurosurgery
Institute for Neurosurgery
Clinical Center of Serbia
School of Medicine
University of Belgrade
Belgrade, Yugoslavia

INTRODUCTION

An introduction of CT and MRI methods resulted in revolutionary changes in the imaging of central nervous systems diseases. The reliability of the use of MRI in the diagnosis of neurological disorders enabled accurate localization, visualization, and anatomical relation and determination of the nature of different pathological processes in the brain and spinal cord.

In the past, it had been very difficult to make such precise diagnosis. A result of this fact is a great improvement of treatment of the patients with C.N.S. disorders. The other advantages are excellent possibilities for an assessment of the results of the therapeutical procedures and accurate follow-up of the cases. This was the resason that the Authors wanted to make a review of the MRI and clinical characteristics of different neurological and neurosurgical conditions from their wide clinical practice and to determine and illustrate the importance of MRI in the diseases of the brain and spinal cord.

THE AUTHORS

A. MAGNETIC RESONANCE IN THE DIAGNOSIS OF THE BRAIN AND CRANIO-CERVICAL JUNCTION PATHOLOGY

Gradimir Dragutinović, Vaso Antunović

GENERAL PRINCIPLES

1. Introduction

Neuroradiologic examinations are very important for the diagnosis of the C.N.S. disorders. Development of the new radiological methods, as well as the improvement of the older ones, have contributed to the accuracy of the neurologic diagnosis.

Examination of the skeletal disorders became possible due to Conrad Roentgens discovery of the X rays in 1885, in Wurzburg. Numerous congenital or acquired disorders of the cranial and facial bones, and spinal vertebrae as well, could be seen in standard or special radiographs (special views, head positions or polytomography).

The application of positive or negative contrast was needed to visualize the soft tissue of the nervous system.

Pneumoencephalography (PEG) is a method of radiological imaging of the brain ventricles and cisterns, following intrathecal injection of the air through a lumbar or suboccipital puncture.

Mini gas cisternography is a variety of PEG, when a single cerebral cistern (pontocerebellar, suprasellar, etc.) is displayed by intrathecal application of 2-5 ml of air. Cisternography and ventriculography can be done using positive (iodine) contrast as well. They were used in the past to reveal intracranial tumors. The diagnosis was based on dislocation and morphological changes of the ventricular system, filled with either positive or negative contrast. They are seldom used nowadays.

Cerebral angiography with iodine contrast enables the direct display of the blood vessels in the brain. Panangiographic catheterization is a useful method to visualize both carotid and vertebral arteries simultaneously.

The computer assisted subtraction of the bone structures, as well as endo- and extracranial soft tissue, have improved angiography a great deal, enabling the smallest vessels to be seen. All three phases of the blood circulation: arterial, parenchymatous and venous, should be recorded during cerebral angiography in order to reveal possible disorders of the arteries and veins, including the tiniest blood vessels. Intracranial expansion should be suspected if pathologic blood vessels or dislocation of the brain arteries are found.

Direct puncture of the carotid or vertebral arteries is no longer used, except in a few small or modestly equipped hospitals, for the emergency diagnosis, if post-traumatic or spontaneous intracranial hemorrhage is suspected, because of the "mass" effect seen in standard radiographs.

Introduction of computerized tomography by Dr. James Ambrous, from Atkinson Morley Hospital in England on October 1st 1971, has revolutionized radiological diagnosis thoroughly. Direct visualization of CNS structures became possible. The inventors of the computerized tomography A. Cormac and G. Hounsfield were awarded Nobel prize in 1979.

Introduction of new techniques have improved computerized axial tomography (CAT) during the past decade. Intravenous administration of the iodine contrast have contributed to the precision of CT diagnosis (23).

Extended scale have enabled better visualization of the finest details of normal and pathologic bone.

Software applications such as Exam, Arrange, etc. have made the reconstruction of the adverse planes possible. Perpendicular, paraxial or oblique planes could be synthesized from the coronal or axial computer tomographs. Pictures obtained by computer reconstruction are of sufficient quality to make a diagnosis of various CNS disorders.

Direct coronal view enables the visualization of the sellar region, without the peril of the radiation damage to the eyes.

Dynamic CT have contributed to the better diagnosis of the tiniest CNS lesions, using computer assisted numeric and graphic analysis of the circulation (5, 9).

CT examination, with the application of the double contrast (intravenous iodine and intrathecal air), have enabled the diagnosis of the smallest tumors in the pontocerebellar angle or "Empty sella" syndrome.

The above mentioned possibilities and additional technological options, such as measurement of the tissue density, delineation, marking or slicing, have made the computerized tomography an indispensable method in radiology.

Contemporary CT scanners can make precise images using finest slices, 3D reconstruction or blood vessel visualization. The examination can be completed in a few seconds which is very important for the patients with head trauma, uncooperative adults or children.

Magnetic resonance is a contemporary method of the direct tissue imaging, without the use of X rays, (NMR - Nuclear Magnetic Resonance; MRI - Magnetic Resonance Imaging; KST - Kern Spin Tomographie).

2. History

The effect of the nuclear magnetic resonance in the molecular bounds was discovered in 1938 by I.R. Rabi. He was awarded Nobel prize in 1944 for his discovery.

Felix Bloch in 1946 performed the first successful spectroscopic experiment by putting his own finger in the middle of the coil, thus enabling spectrometry with intensive proton signal of the magnetic resonance. The following nuclei were used for the magnetic resonance experiments: 31-P, 19-F, 2-H, 13-C, 14-N, 15-N, 23-Na and 24-Si (4).

Gabillard have reported dynamic studies on ordinary glass and different fluids behavior in the magnetic gradient fields. The theory of NMR in inhomogenous fields, developed by Hahn, was the basic principle of the SPIN-ECHO method, used for the measurement of molecular diffusion in fluids, and NMR tomography as well (18).

The first two-dimensional image, caused by the effect of nucleus density in the patient exposed to a magnetic field, was obtained by Damadijan in 1971 (12).

Direct imaging of the neural structures by computed tomography was impetus for numerous investigations and innovations in the imaging techniques, especially in NMR technology.

Principles of CT technique, developed by Hounsfield and Mc Cormmac, were transferred to NMR by Paul Lauterbur in New York in 1973. Practical application of the same planes and views gave the first MR image (6).

NMR tomography was tremendously improved by the application of two-dimensional Fourier transformation (2-D FT) thus obtaining high quality three dimensional images of tissues and organs.

First commercially available NMR machines were very weak, only 0.15-0.3 Tesla (1). Nowadays much stronger machines are used in clinical practice (0.5-1.5 T), while the experimental machines have reached 4.7 T at the moment (Fig. 1).

Patient movements (respiration, heart beat, peristaltic, etc.) could blur the image. Brain and spine imaging were the first applications of Magnetic Resonance in clinical use. Nowadays 75-80% of MR examinations are used for the neurologic diagnosis. The reason for this is the relative inaccessibility of the brain, as compared to other organs and tissues, to any other method of investigation.

Auxiliary techniques can be applied in order to synchronize MRI with the heart beat (**Cardiac triggering**), or respiration (**Respiratory gating**), thus avoiding artifacts. The imaging of the internal organs such as heart, lungs, abdominal or pelvic organs should be done that way.

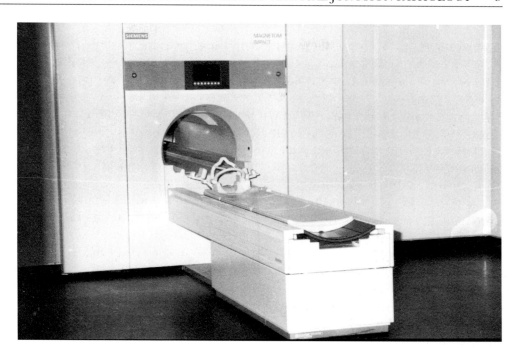

Figure 1. Magnetic Resonance Machine.

3. Operating principles of the Magnetic Resonance

Nuclear particles, protons and neutrons have a spin with mechanical and magnetic momentum. The particle is a dipole, spinning around the axis. Any nucleus with an odd number of protons or neutrons has a spin and nuclear magnetic resonance. Static magnetic field can cause the transfer of spins from one level to another, followed by energy absorption or release. Spin transfer can be induced by oscillating magnetic field provided that the energy of the field corresponds to the difference of the energetic levels induced by a static magnetic field (resonance).

Pulsed radiofrequency (**RF**) can activate the spin system by a short RF signal. When the pulse is discontinued, the spins tend to recover equilibrium, thus inducing electromotor power in the coil around the specimen (head, for example). The signal, proportional to the resultant transversal magnetization, can be detected. Free Induction Decay (**FID**), or transversal relaxation in the homogenous field, is an exponential function of the characteristic time **T2**. The spectrum of a specimen is computed from that signal using Fourier transformation (**FT NMR**) (20).

Once the **RF** pulse is discontinued, the energy, previously absorbed by the spins, is released. The exchange of the energy between the spins and environment is defined by the time **T1** (longitudinal relaxation) (27).

Hydrogen nucleus is essential for the NMR tomography of the human body, because it has one proton and is widely represented all over the body. The term "nuclear" is usually avoided in order to distinguish this diagnostic procedure from the procedures based on nuclear radiation. In Germany the term Kern-spin (Nuclear-spin) tomographie is widely used.

NMR tomography should reconstruct tomographs of different body sections, by location analysis of all the spin signals in the specimen (water protons for example). The space resolution in the homogenous magnetic field is impossible, because each spin has identical resonant frequency. Additional gradient magnetic fields can contribute to the space resolution of the spins, because the resonant frequency is defined by the location and field gradient. Position of a spin can be determined upon the known gradient through frequency and signal phase measurements. Frequency and signal phase are distinguished in time by two- dimensional Fourier transformation (**2D-FT**) of the NMR signal, so that 2D image, like in CT, can be obtained (30).

The CT scan is recorded by detecting the intensity of the narrow band of X-rays, leaving the object, and that is the basic difference between CT and MR. CT is limited to the transversal sections only. Two dimensional image is computed from the volume units - voxels, thus enabling the measurement of the tissue density. The density depends on the slide thickness and can be measured in Hounsfield units.

According to the standard values for normal and pathologic tissue density, a CNS lesion could be defined as either isodense, hypo- or hyperdense, as compared to the normal neural tissue. Inadequate choice of the slide thickness can cause false positive or false negative findings (15).

Software options of contemporary high resolution CT scanners, can reconstruct sagittal and coronal planes upon the image obtained from the axial plane. It takes the experienced neuroradiologist to distinguish between relevant lesions and normal tissue, upon the density values given by a computer.

Magnetic resonance image does not depend on the section plane, direction of a beam or the extent of the examined area, because three orthogonal gradients can be positioned in every possible plane and fully controlled by the operator.

The data obtained from the 3D unit voxel (cm or mm) are transferred to the 2D image consisting of pixels (square). The resolution of the image depends on the matrix size. The bigger matrix is needed for the better resolution. The pixel intensity in CT scan depends only on electron density, while in MRI it depends on proton density, relaxation time T1 and T2, and the water flow as well.

T1 and T2 are determined by the tissue characteristics (water contents, protein and macromolecule quantity, structure, etc.) and the operating frequency as well. T1 depends on the velocity (natural frequency) of the water molecules, influenced by the magnetic field intensity. Different pulse sequences, chosen by an operator, can help to distinguish between two tissues. For example, in the widely accepted Spin-echo sequence the relevant parameters are TR (Repetition time) and TE (Echo time). Adjustment of TR and TE ratio can contribute to the contrast between two tissues with different T1 and T2 relaxation times. The difference in water contents of only 10% can be potentiated by the relaxation time difference of up to 200% (18).

Depending on the TR and TE choice, the MRI can be T1 weighted (T-1W, short TR and TE) or T2 weighted (T-2W, long TR and TE). All the tissues with long T1 will give hypointensive image in T-1W, whereas the tissues with long T2 (which is more often the case) will look hyperintensive in T-2W image (8, 30).

The contrast of the image is influenced by TR and TE ratio that could be combined in different ways, in order to improve diagnostic possibilities.

A lot of different images can be obtained through the combination of sequences, slices, thickness and distance. The interpretation of the gray scale image is influenced by the proton response of a tissue, depending on TR and TE, as well as on the other parameters.

Special sequences, such as FLASH 2D or Inversion Recovery, can be useful for the differential diagnosis of certain lesions. The manufacturers of MR machines and software tend to use different names for such procedures. The names of the sequences quoted in this text are based on the following equipment: Magnetom Imact Expert 1.0 T and Magnetom Siemens 2.0 T (16).

Images of tissues or organs, obtained in different MR sequences, are displayed in the gray scale monitors and defined by a signal intensity. In spite of the signal intensity measurements, individual variability makes the unification of standard normal and pathologic values impossible. This is true, regardless of the tissue or organ involved. It takes an experienced radiologist to interpret the MR findings and evaluate the diverse signal intensities of the lesions, due to different MR sequences (19).

The ratio between the density parameters obtained by CT scan and signal intensity by MR is 1:300, which means that MRI is far more accurate and selective displaying the finest tissue details or lesions whatsoever. Certain MR sequences can reveal some features of the pathologic lesion which can not be seen on the CT scan at al. (12, 13).

The new generation of the MR machines is enriched by 3D reconstruction and MR angiography options. Computer analysis of the MR image enables the neuroradiologist to obtain the best possible differentiation of the lesion from the data stored in the computer, by using optimal planes and slice thickness and changing the conditions long after the patient has left.

Improved software has a lot of advantages for the patient, because of the short examination time as well as for the neuroradiologist, because of the numerous possibilities of image reconstructions and refinements of the data base.

Introduction of the 3D non-invasive MR angiography, have enabled the detailed visualization of the blood vessels, thus avoiding the invasive cerebral or other angiography. However, the need for classic angiography can not be ruled out completely.

MR spectroscopy is done in order to define the specific spectrum of the organic or inorganic components in the tissues or organs. The spectral shift of certain elements, such as sodium or phosphorus, can contribute to the diagnosis of disorders or tissue malfunction. The spectral analysis of phosphorus enables the monitoring of the cell metabolism through adenosine triphosphate, phosphocreatin or inorganic phosphorus. It gives endless possibilities for monitoring of the finest biochemistry changes in tissues and organs, enabling the early diagnosis and analysis of the cellular structure. Its medical application is still experimental at the moment.

4. Magnetic Resonance imaging of the normal anatomy structures

Following sequences have been used in the Magnetic Resonance Center of the Clinical Center of Serbia in Belgrade: **T-1W**, double echo **T-2W**, **Proton Density**, as well as special rapid sequences such as **FLASH** and **FISP**. We would like to explain **Inversion recovery** mode used for the measurement of T1 and obtaining T1 weighted image. It has 180-t-90 pulsed frequency and it is seldom used (29).

The anatomic morphology could be optimally displayed in T-1W sequence, using gray scale (11). It is used for a perfect display of the morphology or topographic relationships, as well as malformations or normal varieties in tissues and organs (Figg. 2-4).

T-2W and **Proton density** are used for obtaining necessary slides, according to the proton density/ T2 ratio, usually 15/90. This sequence takes 2,5-10 minutes, but the images from both sequences can be simultaneously displayed enabling the comparison of the details revealed by **T-2W** and **Proton density** (12).

The characteristic of T-2W sequence is the intensive signal from fluids or pathologic tissue. Most lesions have prolonged T-2W, compared to the normal brain tissue. It could be explained by the fact that T-2W ratio of the normal tissue and tumor, for example, is bigger than T-1W ratio (3).

Decreased signal- to- noise ratio makes T-2W sequence very good for the display of the normal anatomic structure morphology. The signal intensity of the calcifications, iron incrustations, air or even some tumors can be changed, or similar to those obtained in T-1W sequence (Figg. 5, 6).

Relations of the tissue structures in **Proton density** are similar to those in **T-1W** sequence, but pathologic lesions can have more or less enhanced signal intensity, which should be kept in mind during the evaluation of the findings of all applied sequences (Figg. 7, 8).

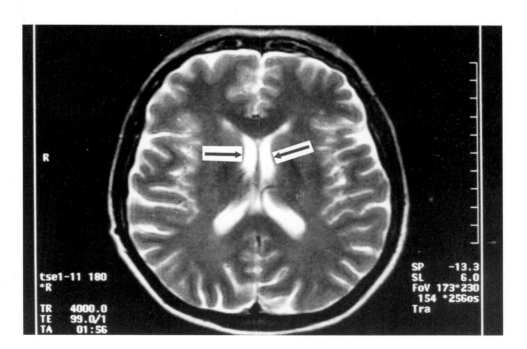

Figure 2. MR image of the normal brain structure, Axial image (SE 560/15). Arrows pointing at lateral ventricles (LV).

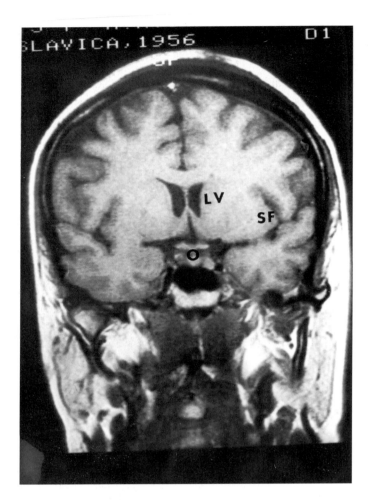

Figure 3. MR image of the normal brain structure. Coronal image (SE 500/15). LV-lateral ventricles, O-optic chiasm, SF-, S- Silvius-Rolandic fissure.

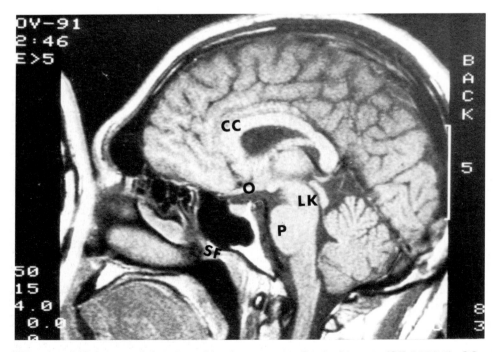

Figure 4. MR image of the normal brain structure. Sagittal image (SE 500/15). CC-corpus callosum, LK- lamina quadrigemina, P-pons, O-optic chiasm, SF- sphenoidal sinus.

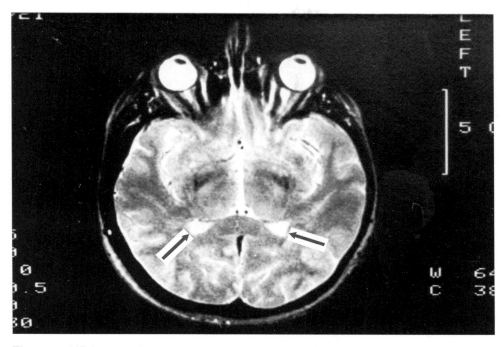

Figure 5. MR image of the normal brain structure. Axial image (SE 2500/90). Arrow pointing at the third brain ventricle - III V. Arrows LK- occipital cornu of the lateral brain ventricles.

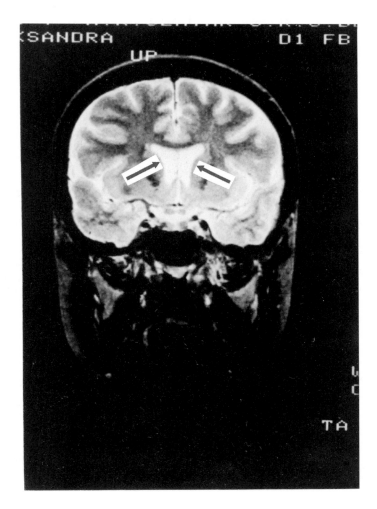

Figure 6. MR image of the normal brain structure. Coronal image (SE 2500/90). Arrows pointing at lateral ventricles- LK.

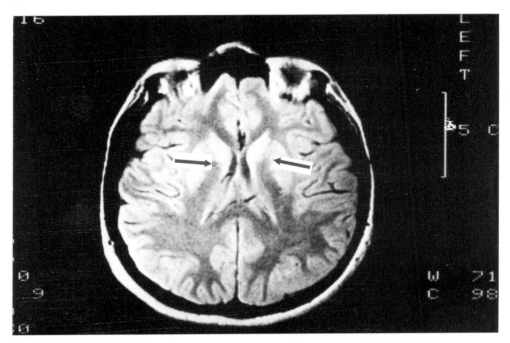

Figure 7. MR image of the normal brain structure. Axial image (SE 2500/15). Arrows pointing lateral ventricles - LK.

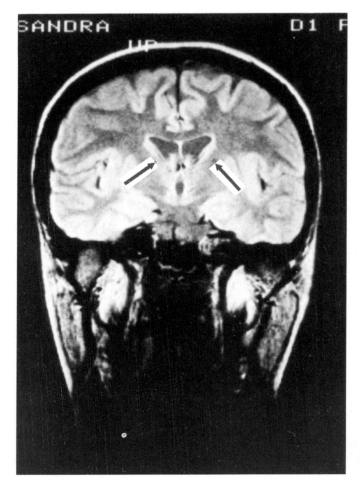

Figure 8. MR image of the normal brain structure. Coronal image (SE 2500/15). Arrows pointing lateral ventricles - LK. Arrow pointing third ventricle- III K.

The different signal intensities of the same tumor obtained by application of three different sequences in the same axial section, show the influence of the technical conditions on the MR image of the normal and pathologic tissue (Figg. 9-11).

Special rapid sequences (GRE), such as **FLASH, FISP** or their varieties can be used to clarify certain pathologic lesions. The names of those sequences depend on the manufacturers of the equipment. Improvement of the basic parameters and introduction of the additional ones have made the application of the rapid sequences used for delineation of certain features of the lesions possible. The imaging can be done in few seconds with a limited number of slices (18).

The comparison of the same blood collection of the left temporal intracerebral hematoma recorded in T-1W and FISP sequences is made to show the possibility of revealing the hemosiderin edge in the neighboring area, the proof of the slow blood flow (Fig. 12).

The blood collection is seen in the coronal plane in T-2W sequence. Differential diagnosis of lipoma, teratoma, etc. should be ruled out.

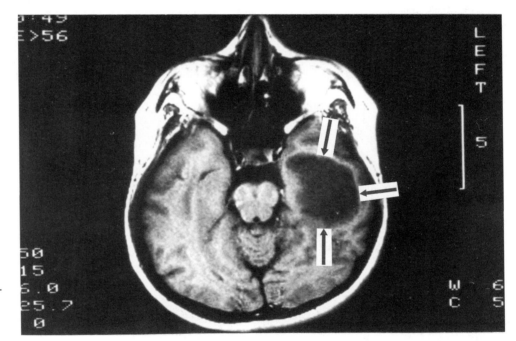

Figure 9. MR image of the brain of the patient B.S. Axial image (SE 500/15) Arrows pointing to the invasive tumor of the left temporobasal region with low signal intensity.

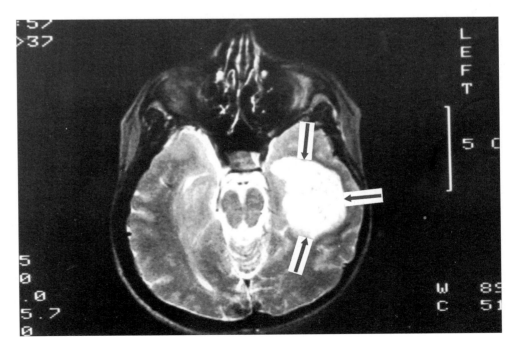

Figure 10. MR image of the brain of the same patient B.S. Axial image (SE 2500/90). Left temporobasal invasive tumor with mixed higher signal intensities (arrows).

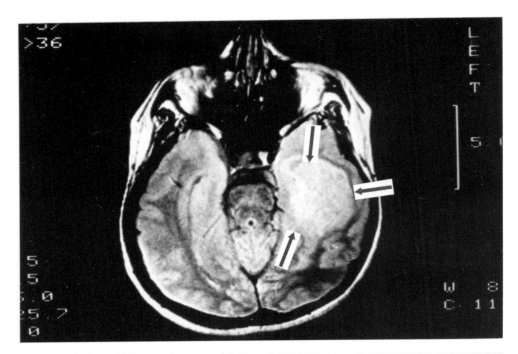

Figure 11. MR image of the brain of the same patient B.S. Axial image (SE 2500/15). Left temporo - basal invasive tumor with higher signal intensities (arrows).

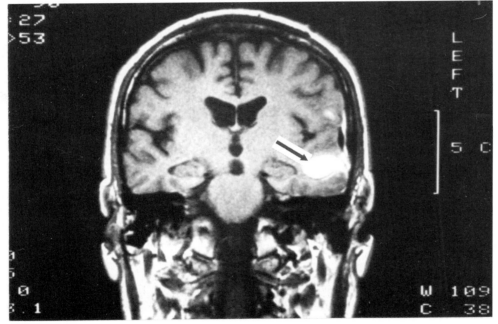

Figure 12. MR image of the brain. Coronal image (SE 500/15). Left temporobasal blood collection with high signal intensity (arrow).

The rapid sequence **FLASH** displays the hemosiderin edge with extremely low signal intensity, and blood collection with high signal intensity. This sequence helps differentiate between blood and other lesions with similar signal intensity, and that is the reason why the rapid sequences are of the utmost importance (Fig. 13) (26).

FLASH sequence can be used for enhancement of the low signal intensity of calcium if the calcification are to be proved. Enlarged field of the low signal intensity can prove calcification excluding any other low intensity signal obtained in standard MR sequences (Fig. 14).

Special rapid sequence **FLASH** for circulation can simulate the angiographic MR examination (**ANGIO MRI**). Enhancement of the high diagnosis signal form blood can display the blood vessel in the certain plane. The application of this sequence is a useful non-invasive tool for the diagnosis of the larger blood vessel disorders such as aneurysms, A-V shunts or hemangioma, but it could not replace the

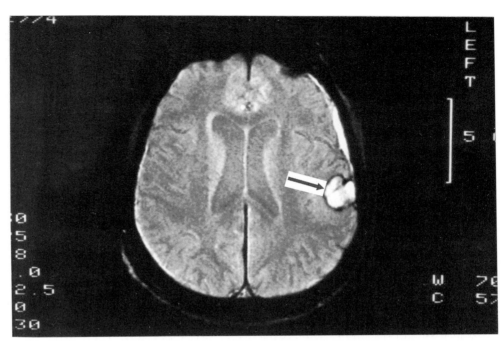

Figure 13. MR image of the brain. Axial image (GRE 250/18/30 degrees). Arrow pointing characteristic hemosiderin edge with low signal intensity surrounding the blood collection in the left temporo-parietal area.

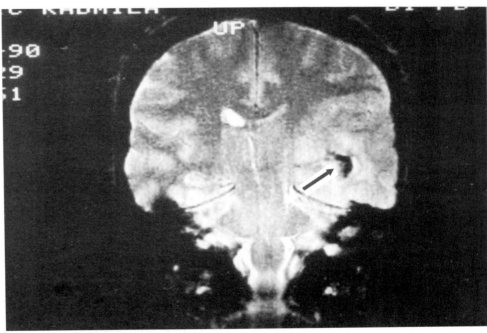

Figure 14. MR image of the brain. Coronal image (GRE 400/18/10 degrees). Marked calcifications in the tumor tissue. Black arrow pointing the low density areas of calcification. White arrow pointing the tumor (oligodendroglioma) causing the compression and dislocation of the third and lateral ventricles.

conventional cerebral angiography. It could be useful for the quick orientation and selection of the patients for the invasive angiography. The differentiation between the slow circulating blood in veins, rapid circulation in arteries or static blood collection can be made upon the parameters chosen for the examination (Figg. 15, 16).

Inversion Recovery sequence takes 15 seconds to complete, but it has no advantage compared to the shorter double echo T-1W sequence. The image is inverted like a negative. It is seldom used in everyday practice because it does not make special contribution to distinguish between pathologic disorders of the CNS (Fig. 17).

Other special sequences can be useful to reveal significant data on, for example, features of the intervertebral discus, bone fragments, adipose tissue, etc. Special sequences should be applied for the confirmation of the diagnosis suspected on the basis of the conventional MR sequences (24).

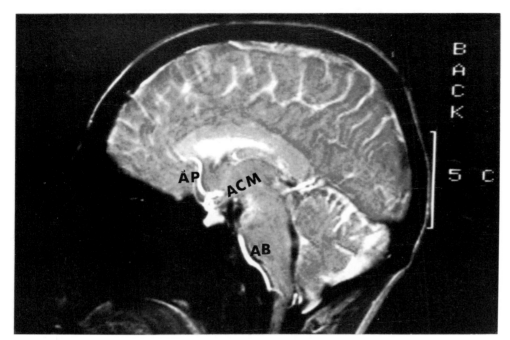

Figure 15. MR image of the brain. Sagittal image (GRE 50/10/80 degrees). (ANGIOFLASH) Medial cerebral artery (MCA), pericallous artery (PA) and basilar artery (BA) are shown.

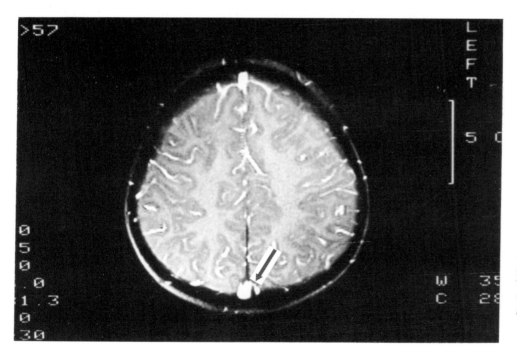

Figure 16. MR image of the brain. Axial image (GRE 50/10/80 degrees). ANGIO-FLASH displays terminal arterial branches in the parietal region as well as the superior sagittal sinus (with high intensity signal as well)- arrow.

5. Artifacts

The neuroradiologist should be well acquainted with natural sciences, especially physics. The artifacts made by X rays must be notified in order to make the correct evaluation of the radiography. The radiologist should be aware of the possibility of artifacts, thus avoiding the peril of the false positive or false negative findings (29).

MR artifacts can change the signal intensity and destroy the morphology of the image. The knowledge on the types and sources of artifacts help prevent the diagnostic error using the correct technology.

Artifacts can be caused by the static or alternating magnetic field, technical features of the signal emitter or recipient in the MR machine, or the complete tissue and organ features in the patient.

Numerous classifications of the artifacts were based on the type and cause of the artifact, as well as its impact on the image quality, or their prevention.

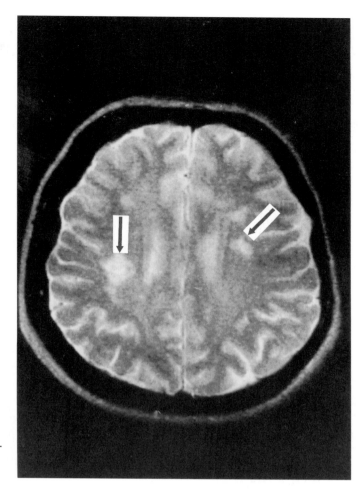

Figure 17. MR image of the brain. Axial image (IR 3000/22/300). Cerebro spinal fluid in lateral ventricles has low signal intensity, white matter high and gray matter low signal intensity. Plaques of the multiple sclerosis have low signal intensity as well (arrows).

The most frequent artifacts are the geometric ones, phantom artifacts caused by the static magnetic field or malfunctioning of the gradient fields, etc. Henkelman have divided artifacts as follows:
- Aliasing artifacts
- Truncation artifacts
- Artifactual black boundaries
- Central artifacts
- Errors in data
- Magnetic field perturbation
- Chemical shift
- Misregistration
- Ghosts

"**Flow phenomenon**" is based upon the signal difference between the flowing fluid (blood, CSF, etc.) and the static tissue and dependent on the section plane. Section plane can be parallel or perpendicular to the blood vessel axis, so that the signal can be either low or paradoxically high depending on the chosen sequence. Signal obtained from the moving hydrogen protons depends on the velocity and direction of the flow, repetition time (TR), echo time (TE), thickness of the slice and applied sequence. Some unusual signals obtained from normal structures can be explained through this phenomenon. For example, the vein in the spinal channel can give extremely high intensity of the signal in sagittal plane in T-1W sequence. "**Flow phenomenon**" can help to obtain MR angiography without the contrast injection.

"**Chemical shift**" based on the resonance difference of the protons in water and lipids is the phenomenon essential to the NMR spectroscopy. That is why there is the edge of the extremely low or high signal intensity between the adipose layers and water containing organs. The choice of the special pulse sequence can select the image displaying single chemical entity (lipid or water) (25).

Artifacts caused by the movements of the patient can deteriorate or destroy the image in conventional radiography and MRI as well. Internal organ movements (heart, lungs, intestine) could significantly influence the quality of the MR image. The application of the special software such as "Cardiac triggering", "Respiratory gating" etc. can help to overcome those problems.

The quality of the image can as well be influenced by the technical features of the machine such as coils, the power of the machine, computer characteristics, etc. Physical and chemical features of the atoms, molecules and tissues are under tremendous influence of the static and alternating magnetic field, so that a lot of artifacts can be expected in the MR tomographs. Different technology adjustment, such as selection of sequences and parameters, are needed to prevent artifacts.

6. Technique of the MR examination

The MR examination is very easy for the patient. It is painless, comfortable and harmless.

The preparation of the patient for the examination is simple. There is no need for the premedication, save for the claustrophobic patients, where the use of a sedative is advisable. Patient can have the meal, water or the medication which he uses regularly, prior to the examination.

The patient should be informed thoroughly about the examination technique.

All the metal objects should be removed (keys, glasses, hearing aid, belt, watch, magnetic cards, hair pins, jewelry, wigs, etc.), because they could disturb the image quality, or damage the powerful magnet inside the MR machine. On the other hand, strong magnetic field can interfere with the functioning of the watch or destroy the magnetic code of the credit cards.

The patients personal clothes are removed, for the practical reasons, and the patient is gowned in the disposable paper gown during the examination. The make-up should be removed, as well as the hair spray, because the tiny metal particles in them could spoil the image quality.

MR examination is completely contra-indicated in patients with cardiac "pace maker" because the powerful magnet can cause its malfunction and accidental death of the patient (Fig. 18).

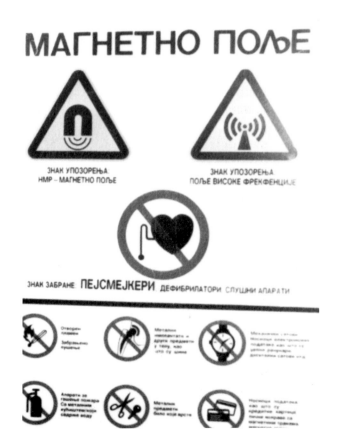

Figure 18. The door of restrictions.
The poster of warnings and restrictions on the special protection door of the MR theater. The warning sign on the powerful magnetic field and high frequency, restriction for the patients with pace maker, metal objects, magnetic cards, watches, metal implants, open flame, etc.

Metal implants, insulin pump, metal foreign bodies, dental prosthesis, ear implants, metal clips, etc. present relative contra-indications to the MR examination. They could become heated or even dislocated, if they are ferromagnetic, by the powerful magnet during the examination. Dislocation of the foreign body can destroy surrounding structures, whereas the dislocation of the vascular clip can cause fatal intracerebral hemorrhage.

Examination of the patients with metal implants became possible after the introduction of new rapid sequence techniques, using the special shields to prevent artifacts.

The effect of the powerful magnetic field on the fetus have not been studied yet, so it would be advisable to avoid the MR examination during the first trimester of pregnancy. No harmful effects on either fetus or the mother have been observed during the later phases of pregnancy.

In the examination room the patient should sign the written consent and confirm that he is fully informed on the details concerning the technique and contra-indications to the examination. The need for the MR examination, as well as the absence of the contra-indications, should be confirmed by signature of three consultants. Final exclusion of the possible contra-indications is done by a neuroradiologist in the Magnetic Resonance Center, based on the interview with a patient and review of a complete medical file prior to the examination.

The claustrophobic patient should be given psychological support and a sedative if it is necessary. Detailed information on the technique of the examination, the alarm knob available to the patient and audio-visual monitoring by a camera, are usually sufficient assurance for the claustrophobic patient to avoid the crisis. A presence of a close relative can be helpful, especially for children.

The female patients with metal IUD are advised to check its position by a gynaecologist after the MR examination in order to prevent unwanted conception.

In patients with known hypersensitivity to certain medication precaution measures should be taken, if the paramagnetic contrast is to be injected. The allergy to the contrast should be tested beforehand and if the patient has proven allergic, he should take protective premedication 24 hours before the examination.

When the patient is prepared for the examination, he should be taken to the theater. Special trolley without the metal parts should be used for the seriously ill or immobile patients (Figg. 19, 20).

Patient is usually in the recumbent position, unless his condition requires compulsive position, laying on a side or on the stomach. The special alarm knob is available, so that the patient can discontinue the examination by a sound alarm any time, when necessary. Talk-over microphone enables the communication between the patient and the physician. Patients condition is audio-visually monitored throughout the examination and surveyed by a radiologist and a technician.

Air conditioning supplies the sufficient amount of fresh air for normal breathing. If the patient feels cold, the additional blanket can be used for warming-up.

Before commencing the examination, patient should be warned to remain perfectly still during the examination, in order to evade MR image blurring.

The patient should be accompanied by MR Center personnel only. Exceptionally, the anesthetist or a close relative could be admitted to the MR room.

The examination usually takes 2-30 minutes, depending on the techniques applied.

During the MR examination a loud noise, made by the metal parts of the electromagnet, can be heard and the patient should be informed about the fact in advance.

High quality MR image is obtained through the coils, special radiofrequency receivers and emitters. Several types of the coils, specially designed for the head, neck, spine, knee, orbits, etc. are available. The brain imaging is done using the head coil, with patient in the recumbent position (Fig. 21).

The spine imaging is done using the oval spine coil. The coil does not disturb the patients comfort. Extended spine coils used nowadays have enabled simultaneous MR imaging of the whole spine.

In uncooperative patients the examination should be done under general anesthesia. Intravenous or rectal application of the anesthetics is desirable. There are special antimagnetic anesthetic machines that could be used in the MR room. Monitoring of the EKG and pulse enables the anesthetist to keep the vital functions of the patient under full control.

Application of the paramagnetic contrast requires the i.v. system with the connectors in the MR room. Intravenous administration of the contrast should take 3-5 minutes in order to avoid possible adverse effects. The MR imaging is commenced after the paramagnetic contrast application.

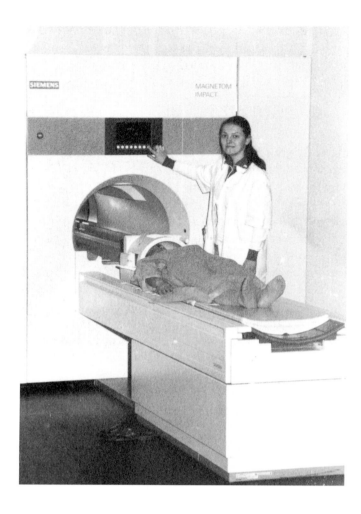

Figure 19. Patients in the theater. The MR theater. Patient laying on the table before entering the tube of the MR machine.

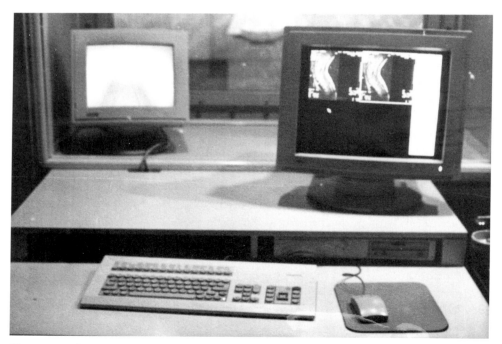

Figure 20. Operators console. Operators table with computer monitors and keyboards outside the MR theater, separated by a protective window.

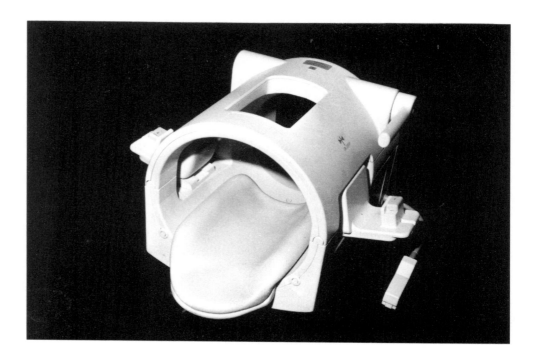

Figure 21. Head-coil.

The patients with metal fillings of the teeth may sense the metallic taste during or after the MR examination. Scintillation can be seen by a patient, because of the effect of the magnetic field on vitreous corpus. In case of the claustrophobic crisis the examination should be discontinued immediately and the patient should be removed from the MR room.

No harmful biological effect of the static magnetic field, currents induced by alternating field or radiofrequency field have been observed yet.

The influence of the static magnetic field on the enzyme activity have not been proved.

Transient decrease of the nerve conduction velocity is neglectable in the commercially available MR machines.

Induced changes to the conduction system of the heart are minimal, as well as the circulatory effects, and no heart pump overload have been observed.

Currents induced by alternating magnetic field can cause scintillation or slightly delayed bone healing.

Impact on the muscle action, especially on the heart muscle, is insignificant in commercially available MR machines (1.5-2.0 T).

Heating effect of the radiofrequency field depends on the applied power and duration of the examination. The elevation of temperature is usually neglectable for a patient, due to the air conditioning in the MR room.

Certain non-magnetic metal objects can be heated to a dangerous extent. That is why any metal implant presents relative contraindication to MR examination.

The MR is completely harmless regarding transient or permanent damage to the patient.

No special treatment is required after the examination.

7. Selection of sequences for the MR examination

A close cooperation of a radiologist and technician during the diagnostic procedures is necessary.

After the detailed browsing through the medical file and the results of previous tests the MR procedure is determined.

Scout examination is the basic tomograph of the brain in sagittal or axial, coronal and sagittal planes in newer MR machines. Three central sagittal tomographs with slice thickness of 8 mm and distance 0.2, or one in each of the three planes, are done in T-1W sequence. Scout examination is done quickly, its duration depending on the central computer. Orientation tomographs can give a lot of information on the head or brain. Information on cranio-cervical junction, posterior fossa, Sylvius aqueduct or hypophysis can be obtained as well.

The selection of the plane for the further examination is based upon suspected pathology. Axial plane is most frequently applied, extending from the top of the cranium to the first cervical vertebrae, with slice thickness 5-10 mm and distance of 0.2 mm in T-2W sequence (26).

Multiplanar imaging in all three planes in T-2W and optional T-1W are suitable for certain pathology.

The imaging of the whole brain (or head) is always done. The number of sections does not affect the time needed for the examination or the artifacts.

The special rapid sequences **FISP** and **FLASH** are useful for the circulation display, detection of the blood collections, calcifications, hemangioma, etc. Special sequences are needed to reveal the specific features of the lesions. The selection of the plane is determined by a location and character of the disorder.

Paraxial oblique planes could be used in cases with incorrect head position, in order to obtain the orbito-meatal line in the axial plane, or other perpendicular planes. They are seldom needed if head position is correct.

Slice thickness can be reduced by up to 1 mm, if required by the size and location of the lesion. For the exploration of hypophysis, slice thickness 2-3 mm with distance less than 1 mm (0.1-0.2) is used. The distance can be reduced to zero, but a lot of artifacts, arising in the contact area of two slices, makes the use of minimal distance much more convenient (17).

Slice thickness of 5 mm and distance less than 1 mm are used for the posterior fossa lesions or orbit examination.

MR imaging is the ultimate diagnostic procedure and should be carefully planned, in order to investigate the whole organ. It is not the emergency examination and the time should not be critical. The patient can be allowed to take some rest between the sequences. Additional sequences can be done later on the same day, or even the next day, when necessary.

The paramagnetic contrast enhancement is always done in T-1W, following previous necessary sequences.

8. Paramagnetic contrast in the magnetic resonance imaging

The application of paramagnetic contrast is required if the diagnosis based on the full range of the sequences is still uncertain, in order to locate the lesion or relationship between tumor and edema, etc. The first commercially available contrast was Gd-DTPA (reg. name Magnevist, Scherring). This gadolinium solution has rather specific properties. There are some other paramagnetic contrast solutions at the moment as well.

The paramagnetic contrast has following chemical properties: Ph 6.5-8.0; viscosity 2.9; osmolality 1.44, etc.

It is manufactured in 20 ml vials; the individual dose being 0.2ml/kg BW. The patient of 70 kg body weight should be given 14 ml of the contrast. The i.v. administration of the contrast should take 3-5 minutes to allow time for possible adverse effects observation.

The peak concentration of the paramagnetic contrast is achieved within 3-5 minutes and maintained up to 90 minutes after administration. The MR imaging should be done within that time span.

Severe hepatic or renal insufficiency is contra-indication to the contrast application.

Possible adverse effects are the sense of heat or slight pain following i.v. administration. Although anaphylaxis and shock are extremely rare, the set of anti-shock medicaments should be available, just in case.

Transient elevation of bilirubin and iron in serum can be observed within 24 hours after the contrast administration. Accidental paravenous injection of the contrast can cause the pain, which should cease within 24-48 hours.

Paramagnetic contrast Gd-DTPA affects the relaxation time of the hydrogen protons in water or other substance. The effect on the normal structures is minimal, whereas the signal intensities of the pathologically vascularized lesions are substantially changed.

The total effect of the contrast application depends on the pulse sequence, the administered dose and the time of the examination. T-1W sequence is always used because of the maximal effect of the contrast on T1 relaxation. The signal intensity change makes the lesion look brighter, in contrast to the normal structures. The lesion is far better differentiated after the contrast application. The longer sequences do not allow the expression of the maximal enhancement effect, like T-1W sequence does. All conventional and special sequences should be done prior to the injection of the contrast for the enhanced T-1W.

The enhancement of the MR image, following paramagnetic contrast injection, is substantially different from the change of the CT scan after the iodine contrast application (19).

The contrast should be administered for carefully selected indications, because of the possible hazards and its high price.

The diagnosis of the brain tumors, different lesions of the gray or white matter, adenoma of the hypophysis, encephalitis, spinal tumors, etc. should be confirmed by contrast injection (2).

The use of the paramagnetic contrast is valuable for differential diagnosis of the poorly defined lesions. The radiologist is personally responsible for the application of the contrast.

The example of the posterior fossa tumor in T-1W sequence before and after the contrast injection is shown in Figures 22, 23 and 24. The signal intensity is enhanced after the Magnevist injection, clearly delineating the tumor from the surrounding edema and normal brain tissue.

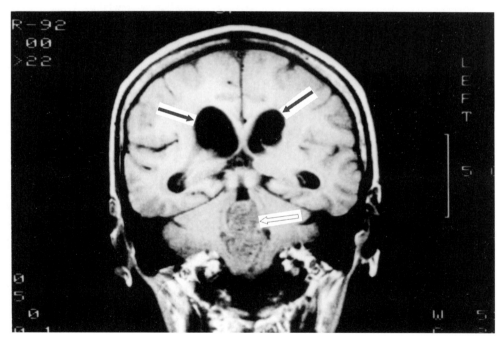

Figure 22. MR image of the brain of the patient K.D. Coronal image (SE 500/15). Irregular oblong lesion of unequal signal intensity can be seen in the posterior fossa, infratentorially, at the level of the IV ventricle. Suspected tumor inside the IV ventricle (white arrow). Supratentorial distention of the lateral ventricles signalize the internal obstructive hydrocephalus (black arrows).

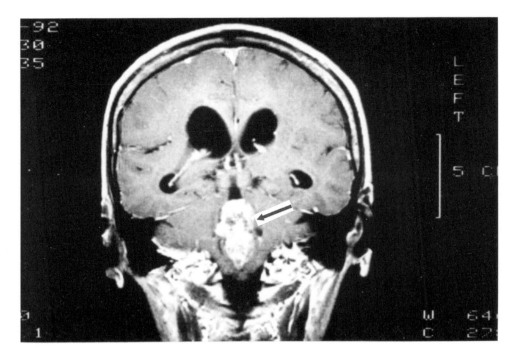

Figure 23. MR image of the brain of the same patient K.D. Coronal image (SE 500/15) after gadolinium-DTPA administration. Posterior fossa tumor with enhanced and mixed signal intensity. The contrast has significantly changed the features of the tumor signal (arrow). Meningioma confirmed by postoperative histology.

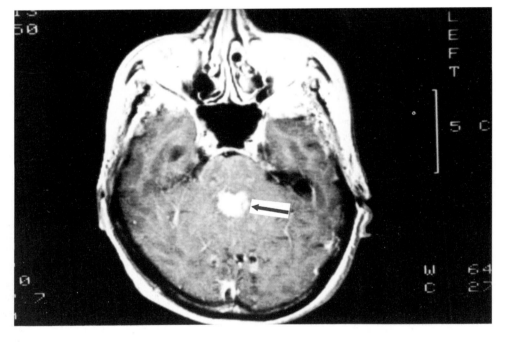

Figure 24. MR image of the brain of the same patient K.D. Axial image (SE 50/15) after gadolinium-DTPA administration. Meningioma with high signal intensity can be seen in the posterior fossa at the level of the IV ventricle. The tumor is optimally delineated and fills the IV ventricle completely.

REFERENCES

1. Andrew ER.: NMR imaging. Chem. Res., 16: 114-122, 1983.
2. Araki T., Inouye T., Suzuki H., Mashida T., Iio M.: Magnetic resonance imaging of brain tumors: Measurement of T-1. Radiology, 150: 95-98, 1984.
3. Bidder GM., Steiner RE.: NMR Imaging of the brain. Neuroradiology, 23: 231-240, 1982.
4. Bloch F.: Nuclear induction. Phys. Rev., 70: 466-474, 1946.
5. Bories J., Derhy S., Chirias J.: CT in hemispheric ischaemic atac. Neuroradiology, 27: 468-483, 1985.
6. Bories J.: Computerized Axial Tomography. Springer-Verlag. Berlin, Heidelberg, New York. 1978.
7. Bradley WG.: MRI Atlas of the Brain. Deutsche Arzte Verlag, Koeln. 1990.
8. Bydder GM., et al.: Clinical use of rapid T2-weighted partial saturation sequences in MR imaging. J. Comp. Assist. Tomogr., 11: 17-18, 1987.
9. Claussen C., Lechner B.: Dynamische Computertomography, Springer-Verlag. Berlin, Heidelberg, New York, Tokyo, 1983.
10. Council on Scientific Affairs: Fundamentals of magnetic resonance imaging. JAMA, 258: 3417-3423, 1987.
11. Council on Scientific Affairs: Magnetic resonance imaging: Prologue. JAMA, 258: 3283-3285, 1987.
12. Damadian R.: Tumor detection by nuclear magnetic resonance. Science, 171: 1151-1153, 1971.
13. Daniels D., Haughton V., Naidich T.: Cranial and Spinal Magnetic Resonance Imaging-An Atlas and Guide. Raven Press, New York, 1987.
14. Gademann G.: NMR-Tomography of the Normal Brain. Springer-Verlag. Berlin, Heidelberg, New York, Tokyo, 1988.
15. Gerhardt P., Fromhold W.: Atlas of Anatomic Correlations in CT and MRI. Thieme. New York, Tokyo, Heidelberg, 1988.
16. Haase A., et al.: FLASH imaging: rapid NMR imaging using low flip angle pulses. J. Magn. Res., 67: 258-262, 1986.
17. Halbsgut A., Lechner B.: Magnetresonanz-Tomographie (NMR),. Springer-Verlag. Frankfurt, 1987.
18. Han JS., Bonstelle CT., Kaufman B., Benson JE., Alfidi RJ., Clampit M.: Magnetic resonance imaging in the evaluation of the brain system. Radiology, 150: 705-712, 1984.
19. Holland GN., Hawkes RC., Moore WS.: Nuclear Magnetic Resonance (NMR) tomography of the brain: Coronal and sagital section. J. Comput. Tomogr., 4: 429-433, 1980.
20. Huk WJ., Gademann G., Friedman G.: Magnetic Resonance Imaging of Central Nervous System Diseases. Springer Verlag. Berlin, New York, Heidelberg, Tokyo, Paris, London, 1989.
21. Kazner E., Wende S., Grumme Th.: Computer und Kernspin-Tomographie intrakranialler Tumoren aus klinischen Sicht. Springer-Verlag. Berlin, Heidelberg, New York, London, Paris, Tokyo, 1989.
22. Lauterbur PC.: Image formation by induced local action examples employing nuclear magnetic resonance. Nature, 242: 190-192, 1973.
23. Leeds NE., Taylor S.: Contrast media in computer tomography. Springer-Verlag. Bremen, 1981.
24. Liessner J., Seider M.: Klinische Kernspintomographie. Enke. Stuttgart, 1987.
25. Matthaei D., et al.: Multiple chemical shitt selective (CHESS) MR imaging using stimulated echoes. Radiology, 160: 791-793, 1986.
26. Pomeranz JS.: Craniospinal Magnetic Resonance Imaging. W.B. Saunders Company. Philadelphia, London, Toronto, Sydney, Tokyo, 1989.
27. Pykett IL.: NMR imaging in medicine. Sci. American., 246: 78-88, 1982.
28. Reiser M., Semmler W.: Magnet-rezonanz- Tomographie. Springer Verlag. Berlin, Heidelberg, New York, Paris, London, Tokyo, Hong Kong, 1989.
29. Stark D., Bradley GWJR.: Magnetic Resonance Imaging. The C.V. Mosby Company. St. Louis, Washington D.C., Toronto, 1988.
30. Van M. Runge: Enhanced Magnetic Resonance Imaging. The C.V. Mosby Company. St. Louis, Baltimore, Toronto, 1989.
31. Zawadcki MB., Norman D.: Magnetic Resonance Imaging of the Central Nervous System. Raven Press. New York. 1987.
32. Zeitler E.: Kernspintomographie. Deutsche Artze Verlag. Koeln, 1984.
33. Zimmerman RA., Bilaniuk LT., Grossman RI., Goldberg HI., Edelstein HI., Bottomley P. and Redington RW.: Cerebral NMR: Diagnostic evaluation of brain tumors by partial saturation technique with resistive NMR. Neuroradiology, 27: 9-15, 1985.

SPECIAL PART

I. MALFORMATIONS

Vaso Antunović, Gradimir Dragutinović, Zvonimir Lević

Congenital malformations of the CNS should be displayed by high quality neuroimaging methods enabling the detailed image of the soft tissue and bone structures as well. Anatomy of the brain should be exposed through multiplanar views in order to distinguish between abnormal structures and normal varieties.

Conventional radiographs of the cranium can show only the bone structures.

Invasive angiography is useful either for the direct display of the vascular anomalies or indirect hint of the other anomalies of the brain.

Computer tomography was the first method ever to enable direct visualization of the brain malformations that could have been proven only post mortem. High resolution CT gives the precise image of the bony malformations of the head. The morphology of the normal, as well as abnormal, structure of the brain is globally displayed. However, some details necessary to confirm certain malformation remain undiscovered by CT scan (8, 9).

Major disadvantages of CT are ionizing radiation, inability of the direct access to all necessary section planes, poor resolution in the reconstructed image, especially in the sagittal plane, insufficient resolution to give the cytoarchitectural details of the brain, a lot of artifacts caused by bony structure superposition, etc. (35).

MRI is a method of choice for the diagnosis of malformation or varieties of the brain and cranial bones.

Congenital malformations are best displayed by MR in the Spin echo sequence. Multiplanar MR gives a realistic image of the numerous developmental disorders of the brain or head. Direct access to the optimal plane for the abnormality imaging is enabled.

T-1W can give the best possible contrast between anatomy details, while double echo sequences (T-2W and PD) are seldom used, to confirm phacomatosis or other malformation, where distinguishing between the CSF cavities and soft tissue lesions is needed.

The perfect knowledge of pathologic anatomy is required for MR diagnosis of the rare malformations unrecognized by a radiologist previously.

W. J. Huk et al. have suggested a very good classification of CNS malformations (14).

1. Midline closure defects (neural tube defects, dysraphic disorders)

a) Encephalocele, meningocele, meningoencephalocele

These malformations are represented by a prolapse of the central nervous system parts through a defect in the cranial bone: meninges with neural tissue (meningoencephalocele) or even with a part of the ventricular system (hydromeningoencephalocele) (14). The term encephalocele engulfs all three groups, because it has been impossible in the past to distinguish between them preoperatively on the basis of neuroimaging. There are also some smaller, non-cystic, dysraphic anomalies, such as rudimentary encephalocela, congenital cranial or scalp defects or dermal sinus, etc.

The incidence of encephalocele is 1:5000 of the newborn children in the western hemisphere and 85% of them are posteriorly located whereas, in the Far East, the anterior localization is far more common (27). Posterior encephalocele are more frequently seen in females, while anterior encephalocele equally affect both genders.

Table 1. CLASSIFICATION OF THE C.N.S. MALFORMATIONS.

1. Midline closure defects (neural tube defects, dysraphic disorders)
    a) Of the brain
        - Craniorachischis
        - Anencephaly
        - Encephalocele and cranial meningocele
            Cranium bifidum occultum
            Occipital encephaloceles
            Parietal meningoencephaloceles
            Anterior encephaloceles
    b) Of the cerebellum
        - Agenesis of the cerebellum
        - Hypoplasia of the cerebellum
        - Hypoplasia of the vermis
        - Dandy Walker syndrome
        - Arnold Chiary deformity
    c) Of the spine
        - Spina bifida occulta
        - Spina bifida cystica
            Meningocele
            myelomeningocele
        - Ventral spinal defects
    d) Of the spinal cord
        - Hydromyelia and syrinogmyelia
        - Duplication of the spinal cord
            Dimyelia
            Diplomyelia
            Diastematomyelia
        - Tethered cord
        - Lipoma
        - Dermoid, epidermoid, dermal sinus
        - Teratoma

2. Malformations of the commissures and midline structures
    -Holoprosencephaly
        Alobar prosencephaly
        Semilobar prosencephaly
        Lobar prosencephaly
    - Agenesis of the corpus callosum
    - Anomalies of the septum pellucidum

- Septo-optic dysplasia
- Cavum septi pellucidi, cavum vergae and cavum veli interpositi

3. Anomalies of cell migration
    - Ectopias and heterotopias
    - Agyria, pachygyria, lissencephaly
    - Polymicrogyria, stenogyria
    - Status verrucosus
    - (Ulegyria)

4. Destructive lesions/ abnormalities
    - Hydraencephaly
    - Porencephaly
    - Schisencephaly
    - Multicystic encephalopathy
    - Hippocampal sclerosis, status marmoratus, status demyelinizatus
    - Ulegyria
    - Hemispheric atrophy
    - Putaminal necrosis

5. Neuroectodermal dysplasias, phacomatosis
    - Tuberous sclerosis
    - Neurofibromatosis (von Recklingahusen disease)
    - Encephalofacial angiomatosis (Sturge Weber syndrome)
    - Von Hippel Lindau disease
    - Other phacomatosis
        Encephaloretinal angiomatosis
        Ataxia teleangiectasia
        Neurocutaneous melanosis
        Linear nevus sebaceous syndrome
        Incontinentia pigmenti

6. Miscellaneous abnormalities
    -Hydrocephalus
    -Microcephaly, microencephaly
    -Macroencephaly
    -Arachnoidal cyst

Neurological deficit caused by posterior encephalocele depends on the degree of the microcephaly, amount of the neural tissue in the sac, the site of lesion and concomitant hydrocephalus. Surgical risk is defined by a vicinity of the vital structures and contents of a sac, because of the lack of the function of the dysplastic tissue. MRI can provide for perfect assessment of the lesion, its relationship with intracranial contents, adverse anomalies, position of the vein sinuses, etc. Additional information on the complete arterial and venous network can be obtained through MR angiography (38).

The patient should be examined under general anesthesia both for CT or MR examination. Computer tomography being easier and shorter, should be applied for the diagnosis of those anomalies (37). Ultrasound is insufficient for preoperative planning, but could be very useful for the prenatal diagnosis of this malformation.

MR gives the most detailed image of those malformation and should be extremely important for the preoperative planning in neurosurgery (Fig. 25).

Besides taking usual precautions in neonatal surgery to avoid hypothermia and hemorrhage, surgery for these anomalies should try to preserve functional brain tissue and obey the esthetic requirements as well.

b) Cerebellar agenesis and hypoplasia

Cerebellar agenesis, or total absence of the cerebellum, is extremely rare. Cerebellar hypoplasia or poorly developed cerebellum is far more common. It could be secondary to the systemic degenerative disorders, perinatal ischemia, etc. (18).

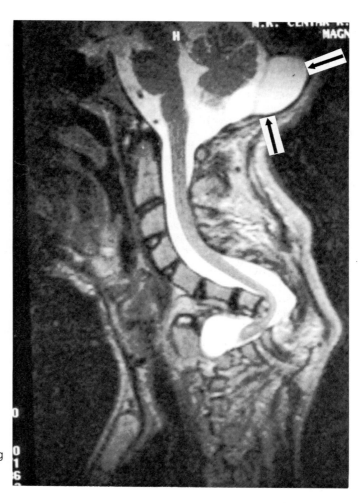

Figure 25. Sagittal image (TSE 7462/112) Arrow pointing at meningocele.

Clinical presentation of the cerebellar agenesis or hypoplasia can be extremely variable. Subjects with normal intelligence have enormous compensation ability for the lost cerebellar function, so that some patients are completely asymptomatic. If there are cerebellar symptoms, such as ataxia, posture or gait disorders, they are non-progressive (13, 35).

In some children with autism the cerebellar hypoplasia was found, but the significance of this finding has not bee explained yet (25-28).

Surgery is not indicated for isolated cerebellar agenesis. If combined with internal hydrocephalus, the shunt CSF drainage is sufficient.

Cerebellar hypoplasia, without the finest details, can be displayed by CT scan. The main disadvantage of CT scan is the inability to display sagittal view of cerebellum.

MR imaging is done in both sagittal and axial views. MR tomograph in sagittal plane in T-1W sequence displays the hypoplastic changes of cerebellar cytoarchitecture (Fig. 26).

c) Dandy-Walker Syndrome

There are structural changes characteristic for Dandy-Walker syndrome such as: agenesis or hypoplasia of vermis, IV ventricle dilation, agenesis of foramina of Luschka and Magendie and cerebellar hypoplasia.

Dandy have assumed that Magendie foramen atresia have caused the IV ventricle dilation, while others have reported the vermis agenesis and rudimentary cerebellar tissue in the cyst wall, explaining this by the failure of cerebellar hemispheres to split and form the cerebellar commissure.

The head is dolichocephalic due to the enlargement of the occipital area.

Dandy-Walker syndrome can be combined with corpus callosum agenesis, Silvius aqueduct stenosis, porencephaly, encephalocelae, etc. Internal hydrocephalus is often found (15).

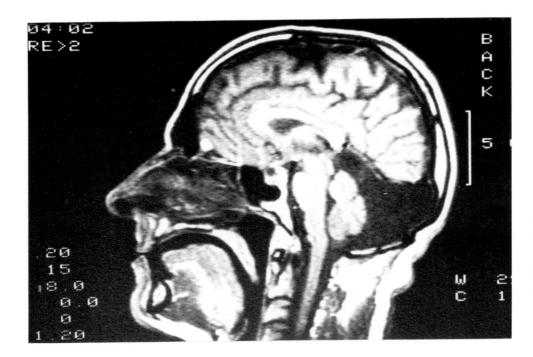

Figure 26. MR of the brain. Sagittal image (SE200/15). Cerebellar hypoplasia with enlarged great cistern, filled with liquor of low signal intensity. Fourth ventricle has normal dimensions.

The syndrome is most often congenital, but it can be acquired due to the infection, chemical agents or other factors as well.

Slowly progressive hydrocephalus used to be responsible for the delayed diagnosis in the past, but nowadays the diagnosis is usually made in the first months of life. Neurologic symptoms are caused by the intracranial hypertension: headache, vomiting, fainting spells, disequilibrium, diplopia, urine incontinence, mental retardation, etc. In some cases the symptoms are occasional. Papillary edema, amblyopia or even blindness, disorders of other cranial nerves, pyramidal signs or respiratory disorders, are rarely seen (23). Ataxia of the gait and extremities as well as dysarthria are characteristic for the advanced stage.

Dandy Walker syndrome can be asymptomatic in some patients.

The symptoms caused by elevated intracranial pressure can be relieved by the VA or VP shunt drainage of cerebro- spinal liquor. Direct resection of the cyst wall is abandoned nowadays. There is still different attitude regarding the cyst or ventricle drainage. In smaller children with moderate hydrocephalus cyst drainage tends to be successful. Some Authors suggest the combined drainage using Y shaped connector (36).

CT scan is insufficient to display the hypoplastic vermis, agenesis of the IV ventricle outlets, stenosis of the Silvius aqueduct, etc. Bigger hypodense lesions located supratentorially can be visualized correctly by CT examination.

MR imaging in sagittal plane using T-1W sequence, with additional axial views can display malformations of both infra- and supratentorial structures in details. Ventricular system is better displayed in T-2W sequence, because it enhances the liquor as well as abnormalities (39, 40). The choice of the plane in T-2W sequence is essential for the imaging of the liquor filled intracranial cavities (Figg. 27, 28).

d) Retrocerebellar Arachnoidal Pouch (Blakes cyst)

Blakes cyst is found either as a single entity or combined with other brain malformation. The enlarged retrocerebellar space is filled with cerebrospinal liquor. Cerebellar tissue is always reduced.

Retrocerebellar cyst is usually asymptomatic, but severe intermittent intracranial hypertension could be seen occasionally. Sometimes the cyst can mimic midline cerebellar tumors (32).

Although CT scan displays the hypodense Blakes cyst, the sagittal image reconstructed from the axial section is insufficient for the precise diagnosis.

MR imaging is a perfect way to expose the retrocerebellar arachnoidal cyst (Blakes cyst) which is frequently associated with internal hydrocephalus. This infratentorial malformation is not so rare as it has

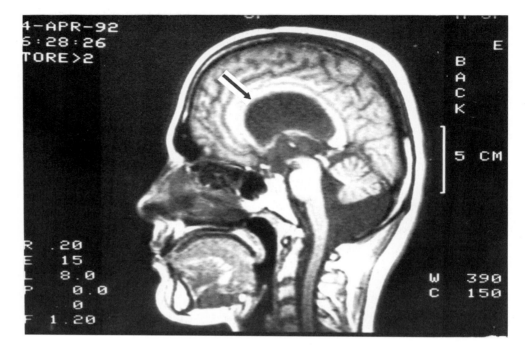

Figure 27. MR image of the brain. Sagittal image (SE 200/15) Dandy Walker syndrome: agenesis of vermis and cerebellar hypoplasia. Fourth ventricle is dilated, especially cisterna magna. Marked internal hydrocephalus - arrow pointing at dilated third ventricle.

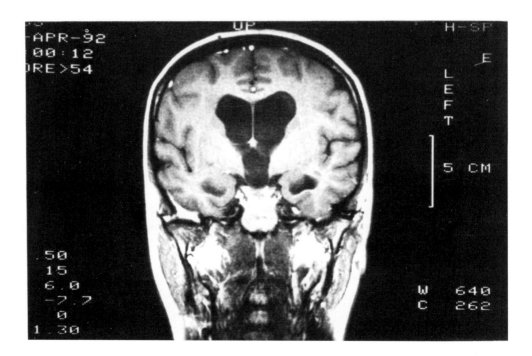

Figure 28. MR image of the brain. Coronal image (SE 500/15) Dandy Walker syndrome: marked internal hydrocephalus, with third and lateral ventricles dilation.

been assumed before. Multiplanar display in both sagittal and axial planes in T-1W or T-2W is needed to reveal the changed morphology (12). Additional imaging planes or *sequences* may be needed for 3D reconstruction and enhancement of certain structures or relationship between cerebellar tissue and ventricular system (Fig. 29).

The cyst, with marked symptoms of the posterior fossa tumor, should be removed surgically. Insertion of the drainage system is usually sufficient (28, 31).

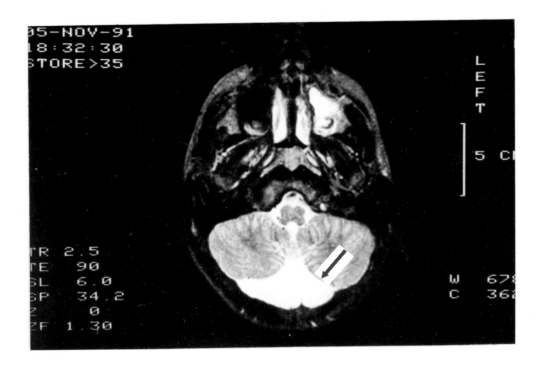

Figure 29. MR image of the brain. Axial image (SE 2500/90). Retrocerebellar arachnoid cyst in the posterior fossa with intensive liquor signal - arrow.

e) Arnold-Chiari Malformation

There are four types of Arnold-Chiari malformation:

Type I   Cerebellar tonsil ectopy with occasional internal hydrocephalus, basilar impression and exceptional hydromyelia or syringomyelia;

Type II   Prolapse of the cerebellar tonsils and vermis, with medullar elongation and extension of the IV ventricle beyond the cranio- cervical junction, through *foramen occipitale magnum.* Consequent venous congestion and leptomeningeal adhesions are usually found. Internal hydrocephalus and meningomyelocelae can be seen as well. Supratentorial internal hydrocephalus, stenogyria, microgyria and *corpus callosum* agenesis is occasionally present (22).

Type III Cervical spina bifida, cerebellar herniation and suboccipital myelo-cerebello-meningocelae are extremely rare.

Type IV   Cerebellar hypoplasia, already mentioned earlier in the text, is included in this entity by some Authors.

Arnold-Chiari type I, without dysraphy signs, can be misdiagnosed in adults as multiple sclerosis, because of the lower cranial nerve, cerebellar or medullar symptoms. Syringomyelic sensitivity dissociation and muscle hypotrophy corresponding to the level of syringomyelic cavity can be seen in this type of malformation as well.

Surgical drainage, after Pudenz, is indicated for the internal hydrocephalus. Syringomyelic cavity used to be treated by drainage, but nowadays the endoscopic method is used to restore the liquor circulation and prevent the further neurologic deficit. Posterior fossa decompression through the suboccipital access, followed by duroplasty, is rarely needed.

Type II has meningomyelocelae with early symptoms of the lower cranial nerves involvement. Cerebellar or other symptoms, found in type I Arnold-Chiari malformation, can be seen as well (1).

Surgery for type II is the decompression cervical laminectomy up to the cerebellar tonsil level, through the suboccipital approach. Arachnoid is preserved and dura reconstructed. Syringomyelic cavity is resected optionally.

Arnold-Chiari type II with cervical dysraphism in children requests complex surgery, consisting of the primary closure of meningomyelocelae, followed by secondary hydrocephalus solution. Craniocervical decompression is still controversial. Some Authors prefer early decompression for the cases with brainstem dysfunction, because of the initial reversibility of the symptoms. Early craniocervical decompression, through suboccipital approach and cervical laminectomy up to the cerebellar tonsil level, followed by plastic reconstruction of dura, is very successful in children. The surgery prevents the compression on the brainstem and subsequent dysfunction of the lower cranial nerves with dysphagia, apnea and food aspiration. Previous attitude that brainstem dysfunction is caused by the congenital structural lesion, has been abandoned nowadays. Contemporary theory explains brainstem dysfunction by a chronic compression effect, which means that the lesions are secondary and possibly reversible in the beginning. The chance for recovery in patients that have already developed the vocal cord paralysis is minimal and their prognosis is generally poor (4).

Computerized tomography is insufficient for the diagnosis of the different types of Arnold Chiari malformation and MR examination should be indicated right away (7, 9).

Sagittal MR tomography in T-1W sequence is optimal for the display of all the features of Arnold Chiari malformation. Coronal and axial planes in T-1W sequence could be used when necessary. T-2W sequence and repeated section planes are not required (39).

MR imaging is indispensable for the precise preoperative assessment of the degree of cerebellar tonsils dislocation, their relationship with major blood vessels, scar tissue, communication between syringomyelic cavity, and fourth ventricle or intraluminar septa inside the syringomyelic cavity. New generation of MR machines provides for the dynamic studies of cerebrospinal liquor (4) (Fig. 30).

2. Malformation of the commisures and midline structures

a) Corpus callosum agenesis

Corpus callosum agenesis (total absence) is a separate entity, but it can be associated with other anomalies as well. Agenesis of the corpus callosum can be either partial or complete (17).

"Disconnection syndrome" is the loss of the communication between the hemispheres due to the corpus callosum lesion. The patient with damaged *splenium corpus callosi* is not able to read or name the colors. Disorder of the anterior third of *corpus callosum* causes well known left hand apraxia. The patient can not perform the task with his left hand, while the right hand functioning is unaffected. The disorder can be caused by cerebral artery occlusion, tumor or surgical resection - callosotomy as well (5).

Agenesis of corpus callosum is partial or complete absence of this commissure. Some patients are asymptomatic and the defect is discovered accidentally. Neurologic deficit can present in a form of epileptic seizures, muscular hypertonia and hyperreflexia, Babinski sign, strabismus, incoordination, character or intellectual changes, psychotic disorder. Hydrocephalus is frequently found. Micro- or macrocephaly are described as well (6).

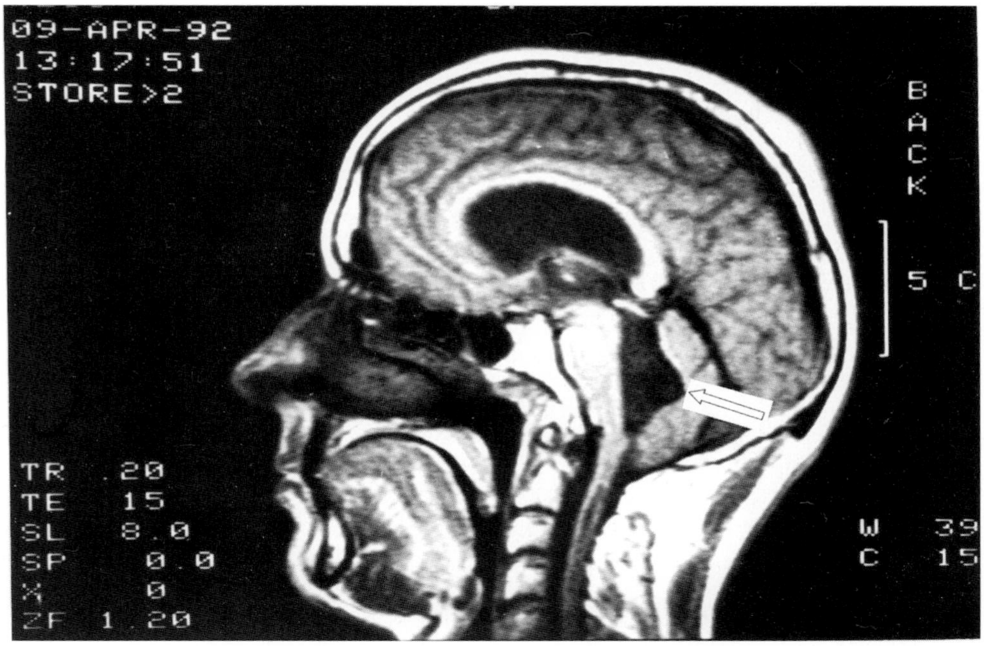

Figure 30. MR image of the brain. Sagittal image (SE 200/15). Arnold-Chiari malformation: prolapse of the cerbellar tonsils - black arrow; syringomyelic cavity in the cervical medullar area - white arrow; cerebellar hypoplasia with gross enlargement of the fourth ventricle, as well as the third and both lateral ventricles supratentorially-white arrow.

Agenesis of corpus callosum, especially if partial, can be easily overlooked on CT scan.

Sagittal MR in T-1W displays the partial or total corpus callosum agenesis. Other views or sequences are not needed (Figg. 31, 32).

b) Cavum septi pellucidi, cavum verge and cavum veli interpositi

Cavum septi pellucidi (*cystis septi pellucidi, ventriculus quintus*) is the cavity inside the septum pellucidum, bounded by glial and ependymal tissue. It is filled with liquor and located either in front or behind the corpus callosum. Liquor system of the cyst of septum pellucidum and ventricles can easily communicate. Exceptionally, foramen of Monroe is closed, thus obstructing liquor circulation.

Cavum verge is posterior limit is the splenium of corpus callosum.

Cavum veli interpositi is the ependymal cavity above the third ventricle filled with liquor. It could com-

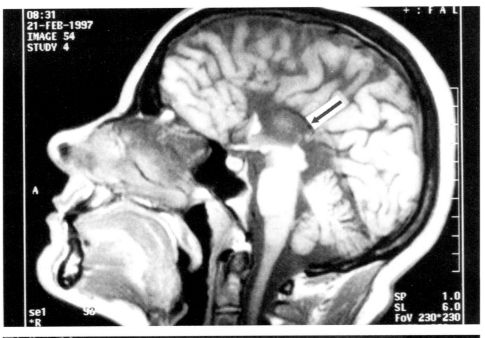

Figure 31. MR image of the brain. Sagittal image (SE 560/15). Corpus callosum agenesis - arrow.

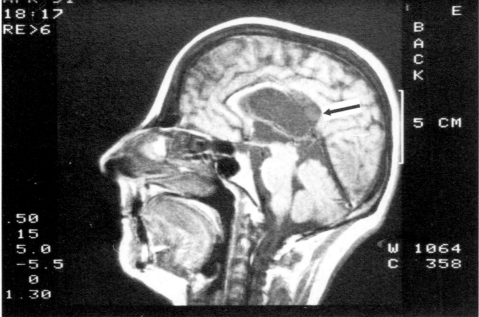

Figure 32. MR image of the brain. Sagittal image (SE 500/15). Partial agenesis of corpus callosum - arrow. Part of the corpus callosum and splenium are missing.

municate with either quadrigeminal lamina cistern or the ventricular system itself. *Cavum veli interpositi* can be combined with *cystis septi pellucidi* and *cavum verge*.

Neuroradiologic imaging usually discovers those malformations by accident. They are asymptomatic and without any clinical significance (16).

Ventriculus quintus is easily displayed by CT.

Cavum septi pellucidi is clearly delineated by MR in T-1W and particularly in T-2W sequence in axial and coronal images. Diagnosis can be based on CT, whereas they are accidentally found in MR image, considering their clinical insignificance (Fig. 33).

3. Anomalies of the cell migration

Anomalies of the cell migration are ectopia, heterotopia, agyria, pachygyria, polymicrogyria, stenogyria and verrucous status. The conditions are extremely rare and seldom reported in the literature.

4. Destructive lesions

Hydroanencephalus, porencephalia, schizencephalia, hyppocampal sclerosis, ulegyria, etc. are extremely rare abnormalities.

a) Porencephaly

Porencephalic cyst can be caused by neonatal infarction and combined with internal hydrocephalus. Some Authors consider it an embryonic disorder (Agenesis) or the sequel of the intrauterine brain tissue destruction.

Liquor filled cyst can easily communicate with ventricular system through a wide or funnel shaped opening.

Porencephalic cysts are usually asymptomatic, but various symptoms can be found as well, depending on the cyst etiology and associated disorders of the brain development. Psychomotor retardation, paresis or paralysis can be present. Porencephaly is frequently found in children with cerebral palsy. Epileptic seizures are rarely caused by retrocerebellar cyst.

CT scan is sufficient for porencephaly visualization.

MR imaging can contribute to 3D display of the porencephalic cyst, which is rarely needed for the specific therapy (Fig. 34) (34).

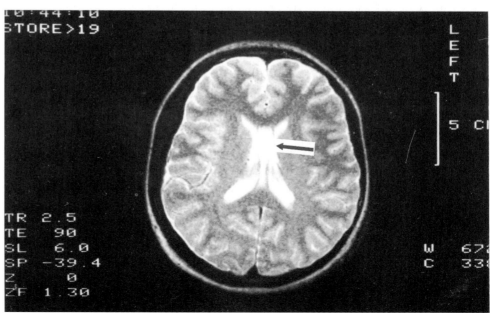

Figure 33. MR image of the brain. Axial image (SE 2500/90). Liquor filled cystis septi pellucidi, with very intensive signal - arrow.

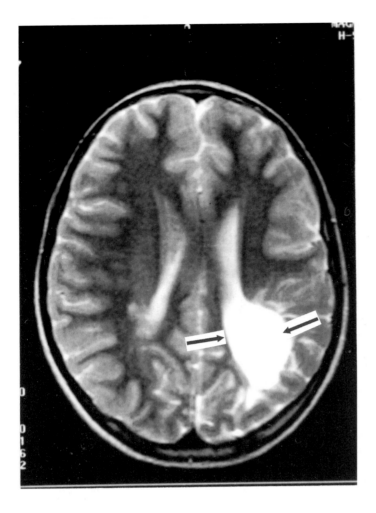

Figure 34. Axial image (SE 4000/99) Porencephaly - arrows.

5. Neuroectodermal dysplasia; phakomatosis

Those malformations are Tuberous sclerosis, Neurofibromatosis, Sturge Webers syndrome, Morbus von Hippel Landau, etc.

a) Tuberous sclerosis - Morbus Bourneville

Tuberous sclerosis, *Morbus Bourneville*, described in 1880, is an autosomal dominant hereditary disorder of cellular differentiation (phakomatous type) of the brain, heart, kidney and other organs. Clinical triad consists of mental retardation, epileptic seizures and sebaceous adenoma. Incidence is around 1 in 100.000 of neonates. Defect of highly penetrating gene, with a lot of spontaneous mutations, is responsible for sporadic cases (10). Various manifestations can be seen, such as sebaceous adenoma, subepidermal fibrosis, subuncal angiofibroma, kidney, liver or lung hamartoma, rhabdomyosarcoma of the heart (50%), epilepsy and oligophrenia, due to glial scars known as tubera. In 6% of children or adult patients, intraventricular subependymal gigantocellular astrocytoma (Gradus I) is found. It originates from the subependymal notch situated near the Monroes foramen in the lateral ventricle wall.

Multiple tumors ("tubera") are built of ecto- and mesodermal cells, situated in the nervous system, kidneys, heart, skin or other organs.

Multiple tumors are found in the brain, usually situated nearby lateral ventricles or in the cortex and, occasionally, in basal ganglia, cerebellum, brainstem or medulla. Sclerosis is microscopically differentiated by the reduction of the nerve cells and increased number of astrocytes.

Hamartomas, calcified tumor notches, are found in the ventricular walls, occasionally protruding into the cavities. If situated in the vicinity of the foramina of Monroe or aquaeductus Sylvii, they can obstruct the liquor circulation, thus causing the internal hydrocephalus (12).

Characteristic hyperdense subependymal calcifications, hypodense cortical hamartomas or intratumoral calcifications can be seen in CT scan. Unlike glioma, which tend to enhance by iodine contrast unevenly, subependymal gigantocellular astrocytoma and multiple tubera are uniformly dyed by iodine contrast. CT is a method of choice for the diagnosis of tuberous sclerosis.

MR imaging is very good in displaying various intracranial tuberous sclerosis manifestations: multiple subependymal notches, cortical architecture disorders and ventricular enlargement. Myelin abnormalities are well shown. Larger subependymal calcifications are seen in MR image as extremely low signal intensity lesions, particularly when special rapid sequences are used (33).

High resolution CT enables discovery of smaller calcification better than MR, and that is the advantage of CT over MR for this entity. Subependymal tumor mass is best displayed by MR imaging, with or without contrast, in coronal plane at the level of Monroes foramen (14). Hamartomas have the signal intensity of a gray matter in T-1W sequence, but in T-2W the signal intensity of a tumor becomes higher, especially after the contrast injection (Figg. 35-37).

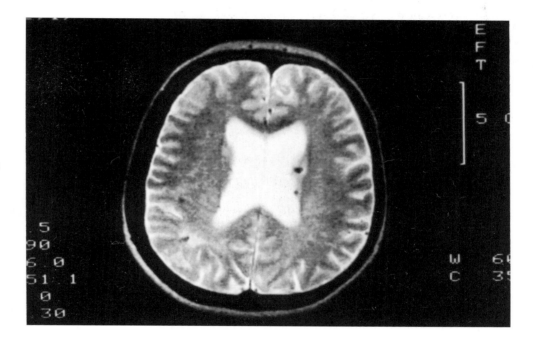

Figure 35. MR image of the brain. Axial image (SE 2500/90). Tuberous sclerosis: arrows pointing at subependymal calcifications shown in low signal intensities. Both lateral ventricles, enlarged due to the internal hydrocephalus, are shown by a high intensity signal of liquor.

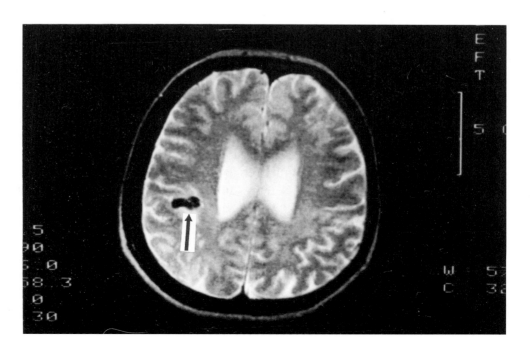

Figure 36. MR image of the brain. Axial image (SE 2500/90). Arrow pointing at calcified tumor in the parenchyma.

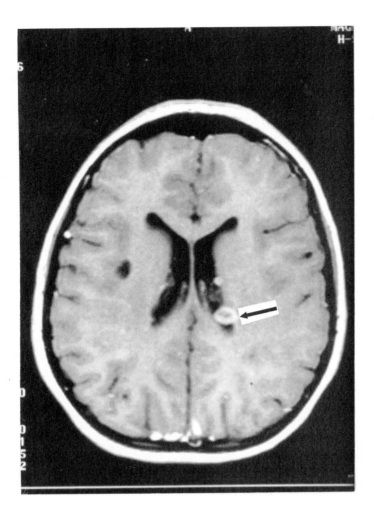

Figure 37. MR image of the brain. Axial image (SE 560/15) after gadolinium-DTPA administration. Arrow pointing at hamartoma of high signal intensity.

From the surgeons point of view those tumors are well delineated, gray or pink in color, and abundantly vascularized. Radical resection is the optimal treatment, but sometimes subtotal resection could be sufficient as well, considering the fact that tumors are slow growing and have low biologic potential. Recurrence of a tumor, although rare and delayed, should be treated by another surgery, for radiotherapy or chemotherapy are completely useless. Disturbed liquor circulation, drainage surgery or its complication can influence the prognosis as well.

b) Neurofibromatosis

Neurofibromatosis is an autosomal dominant hereditary disease (2). There are three types of a disease: neurofibromatosis von Recklinghausen, bilateral acoustic neurofibromatosis and miscellaneous forms different from the first two types. Hormones and growth factors stimulate the proliferation of Schwann cells and fibroblasts, but the basic mechanism is still unknown. Multiple delineated spots and benign skin tumors, as well as neurofibromata of peripheral or autonomous nerves, orbits, paranasal sinuses, paravertebrally or elsewhere are found. Neurofibroma can undergo malignant alteration occasionally (19).

Neurologic deficit depends on the neurofibroma location. Otologic symptoms, headache, vertigo, etc. are the dominant features of acoustic neurofibroma.

CT scan is usually sufficient for the precise diagnosis.

MR imaging, using different sequences and intravenous paramagnetic contrast, can contribute to the precise spatial definition of tumor, which is very important for the surgical treatment. Complete surgical removal of the tumor from the cerebellopontine angle should prevent serious neurologic deficit, or even the death of the patient (Fig. 38).

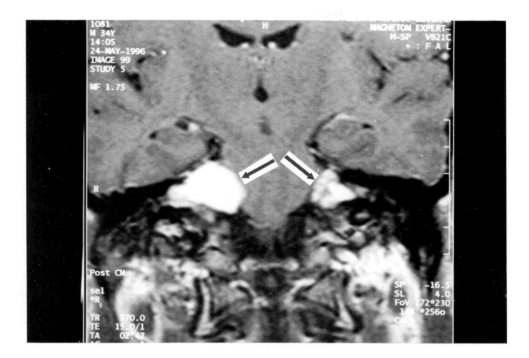

Figure 38. MR image of the brain. Coronal image (SE 570/15) after gadolinium-DTPA administration. Neurofibromatosis - bilateral acoustic nerve neurofibroma - arrows.

6. Miscellaneous abnormalities

a) Hydrocephalus

The abnormality is very important for its high incidence and clinical significance. Ventricular system becomes enlarged due to accumulation of cerebrospinal liquor. Prenatal diagnosis by ultrasound examination is possible nowadays.

In children, characteristic clinical presentation consists of the enlarged head circumference, rapid postnatal growth of the head, tense and widely open fontanels, downwards orientated eyeballs with "sunset" phenomenon and psychomotor retardation.

The first surgical attempt to solve the malformation was made in the ancient Rome. Hydrocephalus can be either isolated, or secondary to the tumor compression on the liquor system, hemorrhage or infection (21).

There are basically three types of causes for hydrocephalus: increased production, disturbed resorption or obstruction to the liquor circulation. According to their objectives, surgical procedures can be divided in to three groups as well: 1. reduction of the liquor production; 2. bypassing of the obstacle using intracranial shunt or 3. extracranial derivation of the excessive liquor to the other body compartments. The last procedure consisting of liquor drainage to the peritoneum, pleura or heart has been frequently used.

MR imaging for hydrocephalus is seldom needed for CT, or ultrasound diagnostic is sufficient, unless the finest details of aqueductal or periventricular lesions is required (29).

It seems that genuine congenital hydrocephalus, unrelated to perinatal trauma, is non-genetic. Concomitant dysraphic malformations, such as Arnold-Chiari or spina bifida, are rarely seen, in less than 2% of hydrocephalus, whereas cranium bifidum with primary aqueductal stenosis (X linked dysraphic anomaly) could be associated with Morbus Recklinghausen (26).

Hydrocephalus is usually acquired. Hydrocephalus is often attributed to intracranial hemorrhage or infection, but there is no substantial evidence. Recent studies have shown that predilection sites of hemorrhage correspond to the gestational age, while the germinal matrix (ependymal and subependymal layer) is particularly prone to the hemorrhage. Viral infections could play a significant role, although numerous healthy newborns have the history of the infection during the pregnancy as well.

Experimental studies have proven that ependyma is susceptible to certain viruses, such as mumps virus. In more than 60% of mothers of the hydrocephalic children, the history of the diseases, drug intake, smoking, hemorrhage, radiation, anesthesia or accidents was recorded, compared to 30% of mothers of healthy children, but no specific agent could be appointed as responsible for hydrocephalus formation. No distinction between isolated and combined hydrocephalus could be made, except for the period when noxious agents are active. Associated or major anomalies occur in early pregnancy, wheres isolated hydrocephalus is found in the later phase (11).

Internal hydrocephalus can have variable clinical course. Cranial diameters can be extremely enlarged. Papillary stasis is seldom seen. Symptoms such as inability to hold the head erect, psychomotor retardation, somnolence, excitation, eventual paraplegia, amblyopia, etc. could be found in hydrocephalic children.

Adults can have headache, vomiting, vision disorders, fainting spells, etc. The symptomatology depends on the age, etiology and evolution of internal hydrocephalus.

CT evaluation is useful for the assessment of hydrocephalus. Nowadays, MR imaging is administered in children in order to avoid ionizing radiation, using rapid sequences for axial, and, optionally, sagittal section to visualize Silvius aqueduct (Figg. 39, 40).

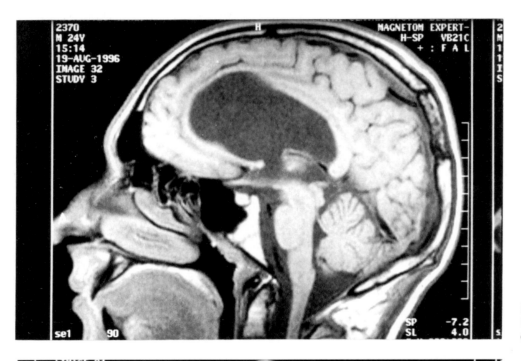

Figure 39. Sagittal image (SE 560/15) - Internal hydrocephalus.

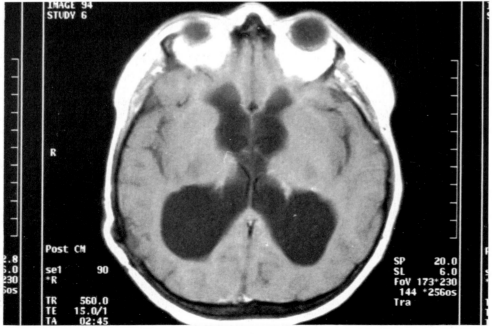

Figure 40. Axial image (SE 560/15) after gadolinium - DTPA administration - Internal hydrocephalus.

MRI could be useful for postoperative assessment in patients with implanted drainage systems, for they are compatible with MR examination. Controls tend to assess the ventricular condition and the position of the drainage system (Fig. 41). MR control can reveal possible endocranial morphological complications, in cases of hydrocephalus combined with other CNS lesions (infection, complications following puncture and porencephalic cyst) (30).

b) Arachnoidal cyst

Medial brain membrane, arachnoid is made of two squamous cell layers of mesenchymal origin. It is adjacent to the internal dural layer, thus forming subdural space and loosely covering the brain surface without entering sulci. That is why there are numerous septa between arachnoid and pia which permit the liquor circulation in the subarachnoid space. In the basal region, arachnoid membrane is thick and separated from pia, thus forming cisterns. Arachnoidal extensions cover the cranial nerves in the posterior cranial fossa. Normal communication between cisterns could be obstructed due to the hemorrhage, inflammation, tumor or developmental disorder of the arachnoidal cysts. Congenital cysts are multilocular, with septa, complicating the surgery (36).

Arachnoidal cysts, both supra- and infratentorial, are frequently seen. Collagen fibers are found in thicker parts of the arachnoidal cyst. Communication between arachnoidal space and cyst can be occasionally seen (3).

Arachnoidal cysts are usually asymptomatic, although they can cause epilepsy. Clinical course depends on the size and location of the cyst. Possible discrepancy between the size and neurologic deficit can exist. Various symptoms could be present, but the diagnosis is more often accidental, during the search for the organic cause of epilepsy. If there is associated malformation, the symptomatology depends on the type of malformation. Hemorrhage inside the cyst is rarely seen, but it could make differentiation between the cyst and subdural hematoma difficult.

CT examination could be insufficient for the diagnosis of the hypodense arachnoidal cyst.

MR imaging, using T-1W and T-2W sequence, in sagittal, axial and coronal planes reveals the details of the arachnoidal cyst (14). Multiplanar display of the symptomatic arachnoidal cyst is important to confirm the diagnosis and plan eventual surgery (Fig. 42).

Symptomatic arachnoid cysts requires surgery (neurologic deficit, marked compression effect, epilepsy beyond control). There are two different solutions to the problem. Cystoperitoneal shunt is suf-

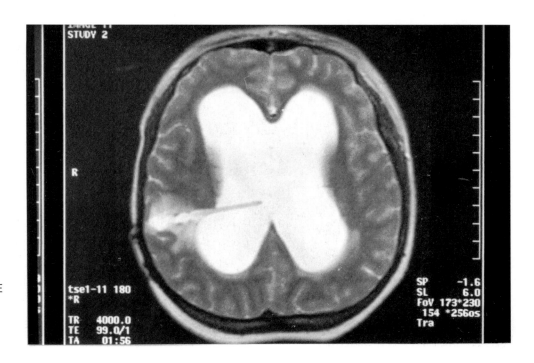

Figure 41. Axial image (TSE 4000/99). Implanted drainage system is displayed.

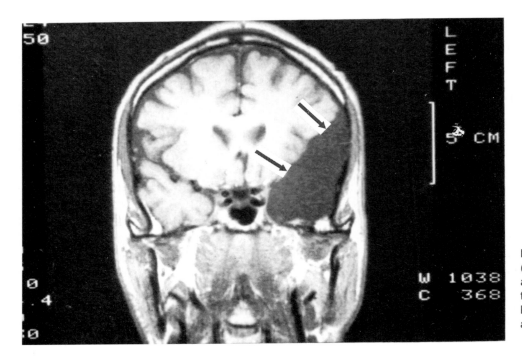

Figure 42. Coronal image (SE 500/15). Enormous arachnoidal cyst in the left temporal region, filled with low signal intensity liquor - arrows.

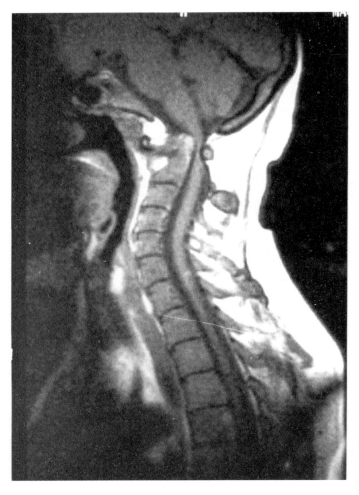

Figure 43. Sagittal image (TSE 700/12). Basilar invagination with spinal canal stenosis.

ficient for cysts without septa, while the cysts with septa should be directly explored and deliberated. Surgical failures in septed cyst could arise because of insufficient preoperative neuroradiologic assessment. MRI could be of the utmost importance. Simple fenestration of the cyst is insufficient and recurrence frequently occurs. There are reports on successful endoscopic surgery for arachnoidal cysts, but the recurrence rate is still pretty high (24, 25).

c) Basilar invagination

Developmental anomalies of the cranial bones and craniocervical junction are best shown by MR examination. Their importance is enhanced by the introduction of new diagnostic or surgical methods for symptomatic anomalies. Surgery should provide for stabilization of the reversible disorders, decompression, if the deformity compresses the neural tissue, or fixation in case of instability. Basilar invagination (prolapse of the cervical vertebra into the cranial base, usually accompanied by atlas occipitalization, incomplete vertebral closure and vertebral fusion, and Arnold - Chiari malformation in 25-30%) belongs to this group of anomalies, as well as basilar impression (acquired basilar invagination because of the bone pathology) and platybasia (abnormal, blunt angle between clivus and anterior basal plane, usually asymptomatic).

Basilar invagination could be suspected on the basis of plain radiographs if the lateral atlantooccipital articulation can not be seen in AP projection of cervical vertebra, through the open mouth. In lateral radiographs, upper projection of dense usually is less than 10 mm above the bimastoid line, and odontoid process 2.5 mm above Chamberlains line (connecting hard palate and posterior edge of the foramen magnum). Cervicomedullar ventral indentation is suspected if Wackenheim line, connecting posterior edge of clivus and spinal canal is dislocated. Anterior decompression is necessary. Disturbed relationship can be optimally visualized by MR examination (Fig. 43) (20).

REFERENCES

1. Adams RD., Victor M.: Principles of neurology. (3rd ed.): McGraw Eiel Bodo Company. New York, 1985.
2. Balomin RL., Le Mastu K.: Neurofibromatosis-2, and bilateral acoustic neurinomas: Distinctions from neurofibromatosis – 1 (von Reciolinghausens disease). Am. J. Otol., 10: 439-442, 1989.
3. Banna M.: Arachnoid cysts in the hypophyseal area. Clin. Radiol., 25: 323-326, 1974.
4. Batzdorf U.: Chiari Malformation and syringomyelia. In Apuzzo M. (ed.): Brain surgery, complication avoidance and management. Churchill Livingstone. New York, Edinburgh, London, Melbourne, Tokio, Vol.2, 1985-2001, 1993.
5. Bogen JE.: The callosal syndromes. In Heilman K.M., Valestein E. (eds).: Clinical Neuropsychology. University Press. New York, Oxford 337-707, 1993.
6. Ettlingar G.: Agenesis of the corpus callosum. In: Vinken PJ., Bruyn GW. (eds): Handbook of Clinical Neurology. North- Holland, Amsterdam, 30: 285-297, 1987.
7. Forbes W., Isherwood I.: Computed tomography in syringomyelia and the associated Arnold-Chiari type I malformation. Neuroradiology, 15: 73-84, 1978.
8. Gademann G.: NMR-Tomography of the Normal Brain. Springer Verlag. Berlin, Heidelberg, New York, Tokyo. 1988.
9. Gerhardt P., Fromhold W.: Atlas of Anatomic Correlations in CT and MRI. Thieme. New York, Tokyo, Heidelberg. 1988.
10. Gomez MR.: Tuberous sclerosis 2nd ed. Raven Press. New York, 1988.
11. Guifre R., Pastore FS., Desantis S.: Congenital (fetal) hydrocephalus-an acquired pathology? Childs Nerv. Syst., 11: 97-101, 1995.
12. Halbsgut A., Lechner B.: Magnetresonanz-Tomographie (NMR). Springer-Verlag. Frankfurt, 1986.
13. Han JS., Benson JE., Kaufman B. et al.: MR imaging of pediatric cerebral anomalies. J. Comput. Assist. Tomogr., 9: 103-113, 1985.
14. Huk WJ., Gademann G., Friedman G.: Magnetic Resonance Imaging of Central Nervous System Diseases. Springer Verlag. Berlin, New York, Heidelberg, Tokyo, Paris, London, 1989.
15. Kalidasan V., Carroll T.: The Dandy Walker Syndrome – a 10 Year Experience of the management and outcome. Eur. J. Pediatr. Surg., 5/1: 16-18, 1995.
16. Liessner J., Seider M.: Klinische Kernspintomographie. Enke. Stuttgart, 1987.
17. Loesor JD., Alvord EC.: Agenesis of the corpus callosum. Brain, 91: 553-570, 1968.
18. Macchi G., Bentivoglio M.: Agenesis or hypoplasia of cerebellar structures. In Vinken PJ., Bruyn GW. (eds): Handbook of Clinical Neurology. North Holland, Amsterdam, 30: 367-393, 1977.

19. McKennan KX., Bard A.: Neurofibromatosis type 2: Report of a family and review of current evaluation and treatment. Laryngoscope, 101: 109-113, 1991.
20. Menezes AH., Van Gilder JC.: Platybasia, Basilar invagination and cranial settling. In Apuzzo M. (ed.): Brain surgery, complication avoidance and management. Churchill Livingstone, Vol. 2, 2029-2049, New York, Edinburgh, London, Melbourne, Tokyo, 1993.
21. Mori K.: Current concert of hydrocephalus: Evolution of new classifications. Childs Nerv. Syst., 11: 523-531 1995.
22. Nishikawa M.: Pathogenesis of Chiari malformation: a morphometric study of the posterior cranial fossa, J. Neurosurg., 86: 40-47, 1997.
23. Pascual-Castronieyo I., Velez A., Pascual–Naschal SI., et al.: Dandy-Walker malformation: analysis of 38 cases. Childs Nerv. Syst., 7: 88-97, 1997.
24. Perneczky A., Tschabitscher M., Resch K.: Endoscopic anatomy for neurosurgery. Georg Thieme Verlag. Stuttgart, New York, 1993.
25. Piven J.: The biological basis of autism. Cur. Opin. Neurobiol., 7: 708-712, 1997.
26. Pomeranz JS.: Craniospinal Magnetic Resonance Imaging. W.B. Saunders Company. Philadelphia, London, Toronto, Sydney, Tokyo, 1989.
27. Raffel C., Mc Comb JG.: Encephalocele. In Apuzzo M. (ed.): Brain surgery, complication avoidance and management. Churchill Livingstone, Vol. 2, New York, Edinburgh, London, Melbourne, Tokyo, 1433-1447, 1993.
28. Rapin D., Katzman R.: Neurobiology of autism. Ann. Neurol., 43: 7-14, 1998.
29. Reiser M., Semmler W.: Magnet-rezonanz-Tomographie. Springer-Verlag. Berlin, Heidelberg, New York, Paris, London, Tokyo, Hong Kong, 1989.
30. Ruge J., McLone D.: Cerebrospinal fluid diversion procedures. In: Apuzzo M. (ed.): Brain surgery, complication avoidance and management. Churchill Livingstone, New York, Edinburgh, London, Melbourne, Tokyo, Vol. 2, 1463-1494, 1993.
31. Trowbridge WV., French JD.: Benign arachnoid cyst of the posterior fossa. J. Neurosurg., 9: 398-404, 1952.
32. Schnizlein HN., Murtagh FR.: Imaging anatomy of the ventricles and cisterns with magnetic resonance. Urban and Schwarzenberg. Medical Publishers. Baltimore-Munich, 1985.
33. Stark D., Bradley GWJR.: Magnetic Resonance Imaging. The C.V. Mosby Company. St. Louis, Washington D.C., Toronto, 1988.
34. Van M. Runge: Enhanced Magnetic Resonance Imaging. The C.V. Mosby Company. St. Louis, Baltimore, Toronto, 1989.
35. Van Hoff SC., Wilmink JT.: Cerebellar agenesis. J. Belge Radiol., 79: 282, 1996.
36. Venes J., Brunberg J.: Cysts. In Apuzzo M. (ed.): Brain surgery, complication avoidance and management. Churchill Livingstone, New York, Edinburgh, London, Melbourne, Tokyo, Vol. 2, 2001-2021, 1993.
37. Wackenheim A., Jeanmart L., Beart A.: Craniocerebral Computer Tomography. Vol. 1, Berlin, Heidelberg, New York, 1980.
38. Warkany J., Lemire RJ., Cohen MM.: Encephaloceles. In Warkany J., Lemire RJ., Cohen MM. (eds): Mental retardation and congenital malformations of the central nervous system. Chicago, Jear Book Medical Publishers Chicago, 158, 1976.
39. Zawadcki MB., Norman D.: Magnetic Resonance Imaging of the Central Nervous System. Raven Press, New York, 1987.
40. Zeitler E.: Kernspintomographie. Deutsche Artze Verlag. Koeln, 1984.

II. CEREBROVASCULAR DISEASES OF THE BRAIN

Gradimir Dragutinović, Zvonimir Lević, Ivan Piščević

Cerebral angiography is the keystone of neuroradiologic diagnosis of cerebrovascular diseases:
- panangiography, after Seldinger, enables imaging of all cerebral blood vessels by catheterization through the aortic arch,
- selective percutaneous carotid or vertebro-basilar angiography is done by direct puncture to the carotid artery, on one or both sides, or to the dominant, usually left vertebral artery, under general anesthesia,
- digital subtraction angiography (DSA) is computer assisted detailed imaging of one or several cerebral blood vessels and their tiniest branches, whether Seldinger technique or direct percutaneous puncture is used.

Invasive cerebral angiography directly displays pathology of cerebral blood vessels, showing a lot of advantages and certain faults. Optimal imaging of blood vessels and pathology such as stenosis, aneurysm, a-v malformation, etc. is possible. Invasiveness, ionizing radiation and technical failure are the basic disadvantages.

CT and MR enable direct visualization of vascular lesions. Being less invasive, CT is done prior to angiography for emergency diagnosis. In a critically ill patient, with cerebrovascular pathology, CT helps to establish the diagnosis, and decide upon conservative or neurosurgical treatment. No iodine contrast enhancement is needed, unless vascular lesions had to be distinguished from other pathology (16).

Angiography should follow the CT examination in emergency diagnosis of vascular pathology, such as aneurysm, internal carotid artery occlusion, a-v malformation, etc.

MR imaging is used in subacute or chronic conditions in order to improve CT and angiographic findings.

Cerebrovascular diseases can be caused by:
- Arterial blood flow disorders
- Venous blood flow disorders
- Hemorrhage
- Vascular malformation
- Other causes (1)

1. Arterial blood flow disorders

Disturbed arterial blood flow is found in A) infarction and B) peripheral angiopathies.

A. Infarction

Infarction group encompasses:
a. Subclinical infarction
b. TIA (transitory ischemic attack)
c. RIND (prolonged reversible ischemia with neurologic insufficiency)
d. progressive infarction - in evolution
e. complete infarction - could not be distinguished in the acute phase

a. Subclinical infarction
MR imaging of subclinical infarction is seldom possible. Mild hypoxia of smaller brain areas caused by circulation disorder, does not change the tissue features enough to be seen by neuroradiologic examination (14).

b. Transitory ischemic attack (TIA)

Transitory ischemic attack (TIA) is caused by short term circulation disorders and brain tissue ischemia with rapid recovery and withdrawal of neurologic symptoms. Various symptoms can be seen in TIA, such as: hemiparesis, hemihypesthesia, dysphasia, dysarthria, hemianopsia, transient blindness (*amaurosis fugax*) or mental confusion. This symptomatology is seen in case of transitory ischemia of the carotid vascular region (38).

Transitory ischemia of the vertebro-basilar region is referred to as vertebro-basilar insufficiency. Vertigo, accompanied by nausea, vomiting, fatigue, disorders of vision (flashes, colors, visual field deficit) or even blindness are seen. Syncope, "drop attack", diplopia, dysarthria, hemiparesis, hemihypesthesia, transitory global amnesia, cranial nerve dysfunction, or headache, are the symptoms of vertebro-basilar insufficiency. "Seesaw" phenomenon, meaning alternative symptoms, such as hemiparesis, of one or the other side, is typical (4).

Symptoms are of short duration, usually for a couple of hours, but no more than 24 hours, and completely reversible.

CT finding is negative.

TIA is rarely diagnosed by MRI. Neurologic examination helps choose the right time for MR imaging. MR angiography (MRA) of the major cervical and cerebral blood vessels is indicated for TIA (37).

c. Prolonged reversible ischemia

Different factors can cause prolonged reversible ischemia of various degrees, with subsequent neurologic deficit due to the disturbed blood circulation and brain tissue oxygenation. Complex biochemical disorders following ischemia can cause dysbalance of intra- and extracellular fluid. Mild brain cell damage, with spontaneous or therapy induced recovery, is followed by minimal nerve cell destruction. Glial proliferation is a sign of regeneration process. Neurologic deficit is characteristic for the first stage of ischemia. *Restitutio ad integrum* is impossible. Ischemic tissue recovery is followed by neurologic symptoms withdrawal (21).

Site and volume of the hypoxic brain mass induce the symptoms of prolonged reversible ischemia. Besides headache and neurologic deficit, disorders of vision, speech, etc. can be found. Different epileptic modalities can arise, depending on location of the ischemic zone. Duration up to several days, neurologic deficit withdrawal after the restitution of ischemia and patient's complete recovery, are the basic features of prolonged reversible ischemia.

Regions of reversible ischemia are seen in CT as hypodense areas (5).

Prolonged reversible ischemia is shown in MR tomographs through a dysbalance of intra and extracellular water, i.e. hydrogen protons. Therapeutic response of ischemic brain tissue can be evaluated by MR controls. Rarely, in cases of complete restitution, withdrawal of the lesion can be confirmed by MRI. MRA of the major endocranial and cervical blood vessels can be useful for the diagnosis.

MR imaging in axial and coronal planes, using T-2W sequence enables the diagnosis of the smallest ischemic lesions, with high signal intensity, more precisely than CT (Fig. 44).

d. Progressive infarction

Evolution of progressive infarction is due either to obliteration of brain blood vessels or to critical decrease of the blood flow, following thrombosis, embolism, etc,. It can cause the death of the brain cells within the vascularization area of the compromised blood vessel. Neighboring tissue remains unaffected, due to collateral vascularization through undamaged blood vessels or CFS (superficial cortical layer, ependyma, subependyma).

Infarction volume depends on the diameter and number of affected blood vessels. Initial edema and ischemia in the infarction zone leads to the cell death. In the next phase, cell disintegration causes necrosis. Cystic cavity formed through colliquation is delineated from normal brain tissue by perifocal edema. White colliquated mass is called white infarction (*Infarctus cerebri albus*). Red infarction, following vein thrombosis and reflux of blood from unaffected cells in the vicinity, has got the red color because of petechial hemorrhage (*Encephalomalacia rubra*).

Ischemic insult has sudden onset. One or several transitory ischemic attacks occasionally precede the complete insult. Wake-up hemiplegia, accompanied by aphasia, is present, if the dominant hemisphere

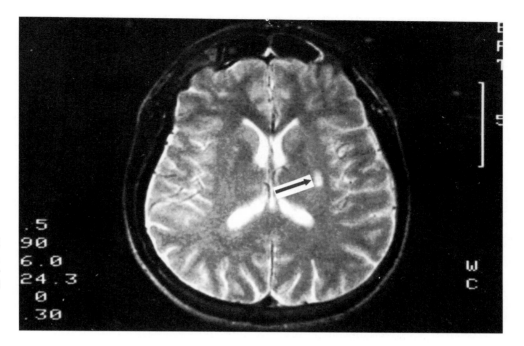

Figure 44. Axial image (SE 2500/90). Small infarction, showing as high signal intensity area in the left temporal region - arrow.

is affected. Sometimes the clinical course is slowly progressive, with oscillatory neurologic deficit, and complete hemiplegia is achieved in a couple of days. Subsequent edema leads to intracranial hypertension and headache. Vomiting and coma can follow during the next few days. Although hemiplegia is considered synonymous to the cerebrovascular insult, neurologic deficit can be extremely variable, depending on blood vessel and brain area which are involved. Hemianesthesia, hemianopsia, alexia, agnosia, dysinhibitory phenomena, confusion, cranial nerve disorders, cerebellar or other symptoms can occur. However, it should be kept in mind that the majority of the brain infarctions are atypical or asymptomatic, found accidentally by CT, MR or autopsy.

CT scan is usually sufficient for the diagnosis of progressive infarction, unless the diagnosis is not clear. Irregular hypodense zone in the vascularization area of the affected blood vessel is seen.

Surrounding bone structures of the cranial base or posterior fossa can cause the artifacts, blurring the picture and thus making CT diagnosis difficult.

The best way to assess progressive infarction is MRI. Multiplanar approach and high resolution of MR imaging provides for differential diagnosis from other lesions and detailed evaluation of the infarction volume and severity (15).

Progressive infarction in the posterior fossa or adjacent to the massive bones of the cranial base, is clearly delineated by MR. Additional MRA should be useful for the precise assessment of the site of lesion and surgery planning (7).

Infarction, with its high signal intensity, is perfectly shown by MR tomographs in axial, coronal, and, optionally, sagittal view, using T-2W sequence. No other sequence is necessary (Fig 45).

e. Complete infarction

Complete infarction is when definitive cyst due to encephalomalacia is formed, with subsequent terminal proliferation of connective tissue cells and macroglia. Cyst wall is built of macroglia and connective tissue cells, separating the cavity from surrounding brain parenchyma. Dark stained hemosiderin deposits, originating from petechial hemoglobin, can be seen in the cyst wall. Shrinking of the cyst can occur due to the fiber retraction, so that cerebral ventricles or cisterns could be dislocated towards the infarction zone.

Complete infarction is definitive lesion of cerebral parenchyma, with maximal perifocal edema regression. Neurologic symptoms, corresponding to the affected brain area, become steady. Conservative treatment and rehabilitation could subdue the sequels of the complete infarction to a certain extent. However, complete recovery is impossible (10).

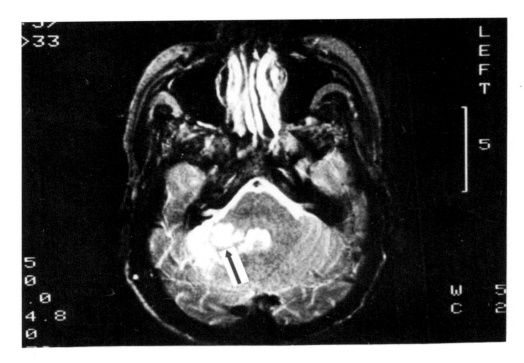

Figure 45. Axial image (SE2500/90). Progressive infarction, of irregular shape and high signal intensity, is seen in the right side of cerebellum, next to the fourth ventricle - arrow.

MR imaging can give precise image of the lesion in case of subacute or chronic complete infarction. CT examination is indicated in subacute phase.

Magnetic resonance is seldom required for the diagnosis, unless differential diagnosis is required, when CT scan and angiography findings are not conclusive. Complete infarction is shown as postencephalomalatic cyst, surrounded by irregular low density edge. Sometimes, it is not easy for the radiologist to distinguish between slowly growing expansive lesion and complete infarction.

Infarction with high signal intensity is best displayed by MR in T-2W sequence using axial and coronal planes (15). Hemosiderin edge has low signal intensity (Fig. 46).

MRA of major endocranial and cervical blood vessels is obligatory.

f. Peripheral angiopathies

Pathologic disorders of precapillary arterioles and capillaries can cause ischemic lesions in smaller regions of the brain.

Hypertensive encephalopathy is found only in malignant hypertension, with diastolic pressure exceeding 130 mm Hg. Malignant hypertension can be seen not only in essential hypertension, but in glomerulonephritis, pheochromocytoma and eclampsia as well. Fibrinoid necrosis of retinal, cerebral and renal arterioles is found. Retinal hemorrhage and effusion, as well as papillary edema of the optical nerve, are seen. Ischemic and hemorrhagic foci and edema are found in the brain (14).

Headache, vomiting, seizures, focal neurologic deficit, such as paresis, palsy, hemianopsia, aphasia, psychological alteration and consciousness disorders, including coma, disturbed mental functioning, and even psychosis, can be found in hypertensive encephalopathy.

Former entity "arteriosclerotic dementia" has been abandoned in favor of "multiinfarction dementia - MID", based on the opinion that the problem is caused by numerous recidivant infarctions, and not by global hypoperfusion, due to diffuse stenosis of the blood vessels.

Multiinfarction dementia decreases cognitive and social functioning. Disorders of memory, orientation, speech and judgment are present.

"Arteriosclerotic pseudoneurasthenia" consisting of constant fatigue, apathy, excitability, melancholy, poor concentration, headache, sleep disorders, forgetfulness, etc. can precede fully expressed clinical entity of MID. Personality features are absurdly enhanced and professional competency is lost. Advanced phase could be characterized by profound dementia. Focal neurologic deficit is observed as well.

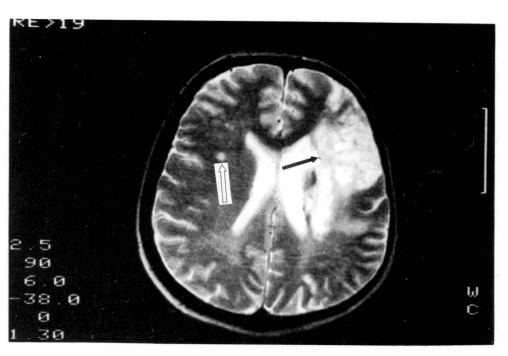

Figure 46. Axial image (SE 2500/90). Complete infarction shown as a large irregular area with high signal intensity, in the left temporo-parietal region, vascularized by arteria cerebri media - black arrow. Few postencephalomalatic cysts of high signal intensity are seen within the infarction zone. Several small infarctions of high signal intensity, are found in the right parietal and left parieto-occipital regions as well - white arrow.

CT scan can be negative in cases with peripheral angiopathy. Infarction and edema are seen as hypodense zones, whereas smaller hemorrhagic foci are hyperdense.

MR image can display numerous non-specific lesions, but they could be recognized only if the complete clinical presentation and other analysis are taken into consideration.

Various manifestations of peripheral angiopathies can be observed during neurologic examination and confirmed by MRI, but no specific feature of this entity, regarding signal intensity, can be outlined.

Multiple microinfarctions are seen, in T-2W using axial section, in MRI of a hypertensive patient. Microinfarctions are lesions with high signal intensity, of variable shape and size (Figg. 47, 48).

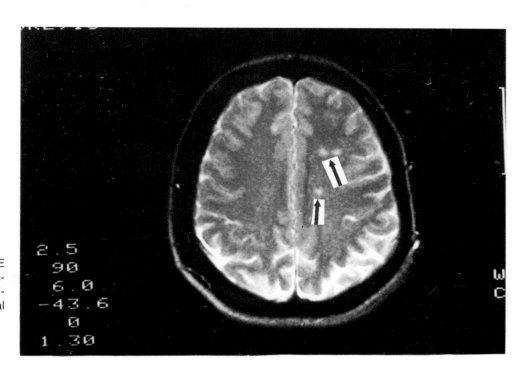

Figure 47. Axial image (SE 2500/90). Punctiform infarctions, with high signal intensity, are seen in the left parietal area - arrows.

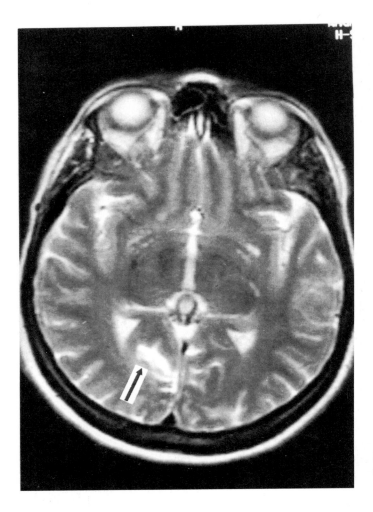

Figure 48. Axial image (TSE 4000/99). Arrow pointing small infarction in the right occipital zone.

2. Venous blood flow disorders

In case of venous blood flow disorder, it is necessary to reveal the changes following either thrombosis of veins and sinuses, caused by infection, trauma, surgery, pregnancy and delivery, or the occlusion of veins due to expansive lesions such as tumor, edema, etc (2).

Sinus thrombosis is usually caused by surrounding infection arising in the middle ear, mastoid, paranasal sinuses, orbit or the soft tissue of the upper part of the face. Apart from local infection signs, the signs of intracranial hypertension, edema of the scalp, venous stasis in the superficial veins, seizures and focal spells, can be seen (33).

In cases of the cavernous sinus thrombophlebitis, edema and suffusion of the eyelids and conjunctiva, accompanied by ptosis, dyplopia and papillary edema are present (13, 18).

Increase of intracranial pressure causes the papillary stasis and vision disorders, despite conservative antiedematous therapy. Lumboperitoneal shunt can help to get intracranial pressure under control.

Thrombosis of the longitudinal or transversal sinus is usually seen in dehydrated and marantic children.

Venous thrombosis or occlusion can cause the red brain infraction, combined meningeal and cerebral infarction, brain edema, etc.

Angiography is a method of choice for the diagnosis of the pathology of cerebral venous system.

CT examination in axial, and eventually direct coronal planes, is insufficient for the diagnosis of the venous lesions. Consequent brain tissue lesions, due to the venous blood flow disorders can be seen in CT, depending on their size and location.

MR can give the detailed image of the venous and sinus pathology. MR tomography is extremely valuable for the diagnosis of the *cavernous sinus* lesions (30).

Thrombosis of the *transversal and sygmoid sinus* is best revealed by MR imaging, in FLASH sequence for slow blood flow, in axial, sagittal and coronal views (implementation of "Flow phenomenon"). Para-axial planes, in the same sequence, can be used as well. Slowly flowing blood has high signal intensity, whereas the thrombi or changed walls of the blood vessel, have lower signal intensities (6).

MR imaging in the sagittal section, using above mentioned sequences, are ideal for revealing the pathologic lesions of the *superior sagittal sinus* (Figg. 49, 50).

3. Hemorrhage

Intracranial hemorrhage can be either intra- or extra-cerebral, spontaneous or caused by trauma. Trauma is the most frequent cause of the cerebral hemorrhage.

Extracerebral hemorrhage can be either epidural, subdural or subarachnoidal.

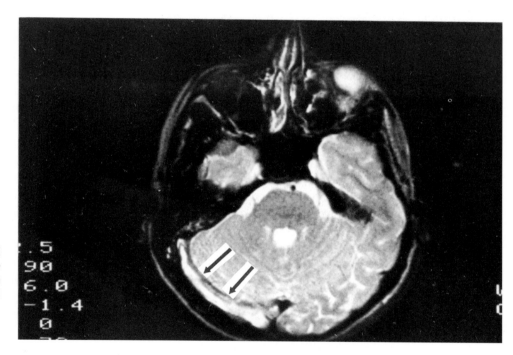

Figure 49. Axial image (SE 2500/90). Thrombosis of the right transversal sinus, shown by high and partly lower signal intensities - arrows.

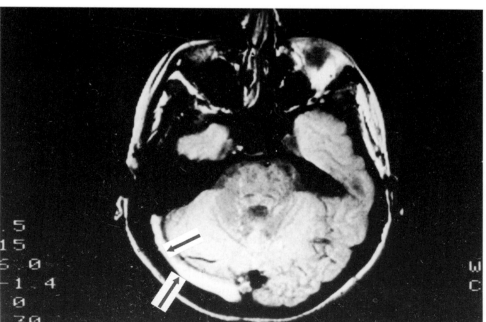

Figure 50. Axial image (SE 2500/15). Thrombosis of the transversal sinus, shown by high signal intensity - arrows.

Epidural hemorrhage is caused by traumatic rupture of the *medial meningeal artery*, and the blood is collected between the cranial bone and dura.

Epidural hematoma is usually caused by the rupture of the *medial meningeal artery*, following fracture of the temporal bone squama. The scull fracture can be proven (by radiography, surgery or autopsy) in 90% of adults and 50% of children suffering from epidural hematoma. Craniogram usually reveals the fracture line across the meningeal sulci and venous sinuses projection. Temporo-parietal location is the most frequent, whereas the frontal, occipital or posterior fossa hematomas are exceptionally rare.

In case of occipital trauma, fracture line cross the venous sinuses, so that such lesion should be suspected if the patient has headache, anxiety, vomiting or abducent paresis.

Typical epidural hematoma caused by ruptured artery, is rapidly progressive: the initial loss of consciousness is followed by transient recovery and later by recurrent unconsciousness, contralateral hemiplegia, seizures and ipsilateral Hutschinson pupil (dilated pupil with no reaction to the light). Epidural hematoma in children can arise without scull fracture. Infants under 2 years of age, have completely different clinical course with pallor, hypotension and vegetative disorders.

Symptoms due to the injury should be differentiated from the complications following the pressure on the brain by hematoma. Local circulation disorder and consequent cerebral edema can cause the dislocation and herniation of the brain as well as intracranial hypertension. Minor trauma can lack the commotion syndrome. Typical course, however, is characterized by the lucid interval after the initial unconsciousness, followed by deterioration of the patients condition due to the hematoma enlargement, with severe headache, vomiting, contralateral paresis, unconsciousness and temporary ipsilateral pupil narrowing, followed by complete dilation (Hutschinson pupil). Further progression of the hematoma leads to the contralateral transtentorial herniation of the midbrain, thus causing the ipsilateral paresis, deep coma, decerebration rigidity and bilaterally dilated pupils. The clinical course, however, can be atypical: i.e. without the lucid interval, in patients with brain contusion, or blurred by trauma to oculomotorius nerve.

Surgical therapy can save the patients life, whereas delayed surgery diminishes the prospects for the patients recovery. Osteoplastic craniotomy, depending on the hematoma location, is followed by blood evacuation and hemostasis.

Epidural hematoma of the posterior fossa can be overlooked, because of atypical clinical course, in the beginning, or rapid progression afterwards, thus endangering the patient by the delayed surgery. In cases with external injuries in the occipital area, with fracture line crossing the venous sinuses, occipital headache, anxiety, abducent paresis, cerebellar signs, neck rigidity, and cardio-respiratory disorders, the occipital epidural hematoma should be suspected. Even in cases with respiratory distress, preceding cardiac arrest, emergency surgery could save the patients life. Exceptionally, epidural hemorrhage can be caused by injury of the dural or cranial bone veins, with the clinical course being atypical due to gradual onset of focal neurologic deficit and slowly progressive consciousness disorder. Neuroradiologic image is identical to the previous entity and surgery is the treatment of choice.

In patients with scull fracture, epidural hemorrhage can be limited to the fracture area. If asymptomatic they don't require surgery.

Diagnosis of epidural hemorrhage is usually made by angiography or CT scan and no MR examination is necessary.

Subdural hemorrhage is caused by trauma, and neurologic deficit either uni- or bilateral is caused by the compression of surrounding structures, in acute, subacute or chronic phase. Acceleration in traffic injuries makes acute subdural hematoma 10 times more frequent than the epidural one. Rupture of pontine or cortical veins, associated with brain contusion, can cause acute subdural hematoma with primary unconsciousness, contralateral palsy and later on, ipsilateral Hutschinson pupil, due to the focal brain compression and herniation. There is no "free interval" regarding consciousness. Surgery is mandatory as it is for epidural hematoma. Osteoplastic or osteoclastic craniotomy should be followed by hematoma evacuation. Emergency surgery can influence the outcome, although the overall results are worse than in epidural hematoma, because of the concomitant brain contusion or intracerebral hemorrhage. Prolonged stay in the intensive care unit increases the risk of the complications, especially in elderly patients. The mortality rate is pretty high, due to the afore mentioned reasons.

Subacute subdural hematoma, following axial head trauma with pontine veins rupture and no associated brain damage, has milder clinical course, resembling epidural hematoma, up to three weeks after the injury. Surgical results are far better. Coagulated, partly organized and seldom colliquated hematoma, without the capsule, is found during the surgery.

Chronic subdural hematoma is caused by minor, often neglected head trauma, that have occurred 1-3 months before. Elderly, alcoholics, with fragile blood vessels, hemophilic patients, or those using anti-coagulant medication are at risk. Venous hemorrhage, following pontine veins rupture, leads to the slow accumulation of blood between *dura mater and arachnoid*. Chronic subdural hematoma can have 1-3 mm thick capsule. The reason why the capsule is formed, instead of the absorption of the hematoma, has not been explained yet. Latent coagulation disorder can prevent hematoma coagulation and resorption. Cellular fibrinolytic activity makes the process of central liquefaction faster than organization of hematoma. The capsule is formed, and the volume increased due to oncotic assimilation of water, secretion or secondary hemorrhage.

Hematoma enlargement causes neurologic deficit, intellectual deterioration, seizures, contralateral and, later on, ipsilateral hemiparesis, due to the brainstem dislocation and compression to the *crus cerebri and tentorium cerebelli*. Intracranial hypertension, with headache, vomiting and papillary stasis, can develop later on, but eventual post-traumatic dementia should be differentiated from the degenerative or vascular one. Ipsilateral Hutschinson pupil can be seen in the terminal stage. Bilateral chronic subdural hematoma can mimic dementia or cerebrovascular insult. Surgery consists of simple craniotomy with hematoma evacuation, resection of the capsule and enabling the liquor circulation in order to prevent recurrences.

Angiography or enhanced CT scan are usually sufficient for the diagnosis, except in cases with bilateral hematoma with confusing findings.

MR imaging is perfect for the diagnosis in such cases because it can make clear distinction between the brain tissue and hematoma (29).

Features of traumatic intracerebral hematoma differ from the spontaneous one. Ruptures of intracerebral arteries are caused by head trauma, usually in the typical brain contusion areas and associated with other injuries. Lucid interval, followed by subsequent deterioration of the patients condition, is typical. Surgery consists of osteoplastic craniotomy, followed by evacuation of hematoma and malatic brain tissue. If there has been free interval, the patient has better prospects. Diagnosis is based on CT scan and MR examination is seldom necessary (26).

Nowadays, cerebrovascular diseases are the cause of death in more than one third of people. Spontaneous subarachnoidal hemorrhage is the cause of death in 5-10% of patients. Subarachnoidal hemorrhage is suspected if the traces of blood are found in liquor, usually following the rupture of the aneurysm into subarachnoidal space. Over one half of subarachnoidal hemorrhage is caused by ruptured aneurysm, but there is still quite a number of unknown etiology(22%). A-V malformation, hypertension or other causes can also lead to subarachnoidal hemorrhage. A-V malformation is the principal cause in patients under 20, while the ruptured aneurysm is more frequent in elderly patients. Ruptured aneurysm is 25 times more frequent than AVM in fifty year olds.

Subarachnoidal hemorrhage attack is a rather dramatic event, that can arise both under stress or during the rest. It can be recognized by the headache, unconsciousness, vomiting and meningeal signs.

Clinical course of the subarachnoidal hemorrhage is rather typical, with sudden occipital pain, spreading to the neck and spine and, sometimes, to the frontal area. Nausea, vomiting and somnolence develop as the intracranial pressure increases. The blood irritates the meninges, thus causing meningeal signs. Focal deficit, such as hemiparesis, ophthalmoplegia, epilepsy etc. can arise, due to the compression by associated intracerebral hematoma to the surrounding brain tissue. Later on, the focal deficit can be caused by vasospasm. Vegetative disorders, especially bradycardia, are usually associated with subarachnoidal hemorrhage (32).

If the blood is found in subarachnoidal space by lumbar puncture, CT scan or rarely MRI, should be followed by panangiography of cerebral blood vessels. MR examination, being non-invasive, can be more appropriate for some patients than classic angiography (20). Treatment depends on the cause of the hemorrhage and clinical presentation. In cases with adjacent intracerebral hematoma, when the patient is in danger, emergency surgery consists of the hematoma evacuation, and the causal therapy should be postponed. If the aneurysm or AVM is proved by angiography, the timing of surgery should be appropriate considering the best prospects, site of lesion and clinical stage. Unless the huge intracerebral hematoma accompanies AVM, there is no need for emergency surgery, and it could be postponed until the patient is stabilized and recovered from hemorrhage (31).

CT scan is an ideal method for the diagnosis of hyperdense extracerebral hemorrhage, as well as for the planning of surgery. Unlike epidural or subdural hematoma, subarachnoid hemorrhage can be easily overlooked on CT scan, except in the acute stage when the blood is clearly seen on the convex surface of the brain or in the basal cisterns. Blood, accumulated in the ventricular system or cerebral cisterns, is hyperdense.

If the chronic extracerebral hemorrhage is suspected and CT scan is negative, MR examination is indicated (19, 28).

Subacute or chronic epi- and subdural hemorrhage can be detected on MR tomographs with accuracy. Extracerebral, i.e epidural or subdural hemorrhage is shown in MRI, done in T-2W sequence using axial and coronal planes, as biconvex or convex-concave area of higher signal intensity. Signal intensity of surrounding brain structures is changed due to the compressive effect of the extracerebral blood collection. Brain lesions are seen as high signal intensity areas in T-2W sequence. Extracerebral blood collection is represented by higher or very high signal intensities, in T-1W sequence, whereas hygroma has low signal intensity (Fig. 51).

Massive subarachnoidal hemorrhage is shown in MRI by characteristic blood signal intensities in the convexity and base of the brain.

Spontaneous intracerebral hemorrhage can be caused either by a) malformation (aneurysm, angioma, etc.) and vascular disorder; or by b) extracranial factors (hypertensive hemorrhage, blood coagulation disorders, infection or intoxication, etc.). Trauma can cause intracerebral hemorrhage, usually accompanied by brain contusion (20).

Pathologist classify hemorrhage either as capillary, caused by diapedesis, or massive, due to the ruptured blood vessel. Capillary hemorrhage has the necrotic edge, with peripheral erythrocytes embedded in surrounding brain tissue. Adjacent brain tissue is edematous. Massive brain hemorrhage (apoplexia cerebri) destructs the brain tissue, thus forming the cavity filled with blood. Moist cerebral edema is found in the vicinity.

Spontaneous intracerebral hemorrhage is usually seen in hypertensive patients, following physical effort. Sudden onset, with hemiplegia, headache, vomiting and unconsciousness, is due to rapidly increasing intracranial hypertension. Hemorrhage in the vicinity of the basal ganglia and *capsula interna*, known as "capsular hemiplegia", is associated with hemianesthesia and hemianopsia.

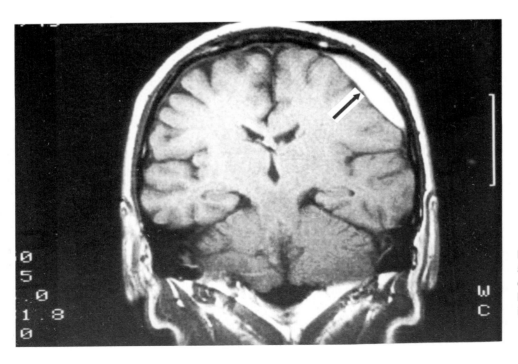

Figure 51. Coronal image (SE 500/15). Left parietal extracerebral hematoma shown as biconvex area of high signal intensity - arrow.

If hematoma is situated in the white matter of the cerebral hemisphere, other disorders such as aphasia, agnosia, apraxia or another cortical deficit can be seen. Conjugated deviation of the eyes and head, contralateral to hemiplegia, is frequently seen. Massive hemorrhage is usually associated with coma, decerebration rigidity and fatal outcome, while minor hemorrhage into ventricular system has no serious neurologic deficit, unconsciousness or poor prognosis.

Surgical procedures for spontaneous intracerebral hematoma in different localizations are studied and discussed by neurosurgeons, because of its high incidence, high mortality rate and varying therapy results reported in literature. According to japanese Authors, 90000 people in Japan die each year because of the cerebrovascular diseases, and, among them, only the patients with spontaneous intracerebral hematoma under 65, with progressive course and clinical deterioration, can benefit from surgical therapy, whereas all the others will do better with conservative treatment. Indications for surgery of the spontaneous intracerebral hematoma have not been clearly outlined yet. Many factors, such as the age of the patient, consciousness level, associated arterial hypertension, hematoma size and location, should be taken into consideration before the surgery (9).

Even the smallest hematoma in the brainstem can cause alternating syndromes, coma and fatal outcome. Cerebellar hematomas are a very serious clinical condition with poor prognosis. Vertigo, vomiting and ataxia are present in the beginning, followed by coma later on. Intracerebral hematoma with compromised liquor circulation requires surgical treatment.

CT scan is absolutely the method of choice for visualizing intracerebral hemorrhage. Hyperdense blood is clearly seen in the native CT scans. CT examination is an ideal method for emergency patients, because of its short duration and resuscitation possibilities. Computerized tomography enables quick diagnosis and proceeding to the angiography in order to define the cause and location of the hemorrhage precisely (40).

MR image is useful for the diagnosis of the basal and posterior fossa pathology, including intracerebral hemorrhage. MR is indispensable for the differentiation from the expansive lesions, artifacts, etc (39, 44).

MR examination, in T-1W and T-2W sequences in axial and coronal planes, can display the blood collection, with high signal intensity, surrounded by perifocal edema, which has low signal intensity in T-1W sequence. MR tomographs of cerebral edema in T-2W sequence shows higher signal intensity.

Hemosiderin deposits, with low signal intensities in all sequences, are found in the vicinity of the blood collection, in the advanced stage of intracerebral hemorrhage. This parameter can be used to determine the chronicity of the hemorrhage (Figg. 52-55).

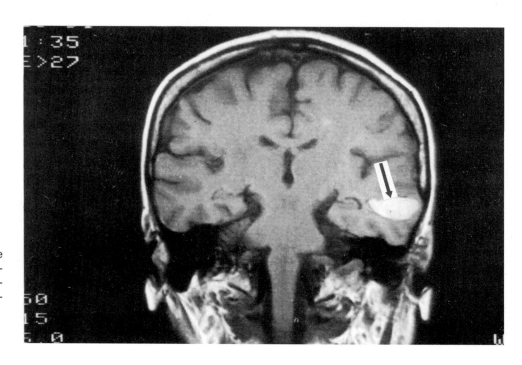

Figure 52. Coronal image (SE 500/15). Small intracerebral hematoma, with high signal intensity, in the left temporobasal region - arrow.

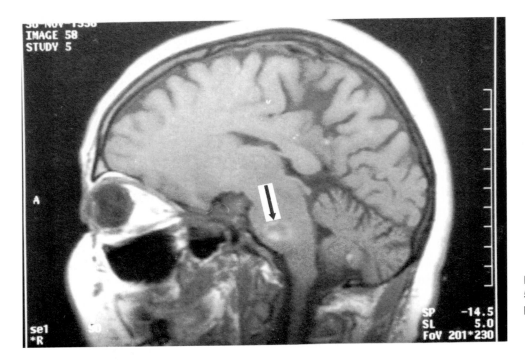

Figure 53. Sagittal image (SE 560/15). Hemorrhage in the pons - arrow.

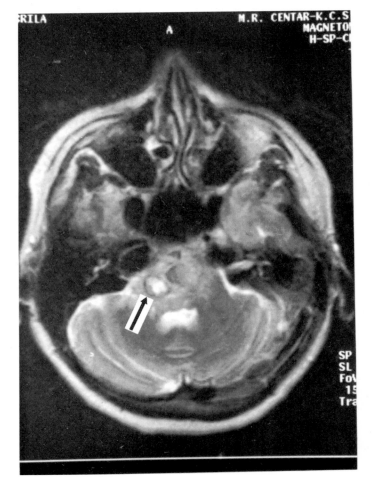

Figure 54. Axial image (SE 2500/90) - Hemorrhage in the pons-arrow.

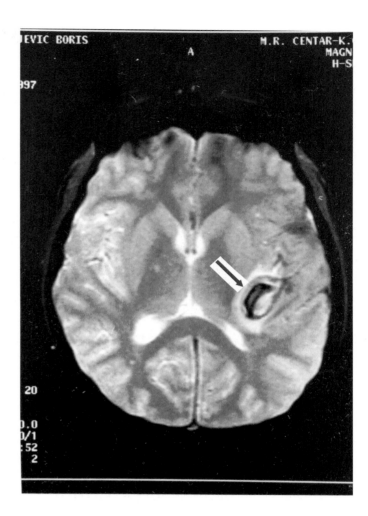

Figure 55. Axial image (GRE 800/26/20 degrees) - Massive hemorrhage in the left temporo-parietal region.

4. Vascular malformations

Vascular malformations are caused by developmental disorders of the blood vessels.
Vascular malformations are:

- A-V malformation
- Aneurysm of the major blood vessels
- Varices of the Galens vein
- Venous angioma
- Capillary telangiectasia
- Cryptogenous, i.e. occult A-V malformation (cavernoma).

Diversity of the pathohistological terms, used for vascular malformations, leads to different classifications. Development and shape of vascular malformation can be explained by irregular structure of the blood vessel walls, their position and relationship between arteries, capillaries and veins, etc.

Vascular malformations of the central nervous system differ from the vascular neoplasms by their specific and easily recognized macro- and microscopic looks. According to WHO classification, based on classic description by Russel and Rubinstein, as well as by McCormick and Boulter, there are four types of vascular malformations of the central nervous system: arterio - 1. venous malformation (AVM), 2. telangiectasia - capillary malformation, 3. venous malformation and 4. cavernous malformation (CM) (31).

a) A-V malformation (angioma)

A-V malformation (angioma) is congenital lesion, usually found in males with family predisposition. They are developed from the aberrant connections within primitive vascular plexus, which covers the developing cortex. At that developmental stage, circulation from the dura, scalp and bones is included in the vascular plexus, so that collateral connections, especially from dura, can be formed. Later on, the aberrant blood vessels become incorporated in the parenchyma, due to the secondary dilation of the veins. Chorioid variety, involving the surrounding venous sinuses, with A-V shunt draining to the major venous sinus in the midline, is seldom seen (aneurysm of the Galens vein) (36).

Intracranial arterio-venous malformation - angioma is a bundle of the tortuous, dilated blood vessels of the various caliber, directly connected to the arteries and veins, without capillary involvement, and surrounded by glial tissue. Abnormal arterial walls, with numerous aneurysms, and hyalinized and fibrous venous walls and a lot of varices, are seen on the microscope. According to the literature data, intracranial hemorrhage is the initial sign of the disease in as much as 30-55%, with minimal risk of the recurrent bleeding, unlike the ruptured aneurysm, and no risk of the blood vessel spasm. Such pathology is rarely candidate for emergency neurosurgery, except when massive intracerebral hematoma endangers the patients life.

In about one half of our patients intracerebral or subarachnoidal hemorrhage presents with hemiplegia, headache, vomiting, meningeal syndrome and unconsciousness. Epileptic seizures are registered in one third, while the focal neurologic signs and headache are the initial manifestation in one fifth of the patients with A-V malformation.

Large A-V malformation can produce progressive neurologic deficit, and even internal hydrocephalus. Some patients with long standing history of migraine have been proven to have A-V malformation in fact.

Angiography is a method of choice for the diagnosis of A-V malformation.

In emergency cases, with rapidly progressive clinical course and neurologic deficit, computer tomography is usually the first neuroradiologic examination. Major vascular malformation such as A-V malformation, bigger aneurysm or capillary telangiectasia can be suspected on the basis of CT scan. Angioma is seen like the hypodense, serpent- like area, in the CT scan and can be enhanced by iodine contrast administration. If CT scan is positive, the angiography is indicated to define the details of the pathologic vascularization, afferent and efferent blood vessels, multiplicity, etc (22, 23, 41).

MR is rarely needed for the diagnosis of angioma. MR examination is however superior to CT for the diagnosis of smaller angiomas, especially if located near the scull base or in the posterior fossa (3, 23).

MR examination, in T-1W sequence with multiplanar projection, can diagnose tortuous blood vessel of changed diameter, with low and high signal intensities ("**Flow phenomenon**"). Apart from low and high signal intensities of the angioma, marked perifocal edema, with higher signal intensity, can be seen in T-2W sequence as well. Possible hemorrhage from angioma shows different densities, depending of the applied sequence. Hemosiderin areas are frequently seen in the vicinity of the bleeding angiomas. Necrosis and calcification can be seen in the angioma as well, with signal intensities varying according to the MR sequence (24).

In **FLASH** sequence, for the slowly flowing blood, A-V malformation is displayed as the tortuous network of various signal intensities, through a combination of tangential and perpendicular effects of the "**Flow phenomenon**" (25, 27). Morphology is characteristic for the A-V malformation. Axial and coronal views are used. Sagittal section can be added, when necessary, to estimate the volume of A-V malformation or to display the afferent and efferent blood vessels (Figg. 56, 57).

Surgery for A-V malformation in the brain should prevent further hemorrhage and "steal phenomenon", enable recovery of neurologic deficit and treatment for poorly controlled epilepsy.

There are several procedures of surgical treatment for angioma, including direct microsurgical exposure, dissection and excision; as well as endovascular procedures of embolization of the afferent blood vessel by various particles, whether alone or combined with microsurgical resection. Angioma can be treated by gamma-knife or proton-ray in stereotaxy as well.

The best way to treat certain A-V malformation is chosen individually, regarding clinical course, neurologic deficit, age and condition of a patient, and surgical risk. According to Spetzler, surgical risk can be estimated for each AVM considering its features: 1. size - less than 3 cm (1 point), 3-6 cm (2), more

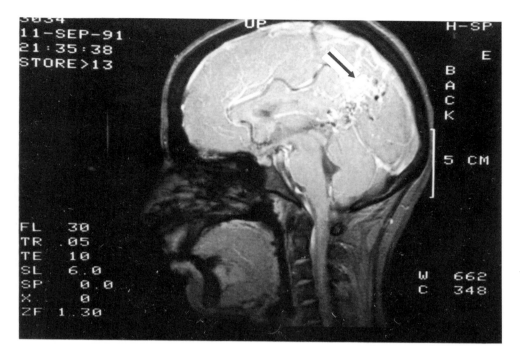

Figure 56. Axial image (GRE 50/10/30 degrees). AV malformation, with high signal intensity and occasional low signal intensity ("Flow phenomenon"), shown parasagittally in left parieto-occipital region - arrow. Irregular vascular network of the AVM is connected to the afferent and efferent vessels. Efferent veins drain to the sinus sagittalis superior.

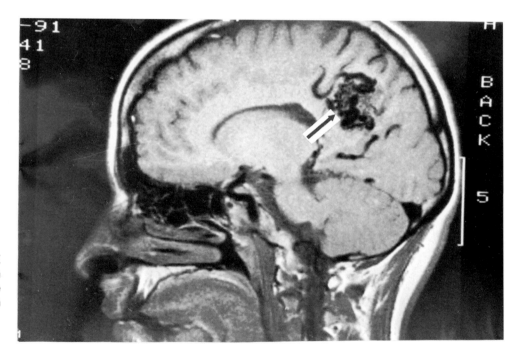

Figure 57. Sagittal image (SE 500/15). A-V malformation presenting as serpentine-like ribbons of varying width, with low signal intensities - arrow.

than 6 cm (3); 2. location - nonfunctional area (0), functional area (1); 3. type of the drainage - superficial (0) or deep (1). Total score of 1- 5 points defines the extent of surgical risk for certain AVM. The patients belonging to the 5th group are at the biggest risk. AVM are seldom considered inoperable nowadays, but if AVM is left untreated, the risk of second hemorrhage is 2-3% and the risk of progressive neurologic deficit 50%, with increasing mortality rate. Generally speaking, 40-50% of the untreated patients with AVM are at risk to be affected by severe neurologic deficit or death (34).

b) Aneurysms

Aneurysm is abnormal dilation of the blood vessel, due to the developmental disorder, atherosclerosis, trauma, etc. Intracranial blood vessels have no *lamina elastica* and muscular layer is insufficient at the branching sites. Aneurysm wall has thick intima and hyperplastic adventitia, with no muscular layer of media whatsoever.

Aneurysms usually belong to the carotid vascular area (80%) and only 20% to the vertebro-basilar one.

The shape of the aneurysm can be saccular, cylindrical, fusiform, navicular, serpiginous, etc. Saccular aneurysms of the branching site are the most frequent and most important from a surgeons point of view. Their fundus is connected to the artery by a neck. Traumatic aneurysms, following penetrating wounds, are extremely rare, as well as mycotic aneurysms which are small, multiple and distally located. Atherosclerotic aneurysms are usually fusiform.

Intracranial aneurysm can remain silent for a long period of time. Sometimes the aneurysm causes neurologic deficit through compression to the surrounding structures. For example, the aneurysm of the internal carotid artery, or, rarely, posterior cerebral artery, can cause oculomotor paresis prior to the rupture; aneurysm of the a. *communicans anterior* can imitate the suprasellar expansion; whereas the aneurysm of the cavernous sinus can damage bulbomotor and superior branch of trigeminal nerves. Aneurysm in the posterior fossa can damage the inferior cranial nerves. Some patients may experience transitory ischemic attack in vascularization area of the artery bearing aneurysm. However, in the majority of cases, severe, life threatening subarachnoidal hemorrhage is usually the first sign of the aneurysm. Intensive occipital pain, irradiating to the forehead, neck, shoulders and spine, accompanied by nausea, vomiting and consciousness disorders, with subsequent coma. Meningeal syndrome is present in typical cases, but focal neurologic deficit can be seen as well.

Emergency diagnosis obtained by CT scan is made if the blood is found in subarachnoidal space, both in the brain base and convexity or inside the ventricular system, but the aneurysm itself is rarely seen in the acute stage. Bigger aneurysms can be seen in CT scan as circular shape, with hyperdense edge and occasional hypodense areas. Differential diagnosis between the aneurysm and expansive lesion is difficult sometimes, especially in the suprasellar region.

Detailed cerebral angiography should follow the CT examination, when aneurysm is suspected and sequels of its rupture confirmed by a CT scan. Angiography helps to assess the details regarding location, shape and size of the aneurysm, width of its neck and position of the fundus, which can be extremely helpful in planning the surgery. Panangiography can reveal concomitant cereberovascular pathology as well.

MR imaging can be a complementary method for the diagnosis of aneurysm (17). Special sequences for rapid and slow blood flow are used. MR can distinguish between the portion of the aneurysm obstructed by the thrombi from the portions patent for the blood flow. Assessment of the aneurysm details by MRI, combined with angiography, can be helpful for choosing the surgical procedures. For example, if there is sufficient blood flow, as proved by angiography, and well organized thrombi in the peripheral parts of the aneurysm, confirmed by MRI, the surgeon may decide to prevent further bleeding by "coating" the aneurysm, if the exclusion by clips is impossible (Figg. 58, 59).

Surgery should be planned individually, based on the recent knowledge on the nature of vascular spasm after subarachnoidal hemorrhage, regarding the risk of secondary rupture and perils of the premature surgery for the ruptured aneurysms. Surgical plan depends on the clinical grade and time elapsed from the hemorrhage, as well as on the international surgical standards. Generally speaking, the anterior aneurysms of the grades I and II, according to Hunt and Hess, should be operated on in the initial phase, within the first 24-72 hours, with reasonable risk, while the patients with clinical grades III and IV should be submitted to the delayed surgery. Results of the therapy of the aneurysm of the terminal V grade are disastrous, both for the conservative treatment and early surgery:

Grade 0   - Non-ruptured aneurysm
Grade I   - Mild headache and slight neck rigidity
Grade Ia - Fixed neurologic deficit without acute meningeal reaction
Grade II   - Severe headache, neck rigidity, without neurologic deficit
Grade III - Somnolence, confusion, mild focal neurologic deficit
Grade IV - Sopor, neurologic deficit, incipient vegetative disorder
Grade V   - Deep coma, decerebration, moribund appearance

Vast majority of the aneurysms, in different locations, can be successfully treated by direct transcranial microsurgery. Pterional access is ideal for the anterior aneurysms, whereas the majority of the aneurysms arising from basilar or posterior cerebral artery should be treated through modified pteri-

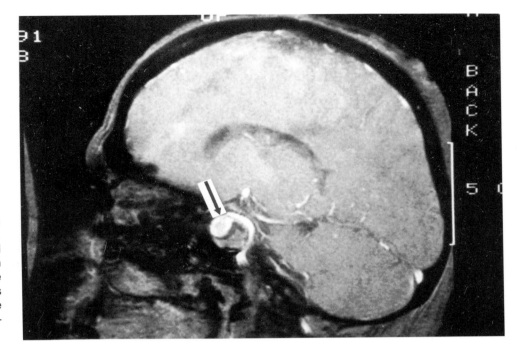

Figure 58. Sagittal image (GRE 50/10/30 degrees). Aneurysm of the internal carotid artery siphon, with high signal intensities, in the projection of the cavernous sinus - arrow. Thrombi inside the aneurysm show lower signal intensities.

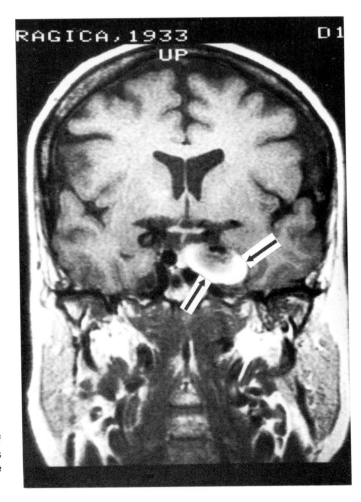

Figure 59. Coronal image (SE 500/15). Huge aneurysm of the left parasellar region, compromising the cavernous sinus, extending to the sellar fossa and dislocating the hypophyseal stalk to the right.

onal or subtemporal approach. Subtemporal, transpyramidal or retromastoid approach should be used for the rest of the posteriorly located aneurysms (9).

Endovascular procedures, for the partial or complete occlusion of the aneurysm, are very good for the aneurysms in specific locations, such as intracavernous or gigantic basilar.

Endoscopic techniques, with specially developed instruments and clips, have been applied for the treatment of the anterior aneurysms recently.

Vascular spasm, which has not been explained in detail yet, can pose a serious problem and jeopardize the surgical results.

MR imaging requires additional angiography for the diagnosis of the vascular malformation, before timing and the type of surgery is decided upon. MR angiography is important for the diagnosis of aneurysm.

c) Varices of the Galens vein

Varices of the Galens vein have not been visualized yet by neuroimaging methods.

d) Venous angioma

Venous angioma are rarely seen. They consist of the major dilated vein surrounded by a bundle of smaller veins in the perfectly normal brain parenchyma. They are usually asymptomatic.

e) Capillary telangiectasia

Although diagnosis is rarely made during the lifetime, the capillary telangiectasia are frequently found during the autopsy. The lesion consists of the pathological and irregular, dilated capillaries connected to afferent arteries and efferent veins. Unlike AVM they have no surrounding gliosis (29).

f) Cavernoma

Cavernoma (occult AVM, kryptogenous AVM, *hemangioma cavernosum*) is tumorlike formation, sometimes without compact structure, or resembling a raspberry. Globally, it belongs to the malformation group. It is built of dilated blood vessels, filled with venous blood, with internal communication. It is therefor called kryptogenous malformation. It can contain various deposits, such as calcium, hemosiderin, cholesterol, etc. No distinction between afferent and efferent vessels can be made, and that is why it is called occult malformation. Under the microscope, the cavernoma wall has a single layered endothelium and stroma containing collagen, elastin, smooth muscles and other elements of the blood vessel structure. Absence of the brain parenchyma is typical. Hemosiderin edge can be seen in the vicinity of the cavernoma. Multiple cavernomas of the brain are frequently found and in 10-30% patients, heredity is proven. It is due to the genetic defect in the long arm of the 7th chromosome. Cavernoma is usually asymptomatic, but it could be accompanied by epileptic fits, massive intracerebral hemorrhage or focal neurologic deficit.

MR imaging is absolutely the method of choice for the diagnosis of the cavernoma. Angiography is negative, because the afferent and efferent vessels are missing, and CT scan is non specific. In less than 50% of cases, the diagnosis is made upon the CT scan findings. If there are additional calcifications, differential diagnosis is even more complicated, so that slowly growing expansion or parasitosis can not be ruled out (8, 11, 12).

Minor intracerebral hemorrhage can be mixed sometimes with cavernoma in the MR image. Histopathology will confirm the diagnosis of cavernoma, made upon MRI, in 80% of patients. Introduction of MR imaging have revolutionized the diagnosis of cavernoma, causing the dramatic increase in the number of discovered cases. It is assumed that cavernoma makes 5-13% of all AV malformations of the brain.

Central portion of the cavernoma shows mixed high signal intensities in T-2W sequence, if multiplanar sections are used, whereas the edge shows lower signal intensity, due to hemosiderin deposits. Perifocal edema, with slightly elevated signal intensities, can be seen in the vicinity of the cavernoma. Inside the cavernoma areas of low signal intensities due to hemosiderin, calcification or thrombi, etc. can be occasionally seen (Fig. 57).

Central portion of the cavernoma shows mixed high signal intensities in T-1W sequence, due to the blood, while the peripheral parts have extremely low signal intensities, so that perifocal edema can hardly can be seen (42, 43). Signal intensity in T-1W sequence depends on the structure of cavernoma, with

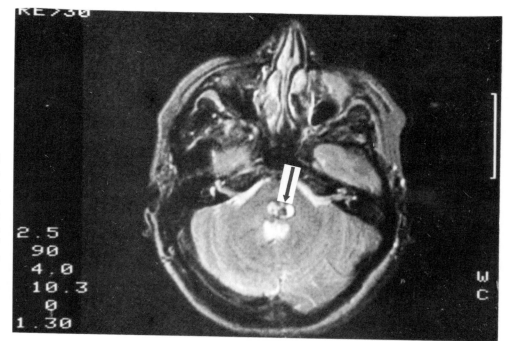

Figure 60. Axial image (SE 2500/90). Well defined cavernoma of the pons, ventrally, adjacent to the 4th ventricle - arrow. Cavernoma shows high signal intensities in general, with occasional areas of low and lower signal intensities of calcification, fibrosis, etc. Hemosiderin edge has low signal intensities.

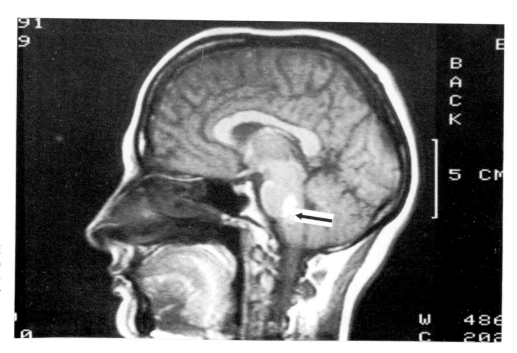

Figure 61. Sagittal image (SE 200/15). Cavernoma in the region of the pons and medulla, with high and mixed higher signal intensities - arrow.

low signal intensities for calcifications, hemosiderin, etc. MR image of cavernoma is specific (Figg. 60, 61).

No substantial evidence of the optimal treatment for cavernoma is available yet, but there are certainly some directions in planning surgical procedures with minimal risk. Surgical risk should be estimated regarding neurologic deficit and peril of the repeated hemorrhage, and compared to the risk in untreated patients. Surgical treatment of patients with solitary, easily accessible, supratentorial or intracerebral lesions, with hemorrhage or poorly controlled epilepsy, has favorable prognosis.

Smaller cavernomas, in the delicate locations, should not be treated surgically.

There are still a lot of controversies concerning clinical significance of the different classifications of the vascular anomalies of the brain. Usual classification, recognizing venous, AV, capillary and cavernous malformation, have proven to be impractical sometimes, especially for the patients showing the features of at least two of those entities. So called mixed anomalies are rare and insignificant for clinical practice, but nonetheless valuable for the study of vascular anomalies pathogenesis.

5. Miscellaneous

Subocclusions and occlusions of the major blood vessels belong to this category.

Angiography shows the change in diameter of the major blood vessels. Echosonography of the major cervical vessels gives reliable estimate of the blood vessels morphology and blood flow, making it indispensable for planning further diagnostic procedures.

CT examination is usual emergency procedure to assess the consequences of the spasm, stenosis, or occlusion of the cervical or endocranial blood vessels.

MR imaging should be used only in terms of special sequences or as MR angiography (see the Chapter *MR angiography*).

MR imaging is important for the diagnosis of arterial dissection, especially in major abdominal and thoracic blood vessels, such as aorta. It enables clear delineation of the dissecant segment, thrombosis or the patent part of a blood vessel (35).

It is believed that plaque qualities, as well as the degree of the stenosis of the commune carotid artery or extracranial segment of the internal carotid artery, could be estimated upon the MR image, thus establishing indications for surgical treatment. Smaller, exulcerated plaque, with minor degree of stenosis could jeopardize the patient more than bigger, "stable" plaque with marked stenosis.

REFERENCES

1. Ad Hoc Committee of cerebrovascular diseases. Classification of cerebrovascular diseases III. Stroke 21: 637-676, 1990.
2. Bausser MG., Barnett HJM.: Cerebral venous thrombosis. In Sturdie M. (ed.): Pathophysiology, Diagnosis, and Management 2nd ed., Churchill-Livingstone, New York, 517-537, 1992.
3. Bidder GM., Steiner RE.: NMR Imaging of the brain. Neuroradiology, 23: 231-240, 1982.
4. Caplan LC: Neurology, 38: 791-793, 1988.
5. Claussen C., Lechner B.: Dynamische Computertomography. Berlin, Heidelberg, New York, Tokyo, 1983.
6. Erdman WA., et al.: Venous thrombosis: clinical and experimental MR imaging. Radiology, 161: 233-235, 1986.
7. Fox AJ., et al.: Magnetic resonance imaging of small medullary infarctions. AJNR, 7: 229-235, 1986.
8. Gademann G.: NMR-Tomography of the Normal Brain. Springer-Verlag. Berlin, Heidelberg, New York, Tokyo, 1988.
9. Grubb Jr R.: Spontaneous Cerebral Hemorrhage. In Apuzzo M. (ed.): Brain surgery, complication avoidance and management. Churchill Livingstone. New York, Edinburgh, London, Melbourne, Tokyo, Vol. 2, 1251-1269, 1993.
10. Hachinski VC., Lassen NA., Marshall J.: Multi-infarct dementia a cause of mental deterioration in the elderly. Lancet, 27: 207-209, 1974.
11. Halbsgut A., Lechner B.: Magnetresonanz-Tomographie (NMR). Springer-Verlag. Frankfurt, 1986.
12. Han JS., Bonstelle CT., Kaufman B., Benson JE., Alfidi RJ., Clampit M.: Magnetic resonance imaging in the evaluation of the brain system. Radiology, 150: 705-712, 1984.
13. Harris FS., Rhoton AL.: Anatomy of the cavernous sinus. J. Neurosurg., 45: 169-180, 1976.
14. Healton EB., et al.: Hypertensive encephalopathy and the neurologic manifestations of malignant hypertension. Neurology, 32: 127-132, 1982.
15. Hect-Leavitt C., Gomori JM., Grossman RI.: High-field MRI of hemorrhagic cortical infarction. AJNR, 7: 581-583, 1986.
16. Heiss WD., et al.: PET CT, and MR imaging in cerebrovascular disease. J. Comput. Assist. Tomogr., 10: 906-910, 1986.
17. Holland GN., Hawkes RC., Moore WS.: Nuclear Magnetic Resonance (NMR) tomography of the brain: Coronal and sagital section. J. Comput. Tomogr., 4: 429-433, 1980.
18. Hosoya T., Kera M., Suzuki T., Yamagushu K.: Fat in the normal cavernous sinus. Neuroradiology, 28: 264-266, 1986.
19. Huk WJ., Gademann G., Friedman G.: Magnetic Resonance Imaging of Central Nervous System Diseases. Springer Verlag. Berlin, New York, Heidelberg, Tokyo, Paris, London, 1989.
20. Karata H., et al.: Subcortical cerebral hemorrhage with reference to vascular malformations and hypertension as causes of hemorrhage. Neurosurgery, 32: 505-511, 1993.
21. Kondstaal PJ., et al.: Tia, rind, minor stroke: A continuum, or different subgroups. J. Neurol. Neurosurg. Psychiatry, 55: 95-97, 1992.
22. Kucharczyk W., et al.: Intracranial vascular malformations: MR and CT imaging. Radiology, 156: 383-386, 1985.
23. Lee BCP., et al.: MR imaging of cerebral vascular malformations. AJNR, 6: 863-867, 1985.
24. Lemme-Plaghos L., et al.: MRI of angiographically occult vascular malformations. AJR, 146: 1223-1235, 1986.
25. Liessner J., Seider M.: Klinische Kernspintomographie. Stuttgart. Enke, 1987.
26. Partian J., Roo PWB.: Nuclear Magnetic Resonance (NMR) Imaging. W.B. Saunders Company. Philadelphia, London, Mexico City, Rio de Janeiro, Sidney, Tokyo, 1983.
27. Pomeranz JS.: Craniospinal Magnetic Resonance Imaging. W.B. Saunders Company. Philadelphia, London, Toronto, Sydney, Tokyo, 1989.
28. Reiser M., et al.: Magnet-rezonanz-Tomographie. Springer-Verlag. Berlin, Heidelberg, New York, Paris, London, Tokyo, Hong Kong, 1989.

29. Riyamonti D. et al.: Cerebral cavernous malformations: Incidence and familial occurrence. Engl. J. Med., 319: 343-347, 1988.
30. Savino PJ., et al.: High field magnetic resonance imaging in the diagnosis of cavernous sinus thrombosis. Arch. Neurol., 43: 1081-1090, 1986.
31. Scharfetten F.: Die subarachnoidal blutung. Schweiz. Randsch. Med. Prax., 79: 1355-1360, 1990.
32. Seiler RW., van Giyn J.: Subarachnoidalblutungen. Ther. Umsch., 53: 585-589, 1996.
33. Southwick FS., Richandson EP., Swartz MN.: Septic thrombosis of the dural venous sinuses. Medicine, 65: 82-106, 1986.
34. Spetzler RF., et al.: A proposed grading system for arteriovenous malformations. J. Neurosurg., 65: 476-483, 1986.
35. Stark D., Bradley GWJR.: Magnetic Resonance Imaging. The C.V. Mosby Company. St. Louis, Washington D.C., Toronto, 1988.
36. Stein BM., Wolput SM.: Arteriovenous malformations of the brain I and II: current concepts and treatment. Arch. Neurol., 37: 1-5, 69-75, 1980.
37. Stevens J.M.: Imaging patients with TIAS. Postgrad Med. J., 70: 604-609, 1994.
38. Took JF., Yuson CP., Janeway R.: Transient ischemic Attacks: A study of 225 patients. Neurology, 28: 746-752, 1978.
39. Van M. Runge: Enhanced Magnetic Resonance Imaging. The C.V. Mosby Company. St. Louis, Baltimore, Toronto, 1989.
40. Wackenheim A., Jeanmart L., Beart A.: Craniocerebral Computer Tomography., Berlin, Heidelberg, New York, Vol. 1. 1980.
41. Wegener OH.: Whole Body Computerized Tomography. Berlin, 1983.
42. Zawadcki MB., Norman D.: Magnetic Resonance Imaging of the Central Nervous System. Raven Press. New York, 1987.
43. Zeitler E.: Kernspintomographie. Deutsche Artze Verlag. Koeln, 1984.
44. Zimmerman RD., et al.: Acute intracranial hemorrhage: intensity changes on sequential MR scans at 0,5 T. AJR, 150: 651-660, 1988.

III. TRAUMA

Miroslav Samardzić, Gradimir Dragutinović, Vaso Antunović

Both extra- and intracerebral post-traumatic hemorrhage have been described earlier in the text.

Brain trauma represents a special chapter in the diagnostic procedures. The patients with both open and closed cranial trauma should be referred to the standard radiographs and CT by attending physician.

CT examination has following advantages for the diagnosis of the head trauma:
it could be performed in a short time
it is comfortable for the patient
resuscitation before, during and after the examination is possible
fracture line and bone fragments are clearly seen
endocranial foreign bodies are easily displayed
hemorrhage and edema are easily recognized
artifacts, due to the patients movement, does not affect the image quality
invalid scan can be rapidly repeated
harmful effect of ionizing radiation is neglectable, as compared to the diagnostic benefit for the vitally endangered patient, etc. (1, 17).

Application of MR imaging in the diagnosis of closed cranial trauma is limited, and for open cranial trauma it is not used at all. Disadvantages of MR imaging are as follows:
MR examination lasts too long
resuscitation of a patient during the examination is impossible
the cost of the examination is too high
artifacts caused by patients movement can blur the image, etc.

In comparison with CT scan, the importance of MR imaging for the emergency diagnosis is practically neglectable (3, 5, 6, 11).

MR examination can be used to differentiate some minor post-traumatic lesions that can not be displayed by a CT scan. Indication for the MR examination is made if neurologic finding is positive and CT scan negative (9, 21).

For example, rare brain trauma, caused by fat or air embolism, can be shown by MR using the classic sequences. Lesions caused by the fat embolism are shown in T-1W and T-2W sequences with signal intensities corresponding to hemorrhagic and ischemic lesions. In cases with air embolism signal intensities correspond to ischemic and demyelination lesions.

Tiniest intra- or extracerebral blood collections, unseen in CT scan, are easily displayed in MRI. This is especially the case with areas inaccessible to the CT scan, because of the numerous artifacts caused by bones, such as scull base, posterior cranial fossa and cranio-cervical junction.

Traumatic brain hemorrhage (intra- and extracerebral) have been described earlier in the text (16).

1. Brain contusion

Cranial trauma is divided into three entities, regarding severity of the injury: commotion, contusion and compression syndrome.

Neurologic deficit is rarely seen in contusion of the brain, so that CT examination is not needed. MR imaging is never required.

Brain contusion means that there is contusion focus, i.e. the region of the damaged brain tissue. Injury to the brain is induced either by direct force (for example in the vicinity of the depression fracture), or by "contre coup" effect of linear acceleration, due to transient contralateral drop of pressure (cavitation), as well as of rotatory acceleration with different amplitudes of deflection, because of various distances of certain brain structures from the central axis. For example, occipital trauma can cause frontal contusion foci.

Head contusion loss of consciousness is seldom seen. Combination of the brain concussion (unconsciousness, vegetative disorders, amnesia) or contusion foci causing neurologic deficit are usually found by CT scan or MRI. Severe head trauma is usually accompanied by the lacerations of the brain, bone fractures, extra- and intracerebral hemorrhage and other complications. The patient is comatose, sometimes for days. Recovery from coma is followed by amnesia and inability to fix the current events.

Brain compression means the morphological destruction of the brain structures, with varying symptomatology depending on the extent and site of lesion. Clinical manifestation of the brain compression can range from mild, with slightly prolonged unconsciousness, to severe, with decerebration and coma. Brain trauma can be either diffuse or focal, with temporal and frontal lobes being injured most frequently, nearby falx cerebri or scull fracture depression.

Permanent neurologic deficit, such as weakness, speech disorder, hemianopsia, cranial nerve disorders, cognitive decline, etc., depends on the site of lesion and extent of the compression injury. Post-traumatic epilepsy is frequently seen in those patients. Recovery can take a very long time, but could be surprisingly good, especially in younger patients.

CT examination is a method of choice in the diagnosis of diffuse brain lesions as well as for localized hypodense contusion lesions. It is indispensable for craniocerebral sclopetary wounds as well as for the war injuries. Smaller lesions, especially in the scull base and posterior fossa, are hard to detect by CT scan (7, 8, 21).

MR imaging enables visualization of the smallest contusion foci, that have remained undetected, because of the artifacts and insufficient resolution of CT scan. MR tomographs can display smaller contusion foci in T-2W sequence, even several weeks after the trauma. Contusion lesions are shown as the areas of higher signal intensities (2, 4, 12, 14, 20). MR imaging can be important for forensic reasons (Figg. 62-65).

2. Brain trauma caused by drowning (Submersio)

Hypoxic encephalopathy can be caused by a variety of accidents, such as submersion, strangulation, cardio-respiratory failure, aspiration of blood or vomited contents, carbon monoxide poisoning, etc.

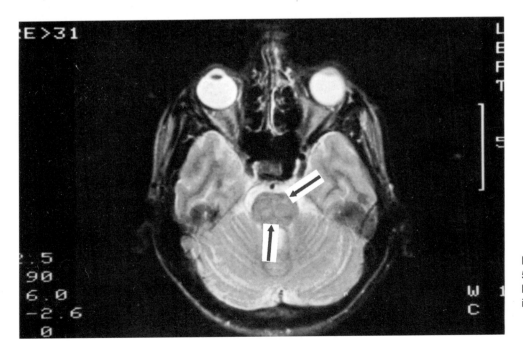

Figure 62. Axial image (SE 500/15). Tiny post-contusion lesions, with higher signal intensities, in pons - arrows.

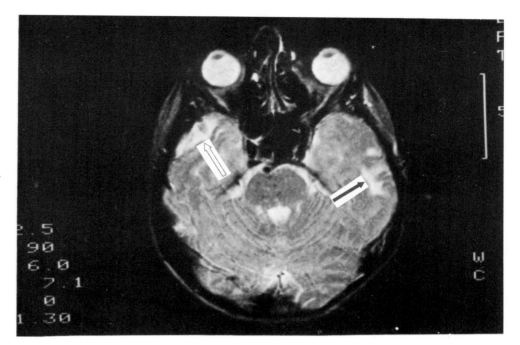

Figure 63. Axial image (SE 2500/90). Sequels induced by the fracture of the left temporo-parietal bone. Left temporal postcontusion lesion of irregular shape and high signal intensities - black arrow. Right temporobasal postcontusion lesion caused by "contre coup" effect. The lesion is also irregular with high signal intensities - white arrow.

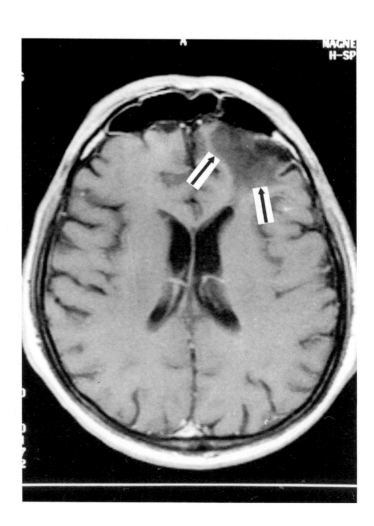

Figure 64. Axial image (SE 570/15) after gadolinium - DTPA administration. Arrows pointing at the postcontusion focus.

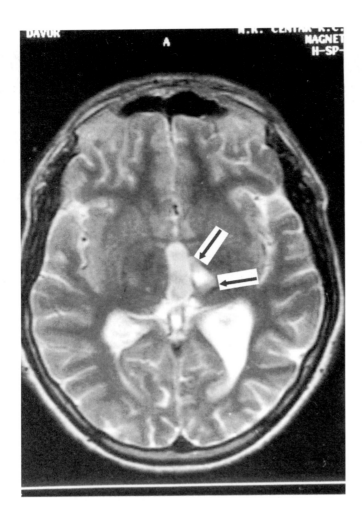

Figure 65. Axial image (TSE 4000/99). Sclopetary wound. Arrows pointing at previous site of the bullet after transventricular extraction.

Brain hypoxia is caused by transient ischemia. Reversible brain damage can be expected if hypoxia (anoxia) has not lasted longer than 5 minutes, whereas long lasting hypoxia leads to irreversible changes or eventual death.

Clinical course depends on the degree and duration of hypoxia. Mild or short term hypoxia can cause transient disorder of attention, thinking or coordination. In serious cases, the loss of certain functions (consciousness, brainstem reflexes, respiration) can induce brain death. Neurologic sequels of post-anoxic syndrome (coma or stupor, dementia, Parkinson disease, choreo-athetosis, myoclonus, visual agnosia, ataxia, Korsakoff amnestic syndrome) are found in recovered patients.

CT scan is capable of detecting bigger hypodense post-traumatic lesions, induced by submersion or suffocation, with substantial neurologic deficit.

MR imaging can reveal the tiniest lesions in the brain of submersion survivors with neurologic deficit, using extremely sensitive T-2W sequence (10, 12, 13). Control MRI enables the assessment of recovery and prognosis of anoxic lesions, corresponding to duration of anoxia. Lesions with higher signal intensities can be found in T-2W sequence in axial and coronal planes, after only three minutes of submersion (Fig. 66).

MR imaging can be useful for the follow-up of patients who have suffered craniocerebral trauma, for the detection of discrete sequels with underlying neurologic deficit or subjective complaints and for forensic reasons, to rule out simulation and aggravation based on the rent motives (15, 18, 19).

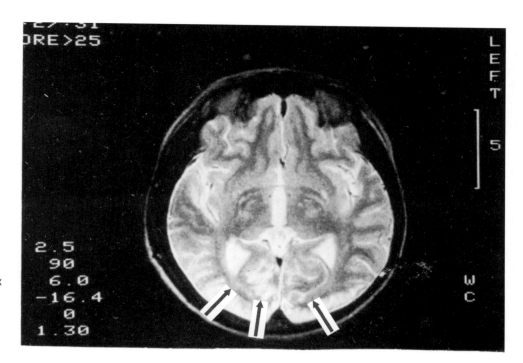

Figure 66. Axial image (SE 2500/90). Bilateral occipital ischemic lesions of the cortex induced by submersion. Lesions have high signal intensity - arrows.

REFERENCES

1. Bories J.: Computerized Axial Tomography. Springer-Verlag. Berlin, Heidelberg, New York, 1978.
2. Bradley WG., Schmidt PG.: Effect of methemoglobin formation on the MR appearance of subarachnoid hemorrhage. Radiology, 156: 99-104, 1985.
3. Chakeres DW., Bryan RN.: Acute subarachnoid hemorrhage: in vitro comparison of magnetic resonance and computed tomography. AJNR, 7: 223-228, 1986.
4. Daniels D., Haughton V., Naidich T.: Cranial and Spinal Magnetic Resonance Imaging-An Atlas and Guide. Raven Press. New York, 1987.
5. Gentry LR., et al.: Prospective comparative study of intermediate-field MR and CT in the evaluation of closed head trauma. AJNR, 9: 91-95, 1988.
6. Gerhardt P., Fromhold W.: Atlas of Anatomic Correlations in CT and MRI. Thieme. New York, Tokyo, Heidelberg, 1988.
7. Halbsgut A., Lechner B.: Magnetresonanz-Tomographie (NMR). Springer-Verlag. Frankfurt, 1986.
8. Huk WJ., Gademann G., Friedman G.: Magnetic Resonance Imaging of Central Nervous System Diseases. Springer Verlag. Berlin, New York, Heidelberg, Tokyo, Paris, London, 1989.
9. Langfitt TW., Obrist WD., Alavi A., Grossman RI., Zimmerman R., Jaggi J., Uzzell B., Reivich M., Patton DR.: Computerized tomography, magnetic resonance imaging and positron emission tomography in the study of brain trauma. Preliminary observations. J. Neurosurg., 64: 760-767, 1986.
10. Liessner J., Seider M.: Klinische Kernspintomographie. Enke. Stuttgart, 1987.
11. Moon KL., Jr., Brant-Zawadzki M., Pitts LH., Mills CM.: Nuclear magnetic resonance imaging of CT-isodense subdural hematomas. AJNR, 5: 319-22, 1984.
12. Partian J., Roo PWB.: Nuclear Magnetic Resonance (NMR) Imaging. W.B. Saunders Company. Philadelphia, London, Mexico City, Rio de Janeiro, Sidney, Tokyo, 1983.
13. Reiser M., et al.: Magnet-rezonanz-Tomographie. Springer-Verlag. Berlin, Heidelberg, New York, Paris, London, Tokyo, Hong Kong, 1989.
14. Rubin JI., et al.: High-field MR imaging of extracranial hematomas. AJR, 148: 813-815, 1987.
15. Stark D., Bradley GWJR.: Magnetic Resonance Imaging. The C.V. Mosby Company. St. Louis, Washington D.C., Toronto, 1988.
16. Van M. Runge: Enhanced Magnetic Resonance Imaging. The C.V. Mosby Company. St. Louis, Baltimore, Toronto, 1989.
17. Wackenheim A., Jeanmart L., Beart A.: Craniocerebral Computer Tomography. Springer-Verlag. Berlin, Heidelberg, New York, Vol. 1, 1980.
18. Zawadcki MB., Norman D.: Magnetic Resonance Imaging of the Central Nervous System. Raven Press. New York, 1987.
19. Zeitler E.: Kernspintomographie. Deutsche Artze Verlag. Koeln, 1984.
20. Zimmerman RA., et al.: Resistive NMR of intracranial hematomas. Neuroradiology, 27: 16-27, 1985.
21. Zimmerman RA., et al.: Head injury: early results of comparing CT and high-field MR. AJR, 147: 1215-1226, 1986.

IV. INTRACRANIAL INFECTION

Branislav Nestorović, Gradimir Dragutinović, Lukas Rasulić

Introduction of CT examination in neuroradiologic practice have improved diagnosis of the infectious diseases of the CNS. Newest CT machinery with HQ resolution have enabled confirmation of the infectious lesions in CNS, for emergencies, as well as for subacute and chronic conditions.

Precise imaging obtained by MRI makes it a method of choice for subacute and chronic infectious lesions of the brain.

Diagnostic doctrine for CNS infections includes CT examination, whilst MRI should be done in cases with poorly defined diagnosis or negative CT findings (7, 9).

Dependent on the extent, infections are classified as *meningitis, meningoencephalitis or meningoencephalomyelitis.*

Brain infections are caused by bacteria, viruses, parasites or fungi.

Bacterial infections are pyogenous (streptococcus, staphylococcus, etc.), lues, non-specific spirochetosis, tuberculosis, etc.

Mumps, poliomyelitis, herpes simplex, etc. are the most frequent viral infections.

Cystiscercosis end echinococcosis are the most frequent parasitic infection in our population, whereas trichinosis is only occasionally seen.

Protozoal infections, such as amoebiasis or malaria are rarely found, whitetoxoplasmosis is not so rare in Europe.

Fungi can cause candidiasis, aspergillosis, actinomycosis, etc.

Neuro AIDS is a separate entity in the CNS diseases.

Meningitis can be caused by pyogenous bacteria or viruses. Streptococcal or staphylococcal meningitis is the most frequent, as well as tuberculous one (24).

Neuroradiologic imaging is seldom applied in cases with CNS infections, unless there is substantial neurologic deficit or long standing poor condition of the patient.

1. Bacterial infections

a) Abscessus cerebri

Brain abscess is a collection of pus inside the brain or cerebellum. Infection causing the abscess, can spread per continuitatem, or be imported from outside in case of the open, penetrant wound or foreign body. Infection can spread localy or due to the metastasized bacteria or infected emboli (18).

Brain abscess is solitary or multiple circumscrypt bacterial infection of the brain. It could be bacterial, fungal, protozoal or viral. Suppurative encephalitis, with local inflammatory necrosis, as well as the septic necrosis of blood vessels, is followed by pus encapsulation and marked edema of the surrounding brain, after a few weeks. In the acute phase, phlegmonous granulocyte infiltration and hyperemia, followed by colliquation, causes the formation of the abscess cavity filled with pus. Perifocal edema is found in the vicinity of the abscess. Abscess wall is built of fibrous cells, glia and neoformated blood vessels, as well as granulation tissue, during subacute and chronic phase. The wall impedes the abscess enlargement. Completely formed abscess has smooth wall and liquid, occasionally clear, contents. Perifocal edema is reduced. Abscess has properties of an expansive process. Exacerbation in chronic abscess depends on the causative agent and immunologic defense of the host (3, 23).

Otogenous abscess is usually situated in cerebellum in children and in the temporal lobe in adults. Frontal abscess is caused by the spread of infection from paranasal sinuses. Abscess is usually solitary, except for the metastatic ones, which are multiple. Progressive headache is usually the first sign of the brain abscess. Nausea, vomiting, papilledema, somnolence, confusion and coma could be seen later on. General signs of the infection, if present, are not prominent. Focal neurologic deficit depends on the site of lesion. Convulsions could be found as well (20).

CT scan is insufficient for the diagnosis of the irregular, hypodense lesion, as seen in the initial phase. Later on, when the liquefaction and demarcation are completed, CT scan with i.v. administration of iodine contrast makes the diagnosis quite clear: the abscess has a hypodense central cavity, surrounded by hyperdense capsule and hypodense perifocal edema. Multiple abscesses can mimic metastases in CT scan (4).

MRI is indicated if the volume assessment is required in preoperative planning or if the abscess is situated near the cranial base or in the posterior fossa. Multiple artifacts make CT scan inadequate for such cases.

In bacterial infections MRI enables the confirmation of the incipient circumscrypt encephalitis and brain colliquation based on the enhanced tissue imbibition.

Initial brain colliquation is seen in MRI, in T-2W sequence, as clearly demarcated zone of high signal intensity.

In MR tomographs, in T-1W sequence after paramagnetic contrast administration, completely formed chronic abscess has a central zone of liquid with low signal intensity, high signal intensity margin and low signal intensity zone of perifocal edema (10, 26). On the contrary, in T-2W sequence, central portion has high signal intensity, capsule has low signal intensity and perifocal edema has irregular higher and high signal intensities. Axial and coronal sections are required (Figg. 67–69).

Surgery is indicated when the abscess and its capsule are completely formed, if the compression effect of the solitary abscess is pronounced. Complete resection of the intact abscess is a method of choice, except for an inaccessible deep abscess, where the partial resection and evacuation, followed by aggressive antibiotic therapy, should be administered to avoid operative risk.

b) Epidural and subdural empyema

Pus collection in epidural or subdural space can arise due to meningitis or spread of infection in case of sinusitis, open injury, osteomyelitis, etc. In subacute or chronic stage of empyema meninges are thickened and the capsule is formed, whereas the content is liquid, more or less. There is marked resemblance between empyema and abscess. Solitary or multiple empyema is usually situated on the convexity, tentorium cerebelli or between the hemispheres. Circumscript encephalitis could be found in the vicinity of empyema.

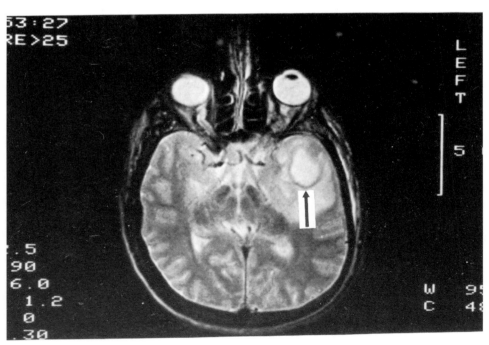

Figure 67. Axial image (SE 2500/90). Left temporo-basal abscess with high signal intensity - arrow. Capsule has low signal intensity. Marked perifocal edema with high signal intensities is clearly demarcated.

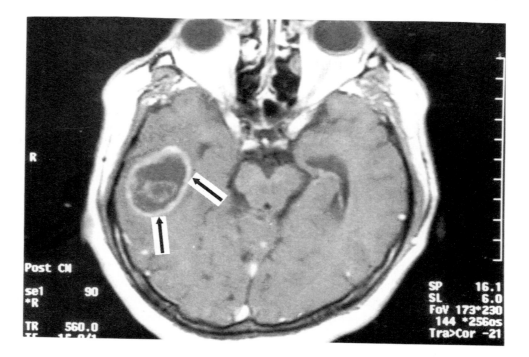

Figure 68. Axial image (SE 560/15) after gadolinium-DTPA administration. Arrows pointing at multiple otogenous abscesses.

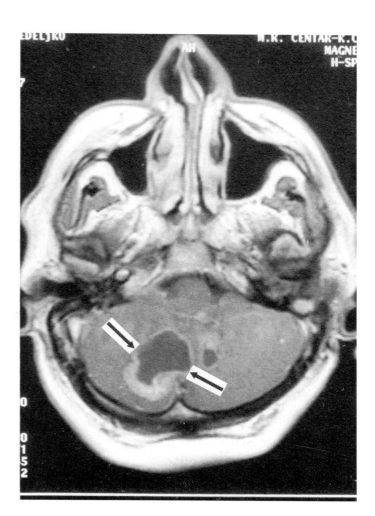

Figure 69. Axial image (SE 560/15) after gadolinium-DTPA administration. Arrows pointing at multiple otogenous abscesses.

Epidural empyema is usually combined with cranial osteomyelitis. Signs of focal inflammation are dominant, with occasional neck rigidity and no focal neurologic signs whatsoever. Focal epileptic seizures are rarely seen. If the temporal bone pyramid is involved, fifth and sixth cranial nerve palsy could arise.

Subdural empyema is accumulation of pus between dura and arachnoid. Bacteria could spread either per continuitatem, for example from the middle ear, mastoid, sinuses, or metastatic from lungs or other regions. Fever, headache, malaise and vomiting can follow exacerbation of chronic sinusitis or mastoiditis. Progression leads to somnolence and coma. Focal neurologic signs include hemiplegia, aphasia, hemianesthesia, focal epileptic seizures, etc. Meningeal signs are present (30).

Surgical treatment include craniotomy with pus evacuation and antibiotic lavage. Antibiotic should be given regarding antibiogram.

CT scan is insufficient for the diagnosis of hypodense subdural empyema. Multiplanar view is required for subdural empyema, depending on the site of lesion. Perifocal edema combined with empyema could not be easily differentiated from tumor in certain cases.

MR tomographs, using triplanar view and T-1W sequence with contrast administration, are the best method for the diagnosis of epidural and subdural empyema.

MRI in T-1W sequence after intravenous administration of contrast, shows subdural empyema as irregular ellipse, with capsular margin with high signal intensity. Central portion of liquid has low signal intensity. Perifocal edema has low signal intensities (16, 17). If the hematoencephalic barrier is damaged, surrounding structures can show higher signal intensities as well (Figg. 70-72).

c) Meningovascular Neurosyphilis

Neurosyphilis is caused by *Treponema pallidum* and could be expressed in various forms. Disease has three stages.

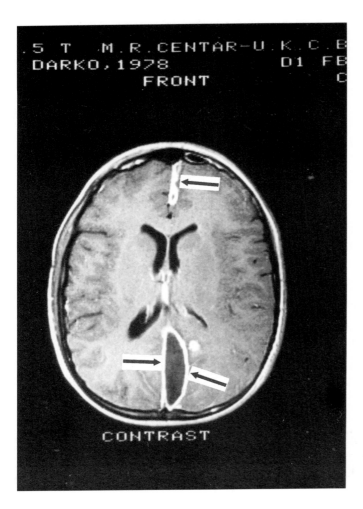

Figure 70. Axial image (SE 550/15) after gadolinium-DTPA administration. Interhemispheric subdural empyema with low signal intensities. Magnevist enhanced capsule show extremely high signal intensity - arrows.

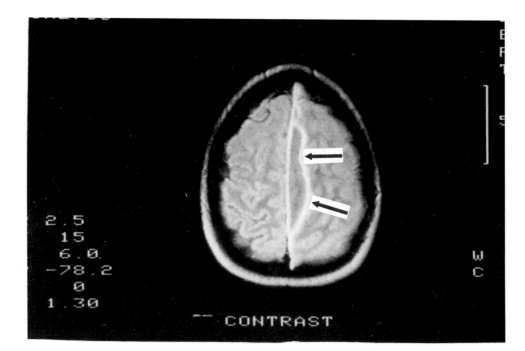

Figure 71. Axial image (2500/15) after gadolinium-DTPA administration. Interhemispheric subdural empyema situated in the upper part of the parietal region, right beneath calota - arrows.

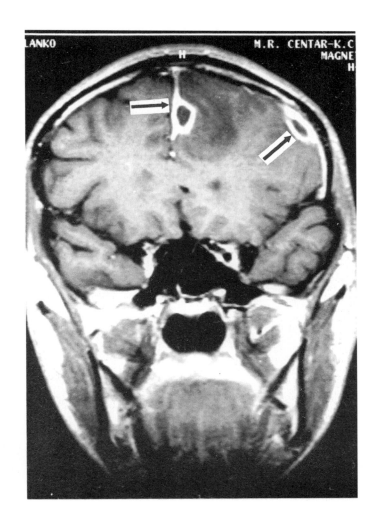

Figure 72. Coronal image (SE 560/15) after gadolinium-DTPA administration. Interhemispherial subdural empyema, found as well in the convexity-arrows.

Meningovascular type of Neurosyphilis could be variable. Recurrent cerebrovascular accidents, accompanied by hemiplegia, aphasia and hemianesthesia in younger patients are frequently seen. Intracranial hypertension with headache, edematous papilla of the optic nerve, convulsions could be seen as well. If the spinal cord is affected, meningomyelitis, progressive spastic paraplegia or radicular motor or sensory impairment, usually in arms, are found (5).

Neurologic finding, clinical appearance, laboratory findings and CT scan are sufficient for the assessment of the condition of CNS structures in meningovascular Neurosyphilis, and enable initiation of the adequate treatment (15, 25).

CT examination reveals nonspecific hypodense lesions of acute or chronic ischemia due to meningovascular Neurosyphilis. Luetic gumma is clearly seen, whereas hypodense areas of demyelination are poorly differentiated (14).

Significance of MRI for the diagnosis of neuro-luetic lesions is purely academic.

MR examination in T-2W sequence merely confirms high signal intensity lesions, corresponding to the areas of ischemia, i.e. infarction. In Neurosyphilis, infarction is caused by specific vasculitis, but in MR tomographs it resembles the infarction caused by any other etiology. We haven't found any luetic gumma in our MR practice so far. Axial view, and eventually additional coronal and sagittal views are used for the MR examination (Fig. 73).

d) Borreliosis

Borreliosis (Lyme disease) is a rare nonluetic spirochetosis caused by *Borrelia burgdorferi*, which is similar to *Spirocheta pallidum*. The infection is transmitted by ixodid ticks. Progressive encephalitis is seen in chronic borreliosis. Ischemic areas of infarctions, due to specific vasculitis, are found in brain parenchyma.

Initial symptoms are present during the second phase of disease, usually in the form of meningitis with fever, cachexia, headache, vomiting and meningeal signs. Peripheral neural lesions with radicular pain, dysaesthesia of the trunk and limbs, facial palsy, impairment of the optic, acoustic or other cranial nerves could be found as well (11).

Central nervous system is involved in the third phase and various neurologic syndromes can mimic multiple sclerosis, brain tumor, benign intracranial hypertension or apoplexy (12).

MRI is better than CT for the diagnosis of this rare non-luetic spirochetal disease. In CT scan borreliosis is seen as several small, hypodense areas.

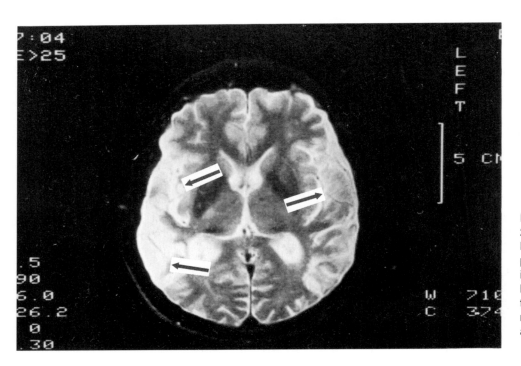

Figure 73. Axial image (SE 2500/90). Bilateral, particularly on the right, temporo-parieto- occipital, large ischemic areas. Ischemic lesions of high signal intensities, caused by specific neuro-luetic vasculitis - arrows.

MRI of borreliosis is specific for the small infarctions, having high signal intensity in T-2W, and low signal intensity in T-1W sequence. Axial view is optimal for the display of the smallest lesions in MRI (22, 24). There is no need for other views or techniques of the MR examination (Figg. 74, 75).

2. Parasytoses

Cysticercosis and echinococcosis are the most frequent parasytosis of the CNS in our country. Brain is the predilection site.

a) Cysticercosis

Neurocysticercosis (*Taenia solium and Taenia saginata*), transferred by a bloodstream, is found in the form of cystic larvae in the brain parenchyma, meninges or ventricular system.

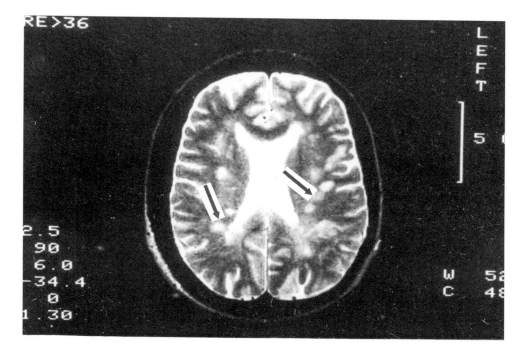

Figure 74. Axial image (SE 2500/90) Numerous ischemic lesions due to specific vasculitis in borreliosis. Smaller areas with high signal intensities are affected, usually clearly defined and occasionally confluent -arrows.

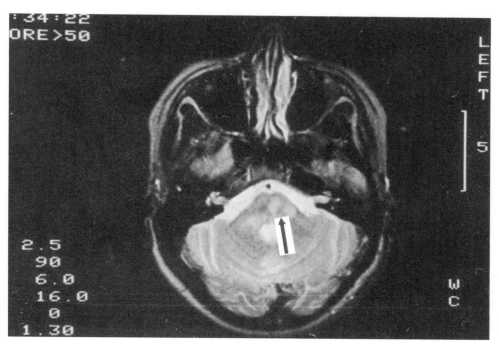

Figure 75. Axial image (SE 2500/90). Numerous ischemic lesions, due to specific vasculitis in borreliosis, in the posterior fossa (pons - arrow).

Acute encephalitic phase of neurocysticercosis is very dramatic due to intracranial hypertension, focal neurologic deficit, epileptic seizures, ocular signs and psychological disorders. Two basic forms are met: diffuse nodular lesions (85%) or localized lesions in the brain parenchyma. Children and adolescents are most frequently affected (65%). Initial phase can take 2-6 months, depending on the number of lesions, general condition of the patient and unrecognized immunologic factors. Severity of the condition depends on the patients age, with youngest patients having the highest mortality rate, as high as 10% (8).

Delayed clinical forms of neurocysticercosis can be classified as follows: 1) meningeal; 2) focal parenchymatous; 3) parenchymatous with intracranial hypertension; 4) ventricular; 5) spinal with compression effect; 6) mixed; and 7) asymptomatic.

Cysticercus in parenchyma, usually in the gray matter and subependyma, are surrounded by perifocal edema. Multiple cysticercus of the meninges can cause non-suppurative leptomeningitis followed by leptomeningeal fibrosis. In the ventricular system, cysticercus can be either intramural or floating in the liquor. In either case they can make an obstacle to the liquor circulation, especially in the vicinity of the foramina or Silvius aqueduct, thus causing partial or complete supratentorial obstructive internal hydrocephalus.

Clinical presentation of the cysticercosis depends on the number and location of cysts, as well as on the phase of their evolution. Cortical cysts usually cause focal epileptic seizures, whereas basal ones can cause cranial nerve impairment or disorders of other neural pathways. Being accompanied by intracranial hypertension it could mimic posterior fossa tumor. Parenchymatous cysts can resemble dementia (27, 35).

CT scan is conclusive in the phase of calcified cysts, occurring 6-8 months after encapsulation inside brain parenchyma. Solitary or, more frequently, multiple tiny zones of calcium high density are seen. In the initial phase of inflammation and fibrosis, it is hard to recognize small non-specific hypodense zones (34).

Meningeal cysticercosis is hard to diagnose by neuroradiology methods. Floating cysts in liquor are almost impossible to recognize, for they are moving along with liquor pulsation, thus causing paroxysmal obstructive internal hydrocephalus (37).

Small zones of high signal intensities are seen in MR tomographs in T-2W sequence in the initial phase of the infection, as well as in the later stages of inflammation and fibrosis. Central cyst with calcium incrustations is shown in low signal intensities, whereas the perifocal edema has high signal intensities. Axial, and eventually coronal views are preferable (Fig. 76).

Surgical treatment is liquor derivation with frequently needed reintervention because of the system

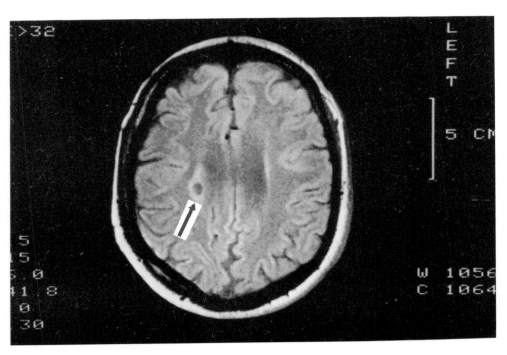

Figure 76. Axial image (SE 2500/15). Right parietal, calcified cysticercus with low signal intensity. It has ellipsoid margin of higher signal intensity, corresponding to perifocal edema - arrow.

obstruction. If there are few, easily accessible, voluminous cysts, they ought to be surgically removed. Specific medical treatment should follow the surgery and serological confirmation of the diagnosis.

b) Echinococcosis

Echinococcosis, affecting both humans and numerous mammals (anthropozoonosis), is a disease caused by the development of the larval, cystic form of Echinococcus granulosus or Taenia echinococcus in men or animals. Man is a transitory host in the developmental chain. Disease is usually transmitted from dog to man, with children being affected 7 times as much as adults.

Taenia echinococcus in the form of eggs, once in the intestinal tract, transforms into the embryo and through portal circulation reaches the "filter" organs: liver and lungs. Few embryos are transferred by arterial circulation to the brain. Once implanted into the brain parenchyma, echinococcus cysts grow and encapsulate. Thick capsule is made of chitin membrane and fibrous layer, underlined by germinative epithelium with buds of new cysts and scolicis. Laboratory findings, supported by clinical appearance and radiological findings make the diagnosis of echinococcosis definitive.

Clinical appearance depends on the size and location of the cyst. Several varieties have been reported, such as: 1) cranial bone location, with cyst without fibrous capsule and eventual rupture and invasion of the subdural space; 2) brain location, with postrolandic area of the left hemisphere, in the vicinity of a. cerebri media, being frequently involved, whilst absence of the surrounding edema and adhesions enabling easier removal of the cyst without rupture. Apart from granulous type with bigger solitary cyst, there is alveolar or multilocular type which can mimic brain malignancies regarding clinical appearance or neuroimage (Switzerland, Tyrol, Siberia) and 3) spinal location, found in adults in the third decade, with discrete symptoms.

Clinical signs of the echinococcus are not typical, often resembling tumor. Focal signs depend on the cyst location, whereas the cyst can cause intracranial hypertension due to its size or interference with liquor circulation. Children with cerebral echinococcus maintain their intellectual abilities and fair general condition for quite a long time.

CT scan is sufficient for the diagnosis of cerebral echinococcosis, especially in the case of the calcified cyst. The cavity is hypodense and the capsule becomes hyperdense after the administration of the intravenous iodine contrast (37).

MR examination is usually done in axial and, eventually, coronal plane. In T-2W sequence echinococcus cyst has high signal intensity, whereas capsule and calcifications have low signal intensities. Perifocal edema has slightly higher signal intensities. In T-1W sequence cyst has low signal intensities (2, 22, 39).

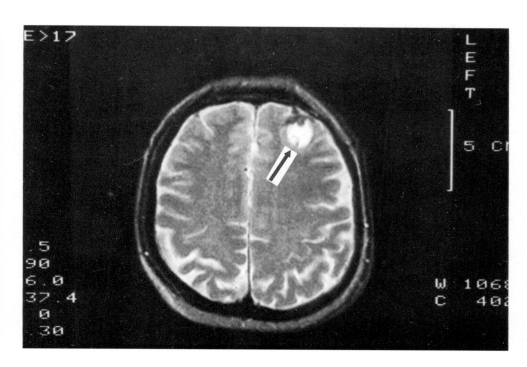

Figure 77. Axial image (SE 2500/90). Left fronto-parietal echinococcus cyst with high signal intensities and marginal calcium deposits of low signal intensity - arrow. Margin of slightly higher signal intensities, corresponding to perifocal edema, is seen around the echinococcus cyst.

Calcifications have extremely low signal intensities (Fig. 77).

In spite of certain advances in the medical therapy, surgical extirpation of the echinococcus cyst remains a method of choice. Bone cyst should be widely resected and bone defects reconstructed by a delayed surgery. Cerebral cysts, being solitary in 98% of cases, should be removed completely and intact. Cyst integrity should be preserved by a careful microsurgical blunt preparation and gentle dissection by fluid injection, to avoid contact of the cyst contents and surrounding brain tissue, which is of utmost importance for future outcome. In case of the intraoperative cyst rupture, lavage with 2% formaldehyde solution is required. Radical resection is extremely important for spinal or vertebral location.

c) Trichinosis

Trichinosis is a parasitosis with complete development inside a single organism, transmitted by larvae of *Trichinella spiralis*. They can be found in the striated muscles of the pig. Parasite can be ingested by a contaminated pork meat and invade skeletal muscles, myocardium, lungs or exceptionally meninges and brain.

Neurological symptoms, such as headache, vertigo, tinnitus, convulsions, meningeal or polyneuritic signs can be found. Reflex impairment, hemiplegia, aphasia, retentio alvi et urinae, etc. are frequently seen (19).

Non-specific meningitis and encephalitis is seen in meninges and brain tissue (Fig. 78). Symptomatic neurologic therapy is indicated.

3. Neuro AIDS

AIDS is a contemporary disease involving CNS as well. Human immunodeficiency virus (HIV) is lympho- and neurotropic.

Neuro-AIDS is caused by a neurotropic HIV. Neurologic syndrome is caused by a direct effect of the virus on the neurons of central and peripheral nervous system. There is HIV dementia complex, HIV menin-

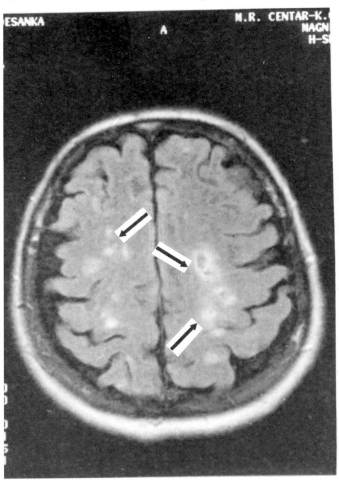

Figure 78. Axial image (TIR 9000/150/2200). Arrows pointing at trichinosis lesions.

goencephalitis, meningitis and myelopathy. The patients are frequently affected by, so called, opportune infection, such as toxoplasmic encephalitis, or malignant tumors, such as lymphoma or Kaposi sarcoma.

Brain infections could be viral or non-viral. *Herpes simplex, herpes zoster, etc.* are usual viral infections, whereas toxoplasmosis, candidiasis, aspergillosis, coccidiomycosis, tuberculosis, lues, etc. are the most frequent non-viral infections (1).

Following diseases are caused by a direct virus action on neural or muscle tissue:

HIV encephalopathy or "AIDS dementia complex" is manifested by subcortical dementia, disequilibrium, leg weakness, epilepsy, extrapyramidal signs, psychosis. Progressive severe psychic and motor deterioration leads to a mute patient in a fetal position (13).

HIV meningitis and meningoencephalitis are similar to the acute infection in infectious mononucleosis with meningeal and focal neurologic deficits.

HIV myelopathy, neuropathy or myopathy have corresponding clinical appearance.

Opportune infections of the CNS are very rarely seen in healthy adults. Toxoplasmic encephalitis, progressive multifocal encephalopathy, Escherichia coli encephalitis, tuberculous abscess, luetic meningoencephalitis, viral or tuberculous meningitis belong to this group (28-31).

CT findings in neuro-AIDS is quite non-specific, depending on the type, location and manifestation of the infection or the disease itself.

MR imaging has advantage over CT for the early and precise diagnosis of the site of lesion (23).

MR image is non-specific and can not define the cause of the CNS lesion. MR image in neuro-AIDS is identical to the findings in certain infections, superimposed to the AIDS.

Lesions of high signal intensities are found in T-2W sequence of MRI in axial and coronal views. MR can show the type of CNS lesion. Laboratory confirmation of the etiology is necessary. Variable forms, size or locations of the cerebral lesions can be seen in MR, depending on the etiology (Fig. 79).

4. Sarcoidosis

Sarcoidosis (Morbus Besnier-Boeck-Schaumann) is chronic granulomatous cyclic disease of unknown origin. Tuberculous etiology is suspected, although tuberculin reaction is usually negative. Etiology has remained unclear until today. Apart from pulmonary, there is also lymphoglandular and milliary type. Sarcoidosis can be found in the spleen, bones, joints, salivary and lachrymal glands and even brain. Among the rare intra- or suprasellar locations, sarcoidosis can be found in the hypophyseal stalk as well (9).

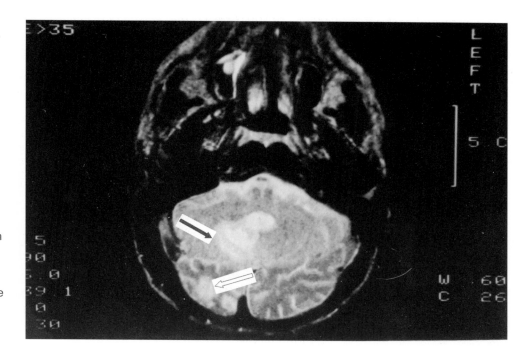

Figure 79. Axial image (SE 2500/90). Multiple AIDS lesions. Big, irregular lesion of the higher signal intensities is seen right to the fourth ventricle - black arrow. Two smaller lesions of the high signal intensity are seen in the right occipital area - white arrow.

Brain sarcoidosis is found in brain parenchyma in the form of non-caseous nodules, made of the radial epithelioid cells. Giant cells and elastic fibers can be found as well. Brain lesions are non-specific and can be proved by biopsy alone.

Granulomatous infiltration of meninges and surrounding neural tissue can cause various neural deficits; epileptic seizure, cranial nerve disorders, paresis, ataxia, hydrocephalus can be found if the basal region is involved. Cranial neuropathy, especially peripheral facial palsy, polyuria, polydipsia, obesity and somnolence are caused by hypothalamic-hypophyseal involvement, whereas visual impairment is seen if optic chiasm and nerves are involved. Spinal cord and peripheral nervous system can be affected as well (6, 20, 29, 33).

CT scan is non-specific and insufficient for the diagnosis of sarcoidosis. Sarcoidosis infiltrations are hypodense, but they could become hyperdense after the contrast administration. Non-specific CT scan or sarcoidosis located in the cranial base, hypophyseal stalk, etc. calls for MR examination.

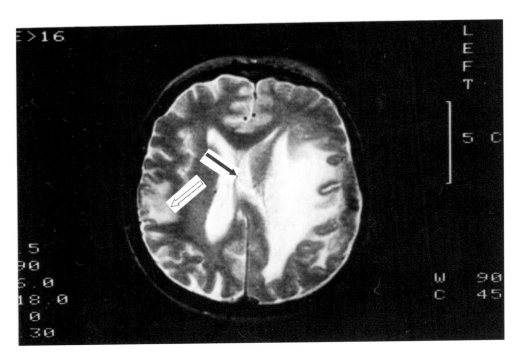

Figure 80. Axial image (SE 2500/90). Left parietal, irregular lesion, causing the left lateral ventricle compression, of the high signal intensities - black arrow. Both lateral ventricles are shifted to the right. Suspect lesion of the lower signal intensities, adjacent to the lesion of high signal intensity, is seen in the left parietal region, nearby tabula interna. Few smaller lesions of higher signal intensity are seen on the right side - white arrow.

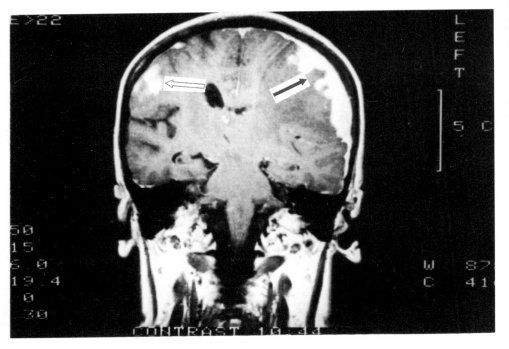

Figure 81. Coronal image (SE 500/15) after gadolinium-DTPA administration. Irregular convex zone of high signal intensity is seen in the convexity of the left temporo-parietal region, corresponding to sarcoidosis - black arrow. The lesion, with slight surrounding edema, cause the compression and dislocation of the lateral ventricles to the right. Irregular berry-like zone of sarcoidosis with high signal intensity is seen on the right side as well- white arrow. Sarcoidosis is considerably enhanced by a contrast (Schering) administration, making differentiation from surrounding edema (retaining low signal intensity) easier.

MR image should be done in axial and coronal views. In T-1W sequence, lesions have low signal intensities, whilst in T-2W they have mixed signal intensities (39).

MR image of sarcoidosis in T-1W is substantially changed after the contrast administration, shown as big zones without perifocal edema. In case of meningeal involvement, the finding is similar to the brain carcinomatosis (41). MR can not provide for the preoperative differentiation (Figg. 80, 81).

Surgery for this rare intracranial entity is indicated only for the symptomatic, tumorlike lesions.

REFERENCES

1. American Academy of AIDS Task Force. Nomenclature and research case definition for neurologic manifestations of human immunodeficiency virus–type (HIV-1) infection. Neurology, 41: 778-785, 1991.
2. Bauer WM., Obermuller H., Vogl T., Lissner J.: MR bei zerebraler alveolarer Echinikokkose. Digitale Bilddiagn., 4: 129-131, 1986.
3. Berlot P., Fedel C., Tornow K., Sdrmiedek P.: Der bakterielle hirnabszesserfahrungen bei 67 patienten. Fortschr. Neurol. Psychiatr., 64: 297-309, 1996.
4. Brant-Zawadzki M., Enzmann DR., Placone RC. Jr., Sheldon P., Britt RH., Brasch RC., Crooks LA.: NMR imaging of experimental brain abscess: comparision with CT. AJNR, 4(3): 250-253, 1983.
5. Burdie JM., Schaberg DR.: Neurosyphilis in the antibiotic era. Neurology, 35: 1368-1371, 1985.
6. Chapelon C., et al.: Neurosarcoidosis: Signs, course and treatment in 35 confirmed cases. Medicine, 69: 261-276, 1990.
7. Davidson HD., Steiner RE.: Magnetic resonance imaging in infections of the central nervous system. AJNR, 6: 499-504, 1985.
8. Del Bruto OH., Sotelo J.: Neurocysticercosis: An update. Rev. Infect. Dis., 10: 1075-1087, 1988.
9. Einzmann RD.: Imaging of Infections and Inflamations of the Central Nervous System; Computerized Tomography, Ultrasound and Nuclear Magnetic Resonance. Raven Press. New York, 1984.
10. Halbsgut A., Lechner B.: Magnetresonanz-Tomographie (NMR). Springer-Verlag. Frankfurt, 1986.
11. Halperin JJ., et al.: Lyme neuroborreliosis central nervous system manifestations. Neurology, 39: 753-759, 1989.
12. Halperin JJ., Volbman DJ., Wn P.: Central nervous system abnormalities in Lyme neuroborreliosis. Neurology, 41: 1571-1582, 1991.
13. Ho DD., et al.: The acquired immunodeficiency syndrome (AIDS) dementia complex. Ann. Int. Med., 111: 400-410, 1989.
14. Holland BA., Perrett LV., Millis CM.: Meningovascular syphilis: CT and MR findings. Radiology, 158: (2), 439-442, 1986.
15. Holwes MD., Brand-Zawadzki MM., Simon RP.: Clinical features of meningovascular syphilis. Neurology, 34: 553-556, 1984.
16. Huk WJ., Gademann G., Friedman G.: Magnetic Resonance Imaging of Central Nervous System Diseases. Springer-Verlag. Berlin, New York, Heidelberg, Tokyo, Paris, London, 1989.
17. Liessner J., Seider M.: Klinische Kernspintomographie. Enke. Stuttgart, 1987.
18. Mampalam Py., Rosenblum ML.: Trends in the management of bacterial brain abscesses: A review of 102 cases over 17 years. Neurosurgery, 23: 451-458, 1988.
19. Mawhoifer SD., Kazma JW.: Trichinosis of the central nervous system. Semin. Neurol., 13: 148-152, 1993.
20. Okasanen V.: Neurosarcoidosis: Clinical presentations and course in 50 patients. Acta Neurol. Scand., 73: 283-290, 1986.
21. Parker JC., Dyer ML.: Neurologic infections due to bacteria, fungi, and parasites. In Davis RL., Robertson DM. (eds.): Textbook of neuropathology. Williams and Wilkins. Baltimore, 632-703, 1985.
22. Pomeranz JS.: Craniospinal Magnetic Resonance Imaging. W.B. Saunders Company. Philadelphia, London, Toronto, Sydney, Tokyo, 1989.
23. Post MJD., et al.: Central nervous system disease in acquired immunodeficiency syndrome: prospective correlation using CT., MR imaging, and pathologic studies. Radiology, 158: 141-147, 1986.
24. Reiser M., et al.: Magnet-rezonanz-Tomographie. Springer-Verlag. Berlin, Heidelberg, New York, Paris, London, Tokyo, Hong Kong, 1989.
25. Rowland LP.: Merritts Textbook of neurology, 9th ed., Williams and Willkins. Baltimore, 1995.
26. Runge VM., et al.: Evaluation of contrast-enhanced MR imaging in a brain-abscess model. AJNR, 6: 139-147, 1985.
27. Scharf D.: Neurocysticercosis. Arch. Neurol., 45: 777-780, 1988.
28. Schroth G, et al.: Early diagnosis of Herpes simplex encephalitis by MRI. Neurology, 37: 179-183, 1987.
29. Scott TF.: Neurosarcoidosis: Progress and clinical aspects. Neurology, 43: 8-12, 1993.
30. Silvaberg AL., Dc Nubile MA.: Subdural empyema and cranial epidural abscess. Med. Clin. North Am., 69: 361-374, 1985.
31. Snider WD., et al.: Neurological complications of aquired immune deficiency syndrome: Analysis of 50 patients. Ann. Neurol., 14: 403-418, 1983.
32. Stark D., Bradley GWJR.: Magnetic Resonance Imaging. The C.V. Mosby Company. St. Louis, Washington D.C., Toronto, 1988.
33. Stern BJ., et al.: Sarcoidosis and neurological manifestations. Arch. Neurol., 42: 909-916, 1985.
34. Suss RA., Maravilla KR., Thompson J.: MR imaging of intracranial cysticercosis: comparison of CT and anatomapathologic features. AJNR, 7(2): 235-242, 1986.

35. Trelles JO., Trelles L.: Cysticercosis of the nervous system. In Vinken P.J. Bruyn G.W. (eds): Handbook of Clinical Neurology. North- Holland, Amsterdam, Vol 35, pp 291-320, 1978.
36. Van M. Runge: Enhanced Magnetic Resonance Imaging. The C.V. Mosby Company. St. Louis, Baltimore, Toronto, 1989.
37. Wackenheim A., Jeanmart L., Beart A.: Craniocerebral Computer Tomography. Berlin, Heidelberg, New York, Vol. 1, 1980.
38. Zawadcki MB., Norman D.: Magnetic Resonance Imaging of the Central Nervous System. Raven Press. New York, 1987.
39. Zeitler E.: Kernspintomographie. Deutsche Artze Verlag. Koeln, 1984.

V. DEGENERATIVE DISEASES OF THE BRAIN

Zvonimir Lević, Gradimir Dragutinović

Degenerative brain diseases could be classified according to different features, such as pathologic iron deposits, etiology, age of the patients, location, etc.

Normal distribution of iron as seen in various MR sequences is well known. Normally, iron deposits are found in globus pallidum, substantia nigra, putamen, nucleus caudatus, thalamus, etc. Brain structures with iron incrustations have low signal intensity, that makes them easily demarcated from normal surrounding structures (Figg. 82, 83).

J. Pomerantz (20) have classified degenerative brain diseases upon the pathologic iron contents:
Neurodegenerative diseases
Parkinson's disease, *Huntingtons* chorea, *Alzheimer's* disease
Diseases of the motor neuron
Demyelinating diseases, such as *Sclerosis multiplex* (possible alteration in signal intensities due to iron deposits),
Degenerative brain diseases following irradiation and chemotherapy.

M. B. Zawadcki (35) have made classification of the white matter diseases or combined white and gray matter diseases, both in children and adults, as follows:
White matter diseases in children:
Multifocal
a. Acute (M.S., anoxia, infection)
b. Subacute (M.S., leukodistrophy, radiation)
2. Diffuse
a. Radiation diseases
b. Leukodistrophy

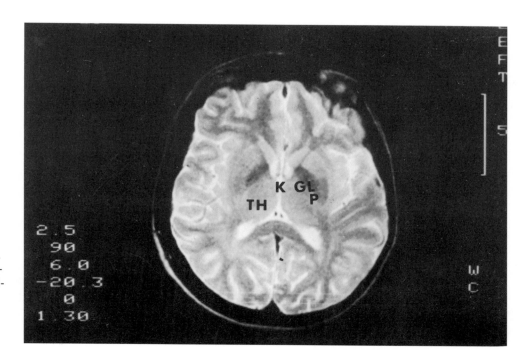

Figure 82. Axial image (SE 2500/90). Normal MR image. G.L.-globus pallidus, P- putamen, III K- third ventricle, TH-thalamus (p. 29 Atlas Daniel's).

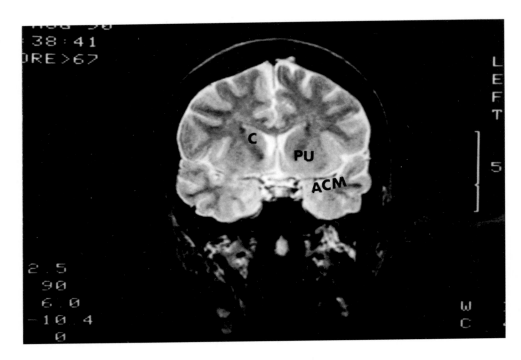

Figure 83. Coronal image (SE 2500/90). Normal MR image. C-nucleus caudatus, Pu-putamen, a.c.m.-arteria cerebri media (p. 47 Atlas Daniel's).

Combined white and gray matter diseases in children:
1. Infection,
2. Anoxia
3. Dysmyelination (Leigh's disease).
White matter diseases in adults:
1. Focal (radiation disease, M.S., ischemia and infection)
2. Diffuse (radiation and infection).
Combined white and gray matter diseases in adults:
1. Ischemia
2. Infection.

Classification of the degenerative diseases of the brain and white matter is after W.J. Huk et al. (11):
Primary neuronal disease (gray matter)
Primary disease of the brainstem and basal ganglia
Primary disease without site of predilection
Myelin disease (white matter).

1. Primary neuronal disease (gray matter)

Primary neuronal diseases (gray matter) are a) congenital, b) acquired and diseases of unknown origin.

a) Congenital diseases are mucolipidosis, gangliosiderosis, lipidosis, etc. They are based on the enzyme deficiency thus obstructing the degradation of certain products and their deposits in the lipozomes of the various tissues. Neuroradiologic experience with those rare neurologic conditions is neglectable.

b) Alzheimer's, Picks and *Creutzfeldt-Jacobs* disease belong to this group.

Common features of all those diseases are delayed psychomotor development and psychomotor deterioration. Palsy, blindness, epileptic seizures, rigidity, opistotonus, ataxia, could be found as well (18).
b) Acquired neuronal diseases (gray matter)
b-1 Alzheimer's disease

Alzheimer's disease is organic lesion of the brain causing dementia. Histopathology findings consist of senile plaques, fibril alteration, neuronal degeneration with destroyed nerve fibers and proliferation of micro- and macroglia. Pigment deposits can be found in the degenerated cells. Diffuse atrophy with cortical iron deposits and loss of the cytoarchitectonics of the brain are typical for the Alzheimer's disease. Alzheimer's disease is usually seen in presenium and therefore it belongs to the group of presenile dementia along with *Huntingtons chorea* and *Picks* dementia. It has been understood nowadays that Alzheimer's dementia and senile dementia are basically the same disease with different time of onset. Alzheimer's disease usually commences before the age of 65, whereas senile dementia begins after that age. It is the most frequent and most significant degenerative disease of the brain.

Initial stage manifestations are loss of memory and intellectual abilities, cognitive deficit, disorientation in time and space, dyspraxia, complex visual disorders, etc. Aphasia, apraxia and agnosia are seen in the later stage. Progression of those disorders, along with development of numerous psychopathological phenomena, can cause enhancement of the previous behavior patterns, apathy or make simultaneous performance of several operations impossible. Hallucinations or compulsive ideas can occur, as well as epileptic fits, delirium or motor deterioration. Gradually complete psychic and motor regression, back to the "fetal" stage, can develop.

CT scan is resolute enough to visualize diffuse atrophy found in this disease. Basic problem with CT is its inability to differentiate smaller lesions and suggest the diagnosis precisely. Iron deposits can not be shown by this examination.

MR tomographs in T-2W sequence show non-specific lesions, such as dilated ventricular system and cortical atrophy. MR is indicated if differential diagnosis is required (23).

Iron deposits in cerebral cortex are shown by extremely low signal intensities in all MR sequences. Cortical reductive lesions in the temporal lobes as well as subcortical reductive changes, along with dilated lateral ventricles are found in MR tomographs in double-echo sequences (**T-2W** and **Proton density**) (9). Complete picture is non-specific for Alzheimer's disease, for subcortical and cortical reductive changes can be caused by several other factors as well (Fig. 84).

b-2 Picks disease

Frontal and temporal lobes are usually atrophic in Picks dementia. Marked circumscript nerve cell destruction, glial proliferation and basal ganglia damage is usually found. Therefor, frontal or temporal symptomatology can predominate. Dysinhibition phenomena, apathy, abulia as well as posture and gait disorders can be seen in "frontal Pick". Gradual deterioration of speech as well as disorders of sexual behavior or bulimia can be found in temporal type of the disease.

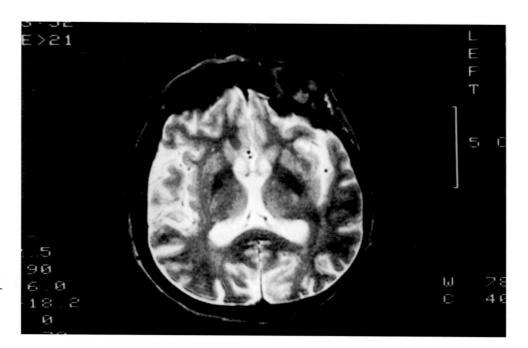

Figure 84. Axial image (SE 2500/90) Alzheimer's disease: dilation of both lateral ventricles and marked bilateral cortical reductive changes.

CT and MR are not specific for morphologic features of Picks disease. MR is better for the detailed display of the lobar atrophy and glial changes in basal ganglia (2).

b-3 Creutzfeldt-Jacobs disease

Creutzfeldt-Jacobs disease belongs to prior diseases. The subacute course is manifested by dementia, ataxia, rigidity and myoclonus. Hallucinations, delirium, stupor and coma can be found as well. Lethal outcome within a year is a rule.

Neuroradiological findings are not specific for this disease (4).

2. Primary diseases of the basal ganglia and brainstem

Primary diseases of the basal ganglia and brainstem are classified as follows:

a) Congenital diseases
    a-1 *Wilson's* disease
    a-2 *Fahrs* disease
    a-3 *Fabrys* disease
    a-4 *Huntingtons* chorea
    a-5 Subacute necrotizing encephalopathy
    a-6 Spinocerebellar degeneration (olivo-ponto-cerebellar degeneration and cerebellar heredoataxy)

b) Acquired and unexplained causes
    b-1 *Wernickes* encephalopathy
    b-2 Central pontine myelinosis

Degenerative diseases of basal ganglia can manifest through hypertonic-hypokinetic and hyperkinetic syndrome. Hypertonic-hypokinetic syndrome or parkinsonism has four major symptoms: rigor, bradykinesis, tremor and postural reflex impairment. Hyperkinetic syndromes can be variable, but not all of them are seen in degenerative basal ganglia disorders. Chorea, athetosis, dystonia, myoclonus and tremor. Dementia and irritability are usual associated psychic disorders.

Degenerative disorders of brainstem can be recognized if there are ophthalmoplegia, glance weakness, postural reflex impairment, dysarthria, dysphagia or ataxia.

Primary degenerative disorders of basal ganglia and brainstem are rare, and their diagnosis has not been significantly improved by neuroradiology or magnetic resonance.

a) Congenital diseases
a-6 Olivo-ponto-cerebellar degeneration

Congenital olivo-ponto-cerbellar degeneration is atrophy of the ventral pons and cerebellum. The condition is usually sporadic, but it could be familiar exceptionally. Etiology is unknown.

Olivo-ponto-cerebellar degeneration is recognized by progressive ascendant ataxia beginning in lower limbs, dysarthria and dysphagia. Numerous neurologic symptoms, such as ophthalmoplegia, retinal degeneration, parkinsonism, hemibalism, athetosis, leg contractures, epilepsy, dementia, etc. have been described (14).

The term multiple system atrophy has been applied to four syndroms striatonigral degeneration, Shay Drager syndrome, parkinson-amyotoaty syndrome and olivo-ponto-cerebellar atrophy- previously considered as distinct and separate entities.

CT is not conclusive for the diagnosis of olivo-ponto-cerebellar degeneration, because of the bone artifacts masking the pathologic lesions in the posterior cranial fossa. Basic axial view, followed by reconstructed sagittal view is insufficient for exploration of the cerebellum. The relationship between white and gray matter could not be judged upon CT scan.

MR image in sagittal and coronal view, in T-1W sequence, can show morphology of olivo-ponto-cerebellar degeneration (11) (Fig. 85).

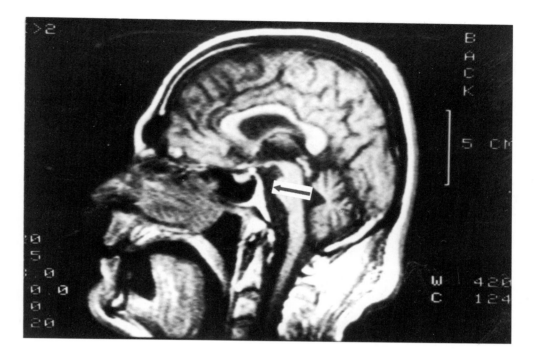

Figure 85. Sagittal image (SE 200/15). Olivo-ponto-cerebellar degeneration - arrow.

b) Acquired and unexplained causes
b-1 Central pontine myelinosis

The condition is seen in potators, patients with ethylic or non-ethylic liver cirrhosis, diabetes, metabolic diseases with electrolyte dysbalance, etc.

Typical destruction of the midline pontine tissue, especially myelin (oligodendroglia) is found, with predominant perivenular inflammatory reaction in the acute and proliferation of macroglia and fibrillar glia in the chronic phase (5).

Variable neurologic deficit can be seen dependent on the size and site of lesion inside the pons.

Smaller lesions of the central pontine myelinosis could not be shown in CT scan, because of poor resolution and artifacts caused by cranial base bones.

MR tomographs in axial, and particularly sagittal view show those lesions as hypointensive area in T-1W sequence or hyperintensive area in T-2W sequence. Those lesions are not typical for their signal intensity and could not be differentiated from multiple sclerosis plaques or ischemic lesions (22).

Complete neurologic symptomatology and laboratory findings as well as affirmative MR image can contribute to definitive diagnosis (Fig. 86).

3. Primary involvement with no sites of predilection

a) Congenital diseases:
   Mucopolysacharidosis
   Farbers disease
   MELAS, MERRF.

b) Acquired and unexplained causes
   Systemic lupus erythematodes
   Neuroradiologic findings, including magnetic resonance, do not contribute to the diagnosis of the diseases belonging to group 3.

b) Acquired and unexplained causes
b-1 Systemic lupus erythematodes
Systemic lupus erythematodes is acquired autoimmune disease (collagenosis) of unknown etiology,

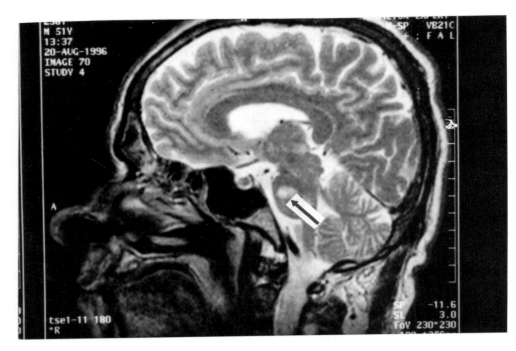

Figure 86. Sagittal image (TSE 4000/99). Arrow pointing at hyperintensive lesion in pons (central pontine myelinosis).

with CNS involvement in 50% of cases. Atrophy and microinfarctions could be seen, but completely negative neuroradiologic finding is not the exception. It has been considered that the atrophy of the brain structures is due to the steroid therapy and is not caused by the disease itself. Damaged arterioles and capillaries are responsible for small solitary or multiple, partly confluent brain or brainstem infarctions. Apart from infarctions, parenchymatous bleeding, as well as subdural or subarachnoidal hemorrhage can be found in patients with lupus.

Neurologic complications of systemic lupus erythematodes (SLE), due either to vascular impairment in peripheral and central nervous system or by the hemorrhage and emboly caused by hypertension or endocarditis, are seen in 75% of patients. Psychic alteration, epileptic fits, cranial nerve disorders, and occasionally chorea, hemiparesis, hemianopsia and aphasia. Polyneuropathy and myelopathy could also be found. In few percent of patients neurologic symptoms arise first, which makes the diagnosis quite difficult (33).

Hypodense infarction zones, hyperdense parenchymatous or subdural hemorrhage and brain atrophy are clearly seen in CT scans (3).

MR image is more selective and precise for the diagnosis of lupus lesions as compared to CT scan (9). Double echo sequence in axial and, eventually, coronal view, displays lesions with high signal intensities, typical for the hemorrhage (Fig. 87).

4. Myelin diseases (white matter)

a) Congenital diseases
   a-1 Metachromatic leukodistrophy
   a-2 Leukodistrophy of globoid cells
   a-3 Ortochromatic leukodistrophies (Adrenoleukodistrophy and *Pelizaeus-Merzbacher* disease)
   a-4 Spongious degeneration
   a-5 Alexander's disease
   a-6 Miscellaneous

b) Acquired and unknown causes
   b-1 Multiple sclerosis (M.S.)
   b-2 Concentric sclerosis
   b-3 Hypertensive cerebrovascular diseases (Binswangers disease and multi infarction dementia MID)

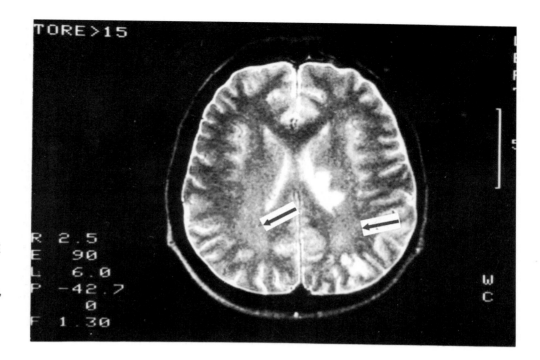

Figure 87. Axial image (SE 2500/90). Multiple brain infarctions caused by systemic lupus erythematodes, with high signal intensities - arrows.

b-4 Progressive multifocal encephalopathy
b-5 Postinfective encephalomyelitis
b-6 Radiation disease
b-7 Necrotizing encephalopathy (brain damage following cytostatic therapy - methotrexate, etc.).

a) Congenital white matter diseases

Magnetic resonance has exceptional selectivity in the diagnosis of congenital white matter diseases. **T-2W** sequence is especially selective for early or advanced stages of the disease, clearly showing distribution, shape and size of lesions in axial and, eventually, coronal views.

The table shows nerve tissue contents of water, lipids, proteins and electrolytes, after B.A. Holand (13).

T-1W and **T-2W** are shorter in the white matter as compared to the gray matter. MR examination makes differentiation of the white and gray matter much easier than CT. Lipids, reach in mobile hydrogen protons, have the particular influence on this differentiation.

White matter pathology could be suspected upon CT scan, but there is a lot of differential diagnostic problems, such as tumor, ischemia, postcontusion focus, etc.

Infratentorial or basal cerebral lesions are poorly visualized by CT examination.

a- 1, 2, 3 Leukodistrophies

Leukodistrophies are genetic, metabolic disorders of myelin, commencing in the first months of life and ending lethally within a few months or years. Blindness, spastic palsy, ataxia and mental retardation or dementia are the most frequent features.

a-1 Signs of metachromatic leukodystrophy are diffuse sclerosis and deposits of non-liposoluble mat-

Table:

Component	Gray matter (%)	White matter (%)	Myelin (%)
Water	82	72	40
Lipids	6	16	30
Proteins	11	11	29
Electrolytes	1	1	1

ter. The matter has tendency towards metachromatic dying, so the condition was named after that. Enzyme deficiency of cerebrosid-sulfatase causes the sulfate brain deposits. Diffuse demyelination, sclerosis and glial proliferation, spongious cavities, "metachromatic lipids", etc. are seen in the white matter. Infantile metachromatic leukodistrophy ends lethally within 12 months, unlike a juvenile form which could last up to ten years. Metachromatic dystrophy is rarely seen in adults.

Laboratory findings in blood and liquor, as well as the peripheral nerve biopsy confirms the diagnosis of metachromatic leukodystrophy.

a-2 *Krabbes* disease or globoid cell leukodistrophy is caused by a lack of the enzyme cerebroside sulfotransferase which should enable transformation of cerebrosides to sulfatides. Protein bound glicolipids are deposited in the cells. Lesions, similar to those seen in metachromatic leukodistrophy, are found in Krabbes disease. All brain lobes are involved in demyelination. The disease has subacute course, ending lethally within 12 months.

Laboratory findings and nerve biopsy in particular, enable the diagnosis.

a-3 Adrenoleukodistrophy, seen in children aged 4 to 12 years, is a combination of adrenal atrophy and diffuse cerebral sclerosis. Apart from symmetric demyelination, axon rarefaction, gliosis, mononuclear perivascular infiltration, etc., could be seen.

a-3 Pelizaeus-Merzbachers disease (sudanophil leukodistrophy) is congenital disease affecting children, with complete myelin absence, although islets of myelin could be found occasionally. Sudanophil lipids are found in perivascular cells (12).

CT scan shows altered density of the brain tissue in leukodistrophies. Hypodensity and distribution of lesions is not sufficient for the diagnosis (30).

MR examination is absolutely a method of choice for the diagnosis of leukodystrophic lesions (1). MR tomographs in T-2W sequence shows periventricular lesions of high signal intensity in leukodistrophies and typical fronto-temporo-parietal lesions of butterfly wings shape. Although signal intensity is not specific, the shape is typical and, along with neurologic and laboratory findings, the diagnosis of this hereditary myelin disease can be made (15, 28, 29).

Typical "butterfly wing" demyelinating lesion in an 8 year old child with metachromatic leukodistrophy is shown by MR examination in T-2W sequence in coronal view (Figg. 88, 89).

Expansive lesion was suspected upon CT scan in 12 year old child with acute unconsciousness spells and neurologic deficit. MR examination in T-2W sequence in axial view confirms the diagnosis of demyelination disease from leukodistrophy group (Fig. 90).

Disturbed hematoencephalic barrier in leukodistrophies enables enormous signal enhancement of

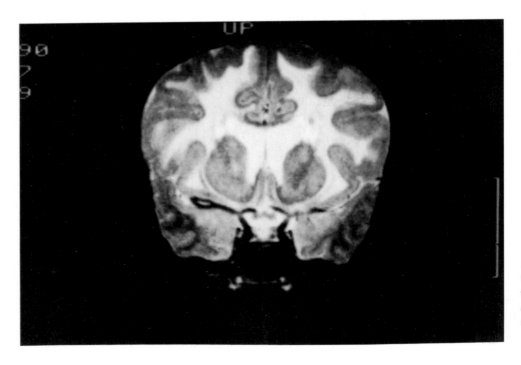

Figure 88. Coronal image (SE 2500/90). Metachromatic leukodistrophy. Bilateral, fronto-parietal, "butterfly wing" demyelination zones of high signal intensity.

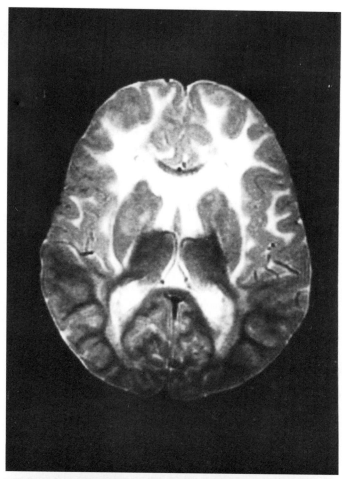

Figure 89. Axial image (SE 2500/90). Metachromatic leukodistrophy. Bilateral, fronto-parietal, "butterfly wing" demyelination zones of high signal intensity.

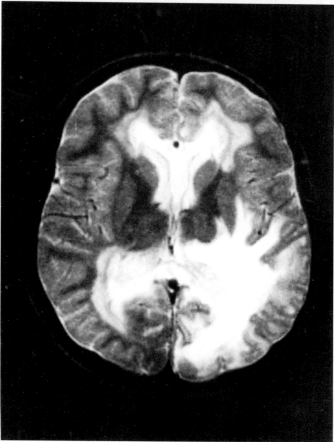

Figure 90. Axial image (SE 2500/90). Lekodystrophy. Bilateral, periventricular and marked left temporo-occipital demyelination zones of high signal intensity.

the margins of demyelination lesions in T-1W sequence, after paramagnetic contrast administration (31). Expansive lesion can be ruled out with certainty (Fig. 91).

Demyelination forms are quite typical in MR images obtained in T-2W sequence. Hereditary white matter diseases are, however, diagnosed upon clinical and laboratory findings and eventual biopsy.

b) Acquired and unknow causes
b-1 Sclerosis Multiple

Multiple sclerosis (M.S.) is the most frequent representative of a group of acquired demyelinating disease of the CNS in which myelin is the target of autoimmune inflamatory process. Multiple demyelination lesions are found in the white matter and cortex as well. Periventricular location of M.S. lesions is frequently seen. Infratentorial or intramedullar M.S. lesions can be also found. Ventricular system dilation, subcortical reductive changes and cortical reduction are usually found in patients with M.S. (32).

Diameter of M.S. foci could vary from microscopic up to several centimeters. There are usually several dozen of M.S. foci at a different developmental stage. Etiology is still unclear with environmental, probable virus or genetic abnormality of the immune system, being a possible cause.

Clinical manifestation is not always proportional to the location or size of the plaques. Some of the plaques are asymptomatic, others have minimal or severe neurologic deficit. M.S. is clinically defined as "disseminated in time and space". Dissemination in time means that it has relapses and remissions, and dissemination in space regards the scattered foci. The course can be remittent, with long-standing remissions from one month up to four decades, progressive from the beginning or becoming progressive after several remissions and exacerbations.

Clinical symptoms are variable, so that there is virtually no neurologic deficit that could not be associated with M.S. Pyramidal, and cerebellar signs are frequently found, as well as various sensory deficits, retrobulbar neuritis or other cranial nerve impairment, disturbed sphincter control, cognitive or emotional disorders.

Evolution can vary from the frust forms, found accidentally to acute ones ending lethally within sev-

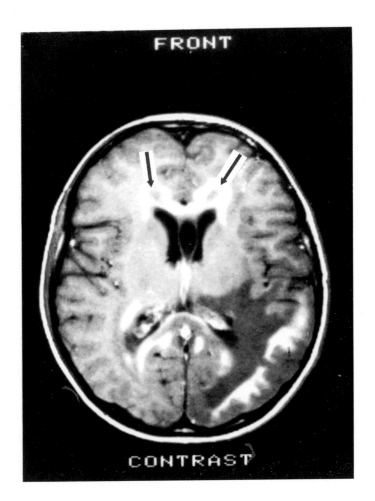

Figure 91. Axial image (SE 500/15) after gadolinium-DTPA administration. Lekodystrophy. Demyelination zones of lower signal intensities. Magnevist enhances signal intensities considerably in regions of acute disturbance of hematoencephalic barrier - arrows.

eral months. Average evolution of M.S. takes 20 to 25 years.

Clinically evident M.S. meets criteria of "dissemination in time and space". The most important laboratory findings that support the diagnosis are abnormal evoked potentials, intrathecal synthesis of oligoclonal immunoglobulins G and positive MR image. Those findings, however, are not specific and the clinical picture is the only way to establish the diagnosis.

CT examination reveals hypodense periventricular M.S. plaques in the cerebrum. Mature lesions does not alter after the contrast administration, whereas the recent plaques become marginally hyperdense.

Disadvantages of computer tomography include inability to discover infratentorial, basal or spinal lesions (because of the artifacts caused by massive bones of cranial base and spine), with lesions being atypical and hard to tell from infarction, tumor, etc.

The neuroradiologic aspect of M.S. includes probable and possible diagnosis of M.S.

Clinically definite M.S. is a form where laboratory findings are sufficient for the definition of the disease. Neuroradiology is of purely academic importance for patients with M.S. CT scan confirms multiple hypodense lesions, mostly periventriculary. MR examination is not indicated for this form of M.S.

MR examination is indicated for probable and possible forms of M.S. Probable form of M.S. is a disease where probable M.S. is suspected upon clinical course, neurologic and laboratory findings, but there is still no absolute certainty. CT scan can reveal one or more suspect M.S. plaques. Magnetic resonance is absolutely indicated for this form of M.S., for it could prove solitary or multiple plaques in different locations and confirm the diagnosis.

Possible M.S. is a condition of the patient following first attack with discrete neurologic deficit and inconclusive laboratory findings. CT scan is negative in possible M.S. MR imaging is mandatory, because of its ability to prove the tiniest M.S. plaques and discover the disease in the earliest stage.

MR image in T-2W can reveal the tiniest M.S. plaques, regardless of location. Lesions are seen as foci of high signal intensity. Same lesions are not perfectly seen in T-1W sequence; smaller foci of low signal intensity located nearby sulci, cranial base or in the posterior fossa could be easily overlooked. MR image is not absolutely conclusive for the disease, so that clinical and laboratory findings are needed to confirm the diagnosis (21).

The use of the magnetic resonance imaging (MRI) has provided a powerful approach to the visualization of central nervous system lesions in multiple sclerosis (MS). Therefore, MRI was shown to be of special value in the diagnosis of MS and several MRI diagnostic criteria were recommended up to now.

Paty et al. (17) suggested that lesions considered typical of MS were those of high intesity on T-2W images, greater than 3 mm in diameter and located predominantly in the white matter. The following MRI diagnostic scale was established:

MRI strongly suggestive of MS:
A) four lesions present;
B) three lesions present, one periventricular
MRI suggestive of MS:
A) three lesions present;
B) two lesions present, one periventricular.
MRI possibile MS:
A) two lesions present;
B) one lesions present in a periventricular location.

Fazekas et al. (7) recommended that optimal specificity of MRI findings for the positive diagnosis of MS could be obtained if at least three areas of increased signal on the T-2W images were present, in addition to at least two out of the following three MRI features:
a) a lesion exceeding 6 mm in diameter;
b) periventricular lesion;
c) infratentorial location.

According to the criteria of Barkhof et al., the specifity of MRI findings in MS could be increased if eight areas of increased signal on T-2W images, and a gadolinium enhancing lesion or an infratentorial lesion, are required for the positive MRI diagnosis of MS.

There is a typical example of MR tomograph in T-2W sequence, in axial view, with bilateral parietal, periventricular, multiple plaques of high signal intensity. M.S. has been confirmed upon clinical and laboratory findings (Figg. 92, 93).

Solitary M.S. plaque is shown in T-2W sequence in a 25 year old female with pontine neurologic symp-

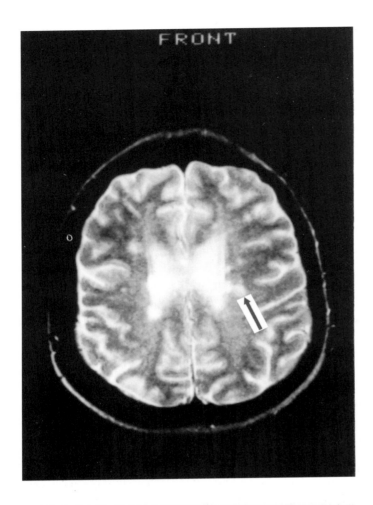

Figure 92. Axial image (SE 2500/90). Bilateral parietal, periventricular M.S. lesions of high signal intensities - arrow.

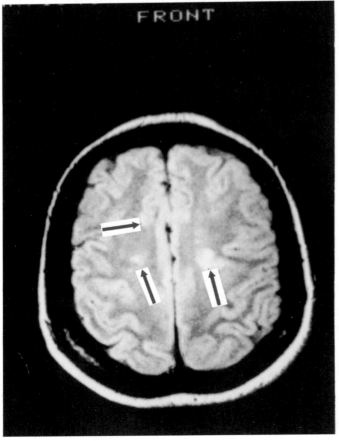

Figure 93. Axial image (SE 2500/15). Bilateral parietal M.S. lesions of high signal intensities - arrows.

tomatology. Small demyelination zone have not been seen in CT scan. Neurologic and laboratory findings have confirmed the diagnosis of M.S. (Fig. 94).

CT scan have revealed hypodense lesion in the left parietal, periventricular area in a 23 year old female, following first generalized epileptic seizure. Tumor has been suspected. Neurologic and laboratory findings have suggested recent M.S. plaque. MR tomographs in T-2W sequence have shown irregular, spherical lesion of mixed signal intensities in the left periventricular region (Fig. 95).

Recent M. S. plaques in exacerbation, with disturbed hematoencephalic barrier, have specific features in T-1W sequence after paramagnetic contrast administration (11). Wide margin of a plaque is shown by high signal intensities. This feature is significant for the estimate of the age of M. S. plaque, i.e. the phase of the disease (Fig. 96).

Paramagnetic contrast Magnevist enhances signal intensities in cases with disturbed hematoencephalic barrier, thus enabling diagnosis of recent M.S. plaques. This feature is used for differentiating solitary plaque from ischemia, tumor, etc. Neurologic and laboratory findings can contribute to differential diagnosis of a solitary M.S. plaque and suspected expansive lesion in the initial phase (24).

b-3 Hypertensive cerebrovascular disease (Binswangers disease and Multiinfarction dementia)

Binswangers disease is caused by a decreased circulation through arteriosclerotic vessels, in hypertonic and normotonic patients, and microembolization causing infarctions and hemorrhage. Generalized pathologic lesions can be confluent as well. Lesions are situated periventriculary in the white matter and in semioval center.

Binswangers disease commences gradually, with progressive course and occasional exacerbation in a form of acute focal neurologic deficit. Psychic alteration have been noticed in all of the patients, usually as intellectual deterioration. Character changes, apathy, loss of interest for everyday activities, paranoia, memory deficit, disorientation, behavior disorders, euphoria, aggression, depression, etc. can be

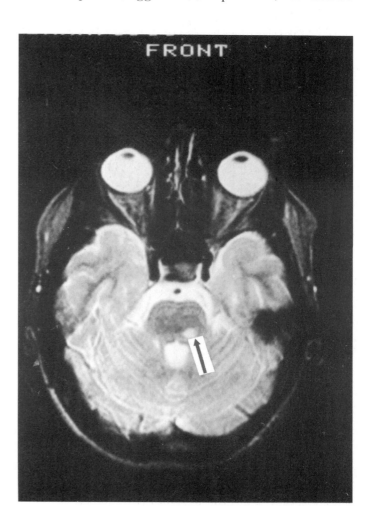

Figure 94. Axial image (SE 2500/90). Parasagittal left pontine M.S. plaque shown as round zone of high signal intensity - arrow.

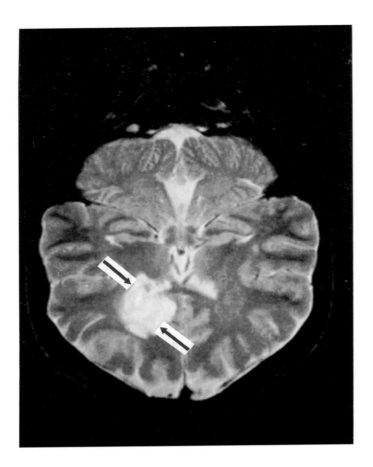

Figure 95. Coronal image (SE 2500/90). Bigger irregular zone of mixed higher and high signal intensities, without compression effect, is shown in the left periventricular area - arrows.

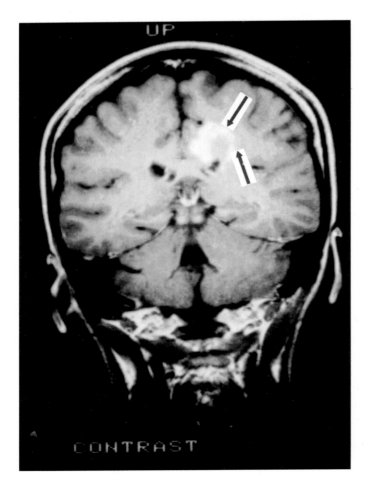

Figure 96. Coronal image (SE 500/15) after gadolinium-DTPA administration. Arrows pointing at recent M.S. plaque.

found in those patients. Aphasia, hemianopsia, apraxia and other signs of cortical damage are rarely seen (23, 26).

CT scan can reveal bigger hypodense infarctions, demyelination zones and hyperdense brain hemorrhage. MR tomographs in T-2W sequence in axial view can show pathologic lesions precisely as compared to the poor resolution of CT scans.

MR image reveals bilateral, diffuse, particularly periventricular, confluent, diffuse or circumscript demyelination lesions in a white matter (Fig. 97).

Multiinfarction dementia (MID) is a condition which could not be easily differentiated from Binswangers disease, because it is caused by arteriosclerotic process in cerebral blood vessels as well. Arterial hypertension and diabetes mellitus are usual underlying conditions. The disease affects mainly elderly patients.

Previous term "dementia arteriosclerotica" has been replaced by multiinfarction dementia, for it has been understood that the condition is not due to global hypoperfusion through uniformly stenosed blood vessels, but caused by numerous focal ischemia and multiple infarctions of varying size.

Apart from multiple infarctions, both cortical and subcortical reductive changes are seen bilaterally.

MID is clinically presented by a loss of cognitive functions and reduced social competency. In the beginning, clinical appearance resembles neurasthenic neurosis ("pseudoneurasthenia arteriosclerotica") with symptoms, such as fatigue, irritability, apathy, reluctance, headache, insomnia or hypersomnia, loss of concentration. Loss of memory and efficiency is obvious. Speech, judgment and orientation disorders could arise in a later phase. Dementia could vary from slight to deep, when patient becomes helpless and reduced to a "digestive tube".

CT scan could be sufficient for the diagnosis of lesions, although it is incapable to reveal microinfarctions in all locations. Discrepancy between negative or inconclusive CT scan and positive neurologic and laboratory findings is not exceptional. Discrepancies between CT scan and clinical appearance are considerably higher as compared to positive correlation between MR image and neurologic and laboratory findings.

MR image is not specific, showing numerous small infarctions, of varying size and shape, in cortex,

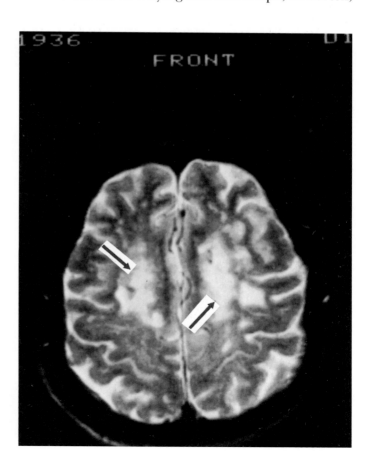

Figure 97. Axial image (SE 2500/90). Binswangers disease - bilateral parietal numerous solitary, mostly confluent infarctions with high signal intensities - arrows.

white matter, basal ganglia, etc. (25, 34). Cortical and subcortical reductive changes are seen in MR tomographs (Figg. 98, 99).

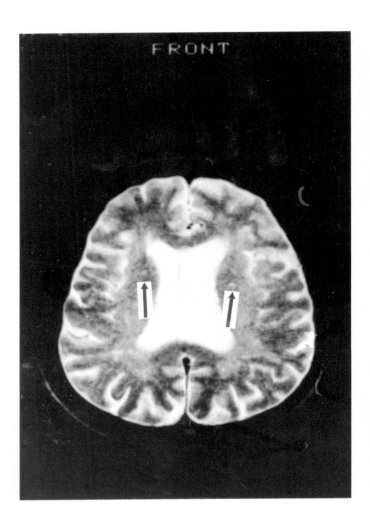

Figure 98. Axial image (SE 2500/90). MID. Numerous small, partly punctiform infarctions shown as zones of high signal intensity - arrows. Dilation of both lateral ventricles, particularly the left one.

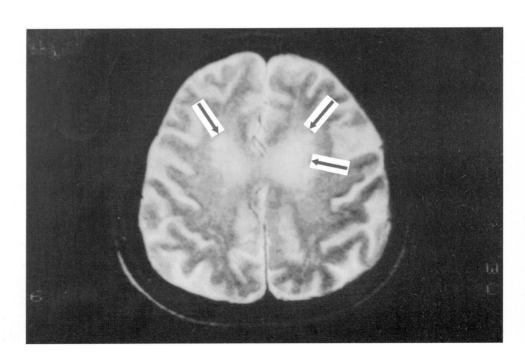

Figure 99. Axial image (SE 2500/90). MID. Numerous small, partly confluent infarctions located high under the chalet, supra- and periventriculary - arrows.

b-5 Postinfective encephalomyelitis

Acute disseminated encephalomyelitis (post-parainfectious encephalomyelitis, postvaccinal encephalomyelitis) could occur in the course of different infections, especially the acute exanthematous diseases, and following vaccinations.

Clinically and pathologically all these cases are similar, regardless of the nature of the precipitating infection disease or vaccination.

Pathohistologic features are edema, hyperemia, petechial hemorrhage, colliquation and necrosis zones in cortex, subcortical white matter, basal ganglia, brainstem, etc. Perivascular lymphocyte infiltrations are usually present. Pathohistologic changes depend on the causative agent, severity and duration of illness. During the recovery phase, apart from dead cells, altered cells can partly regenerate, perivascular infiltration vanish or subdue, and glial proliferation leads to gliosis. Demyelination changes in white matter are focal, and, sometimes, confluent. Periventricular location is the most frequent one.

Postinfective encephalomyelitis is manifested by a headache, confusion, meningismus or recurrent hyperpyrexia with convulsions and coma. Hemiplegia, ataxia or transversal myelitis are rarely seen, and choreathetosis is exceptional. Encephalomyelitis following morbilli is 10-20%, and various sequels could be seen as well.

CT examination with low resolution can show non-specific pathologic changes of postinfective encephalomyelitis in the brain. The lesions are hypodense and they don't change after iodine contrast injection.

MR image in this condition is also non-specific. MR tomographs, regardless of sequence, show the lesions similar to multiple sclerosis in various modalities (13, 19). MR can help to assess the size and location of non-specific lesions, which can be defined upon complete clinical appearance and laboratory findings (Figg. 100, 101).

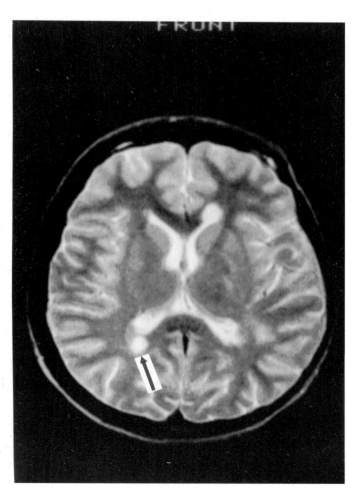

Figure 100. Axial image (SE 2500/90). Postinfective encephalomyelitis: bilateral periventricular multiple demyelination lesions of high signal intensity - arrow.

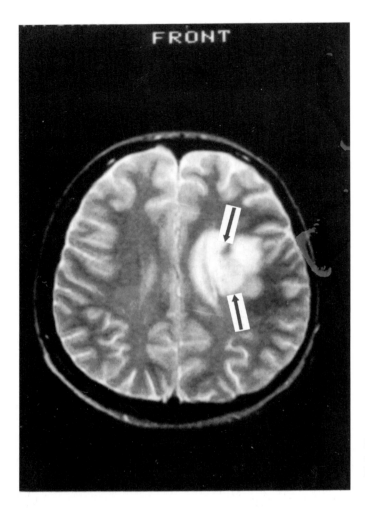

Figure 101. Axial image (SE 2500/90). Postinfective encephalomyelitis: left parietal, confluent, demyelination lesions of high signal intensity - arrows.

b-6 Postirradiation sequels

Radiotherapy for expansive lesions of the CNS can cause adverse effects on the brain structures. Type of radiotherapy, radiation fields and dose have favorable effects on expansive lesion, but could cause possible damage to the adjacent structure, as well as to healthy tissues affected by ionizing rays. Adverse effects of radiotherapy can be classified according to the type and degree of lesions: acute radionecrosis; early changes arising from 3. to 6. week with hematoencephalic barrier disorder and subsequent brain edema; transitory radiation injuries in form of demyelination and late radiation injuries manifested by infarction, hemorrhage, demyelination and necrosis.

Clinical appearance of a patient after radiotherapy depends on the type, degree and location of postirradiation lesions. Progression of neurologic or endocrine symptomatology, during or following radiotherapy, makes an indication for MR examination.

Larger hypodense postirradiation lesions of CNS can be seen in CT scan. There are certain limitations of CT scanners, especially of those with low resolution, regarding sensitivity in diagnosis of smaller lesions, such as edema, demyelination, infarction, hemorrhage, necrosis, etc., as compared to MR machines.

Postirradiation pathologic alterations in CNS are seen in MR image in focal necrosis, vascular proliferation and atypical gliosis signal intensities. Postirradiation changes of white matter include demyelination and necrosis (6, 16).

MR image is not specific and diagnosis is based upon neurologic clinical appearance, and data regarding radiation dose, field and type, etc. (Figg. 102-104).

In patients who have undergone surgery and postoperative radiation, lesions induced by surgery and radiation could be superimposed. Combined lesions can create a diagnostic problem.

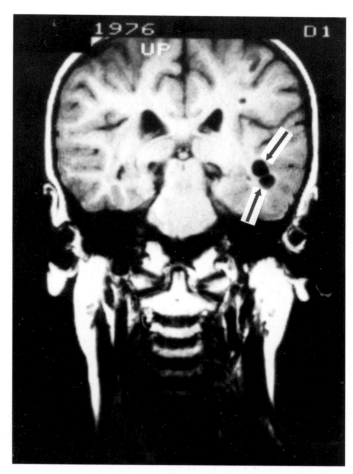

Figure 102. Coronal image (SE 500/15). Left temporal and parietal postirradiation lesions following irradiation for posterior fossa tumor. Lesions have low signal intensities - arrows.

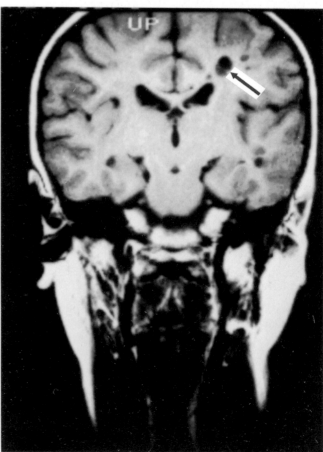

Figure 103. Coronal image (SE 500/15). Left temporal and parietal postirradiation changes following irradiation for posterior fossa tumor. Lesions have low signal intensities - arrow.

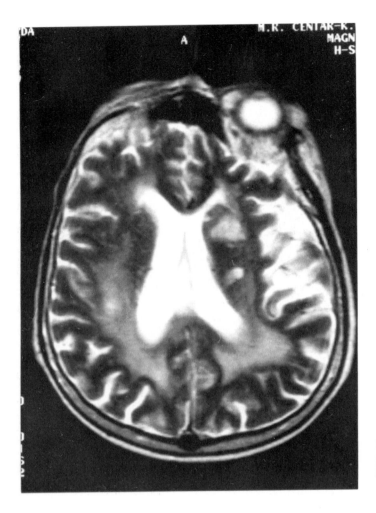

Figure 104. Axial image (TSE 4000/99). Bilateral periventricular postirradiation lesions of high signal intensity, following irradiation for posterior fossa tumor.

b-7 Necrotizing encephalopathies

Certain medication used for polychemotherapy (oral, intravenous or intrathecal), such as Methotrexate, can cause neurologic complications or conditions. Cytostatic drugs can cause the damage to the CNS by their toxic effect. Harmful adverse effects of polychemotherapy should be monitored neurologically and radiologically in order to adjust the treatment, i.e. doses of drugs, etc. Pathohistology changes induced by certain drugs are edema, focal or confluent demyelination, infarction, hemorrhage, gliosis, necrosis, etc.

Diseases induced by harmful effects of polychemotherapy are called necrotizing encephalopathy.

Necrotizing encephalopathy can be recognized by gradual onset of dementia, pseudobulbar paralysis, ataxia and cortical focal deficits.

CT scan can reveal a bigger hypodense lesion, usually supratentorially.

MR image has higher precision and selectivity than CT scan, for discovering initial, discrete lesions of a white matter. Necrotizing encephalopathy in demyelination form can be seen in MR tomographs after chemotherapy with high doses of methotrexate in patients with acute lymphatic leukemia. Bilateral, periventricular, marked demyelination lesions have altered, i.e. higher signal intensities (Fig. 105).

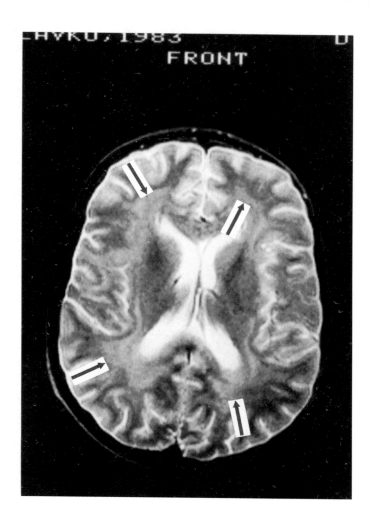

Figure 105. Axial image (SE 2500/90). Methotrexate necrotizing encephalopathy: bilaterally periventricular intensified signal of the white matter (demyelination) - arrows.

REFERENCES

1. Bewermeyer H., et al.: MR imaging in adrenoleukomyeloneuropathy. J. Comput. Assist. Tomogr., 9: 793-800, 1985.
2. Bidder GM., Steiner RE.: NMR Imaging of the brain. Neuroradiology, 23: 231-240, 1982.
3. Bories J.: Computerized Axial Tomography. Springer-Verlag. Berlin, Heidelberg, New York, 1978.
4. Brant-Zawadzki M., Fein G., Van Dyke C., Kiernan R., Davenport L., de Groot J.: MR imaging of the aging brain: patchy white-matter lesions and dementia. AJNR, 6: 675-682, 1985.
5. Brunner EJ., et al.: Central pontine myelonolysis and pontine lesions after rapid correction of hyponatremia: A prospective magnetic resonance imaging study. Ann. Neurol., 27: 61-66, 1990.
6. Dooms GC., Hecht S., Brant-Zawadzki M., Berthiaume Y., Norman D. Newton TH.: Brain radiation lesions: MR imaging. Radiology, 158: 149-155, 1986.
7. Fazekas F., et al.: Criteria for an increased specificity of MRI interpretation in eldery subjects with multiple sclerosis. Neurology, 38: 1822-1825, 1988.
8. Grossman RI., Gonzales SF., Atlas SW., Galetta S., Silberberg DH.: Multiple sclerosis: gadolinium enhancement in MR imaging. Radiology, 161: 721-725, 1986.
9. Halbsgut A., Lechner B.: Magnetresonanz-Tomographie (NMR). Springer-Verlag. Frankfurt, 1986.
10. Holland BA.: Diseases of wite matter. In Brant-Zawadzki M., Norman D. (eds): Magnetic resonance imaging of the central nervous system. Raven Press. New York, 259-277, 1986.
11. Huk WJ., Gademann G., Friedman G.: Magnetic Resonance Imaging of Central Nervous System Diseases. Springer Verlag. Berlin, New York, Heidelbeg, Tokyo, Paris, London, 1989.
12. Journel H., et al: Magnetic resonance imaging in Pelizaeus-Merzbacher disease. Neuroradiology, 29: 403-405, 1987.
13. Kesselring J., et al.: Acute disseminated encephalomyelitis MRI findings and the distinction from multiple sclerosis. Brain, 113: 291-302, 1990.
14. Konigswark BW., Weina LP.: The olivopontocerebellar atrophies: A review. Medicine, 49: 227-230, 1970.
15. Kumar AH., et al.: Adrenoleukodystrophy: correlating MR imaging with CT. Radiology, 165: 497-499, 1987.
16. Liessner J., Seider M.: Klinische Kernspintomographie. Enke. Stuttgart, 1987.
17. Paty DW., et al.: MRI in the diagnosis of MS: A prospective study with camparison of clinical evaluation, evoked potentials, oligoclonal banding, and CT. Neurology, 38: 180-185, 1988.

18. Pendlebury WRW., Soloman PR.: Alzheimers Disease, Clinical Symponsia. CIBA, 48(3): 1-32, 1996.
19. Pennock J., et al.: Magnetic resonance imaging of the brain in children. Magn. Reson. Imaging, 4: 1-12, 1986.
20. Pomeranz JS.: Craniospinal Magnetic Resonance Imaging. W.B. Saunders Company. Philadelphia, London, Toronto, Sydney, Tokyo, 1989.
21. Poser CM., et al.: Neuroimaging and the lesion of multiple sclerosis. AJNR, 8: 549-555, 1987.
22. Price DB., et al.: Central pontine myelinolysis: report of a case with distinctive appearance on MR imaging. AJNR, 8: 576-582, 1987.
23. Roman GC., et al.: Vascular dementia: diagnostic criteria for research studies. Report of the ninds-airen international workshop. Neurology, 43: 250-260, 1993.
24. Runge VM., Price AC., Kirschner HS., Allen JH., Partian CL., James AE. Jr.: The evaluation of multiple sclerosis by magnetic resonance imaging. Radiographics, 6(2): 203-212, 1986.
25. Stark D., Bradley GWJR.: Magnetic Resonance Imaging. The C.V. Mosby Company. St. Louis, Washington D.C., Toronto, 1988.
26. Tatemichi TK., Sadator N., Mayeny R.: Dementia associated with cerebrovascular disease, other degenerative diseases, and metabolic disorders. In Terry RD., Katzman R., Bick L., (ed.): Alzheimers Disease. Raven Press. New York, 1994.
27. Van M. Runge: Enhanced Magnetic Resonance Imaging. The C.V. Mosby Company. St. Louis, Baltimore, Toronto, 1989.
28. Valk J., Van der Knaap MS.: White matter and myelin. In Valk J., Van der Knaap MS., (eds): Magnetic resonance of myelin, myelination, and myelin disorders, Springer-Verlag. Berlin, 9-21, 1989.
29. Volkow ND., et al: Adrenoleukodystrophy: imaging with CT, MRI and PET. J. Nucl. Med., 28: 524-529, 1987.
30. Wackenheim A., Jeanmart L., Beart A.: Craniocerebral Computer Tomography., Berlin, Heidelberg, New York, Vol. 1, 1980.
31. Waltz G., Harik SI., Kaufman B.: Adult metachromatic leukodystrophy: value of computed tomographic scanning and magnetic resonance imaging of the brain. Arch. Neurol., 44: 225-232, 1987.
32. Whitaker JN., Mitahell GW.: Clinical features of multiple sclerosis. In: Raine CS., McFarland HF., Tourtellotte WW. (eds): Multiple sclerosis clinical and pathogenetic lavis. London. Chapman Hall Hedical, 3-19, 1997.
33. Wong KL., et al.: Neurological manifestations of systemic lupus erythematosus. QY Med., 88: 857-870, 1991.
34. Young IR., et al.: Nuclear magnetic resonance (NMR) imaging in white matter disease of the brain using spin-echo sequences. J. Comput. Assist. Tomogr., 7: 290-298, 1983.
35. Zawadcki MB., Norman D.: Magnetic Resonance Imaging of the Central Nervous System. Raven Press. New York, 1987.

VI. BRAIN TUMORS

Miodrag Rakić, Vaso Antunović, Ljiljana Djordjić, Gradimir Dragutinović

There are several different brain tumor classifications. They could be sorted according to malignancy (benign or malignant), localization (midline, cranial base, arising from certain area or structure, etc.). They could be congenital or acquired. Acquired tumors can be either primary (glioblastoma, etc.) or mixed (intraventricular tumors) or exogenous (meningioma, hypophyseal adenoma, epidermoid, teratoma, lipoma, etc.). Carcinoma, melanoma etc. are secondary tumors.

Tumors are classified according to the degree of malignancy, regarding survival time, malignancy grade and incidence in our population. There is a classification dividing tumors in intra- and extracranial, with modalities concerning tumor spread (such as. intracranial with extracranial propagation or vice versa).

Subclasses within tumor classification include varieties such as hemorrhage and necrosis inside tumor, its hormonal activity, pseudotumors, etc.

Tumors can be classified regarding origin of the neoplastic cells (11, 25):

Tumors:
  Neuroepithelial
  Of neural sheath origin
  Meningeal
  Vascular
  Germinal cell
  Malformation or other
  Primary malignant lymphoma
  Metastasis

Hypophyseal or sellar tumors, as well as cranio-cervical junction or extracranial tumors with endocranial spread are separately classified.

Endocranial spread of different expansive neoplasms with aggressive features makes separate entity. Destruction of the bones, usually cranial base enables the endocranial spread with subsequent lesion of the brain tissue either by compression or infiltration.

Pseudotumors are tumorlike formations classified along with expansive lesions although they don't have tumor features (25).

Metastatic growths differ by the type of primary location or common features of secondary deposits, etc.

There are many classifications, but all of them are insufficient. World Health Organization classification of the central nervous system tumors published by Zuelch in 1979 became insufficient when new methods of tumor identification were developed (38).

Kepes have revised the WHO classification in 1990, according to latest achievements in this field (27).

According to this revised classification brain tumors in adults are:

tumors of neuroepithelial origin (astrocytal, oligodendroglial, ependymal, mixed, chorioidal plexus tumors, neuroepithelial tumors of unknown origin, neuronal, mixed neuronal-glial, pineal, embryonic)

  tumors of cranial and spinal nerve origin

  tumors of the brain membranes origin (meningothelial and non-meningothelial)

  hematopoetic tumors

  germinal cell tumors

Childhood tumors are classified as follows:
tumors of neuroepithelial origin (glial, neuronal, primitive neuroepithelial, pineal)
tumors of the brain membranes origin
primary malignant lymphoma
tumors of vascular origin
germinal cell tumors
malformation tumors
tumors of neuroendocrine origin
local spread of the regional tumors
metastatic tumors
unclassified tumors

Supratentorial:
lobar tumors
deep structure tumors
medial tumors
meningeal

Transtentorial

Infratentorial:
medial
cerebellar tumors
brain stem tumors
extracerebellar tumors

Craniocervical and cervicocranial tumors

During the last decade tremendous improvement of histologic diagnosis due to immunohistochemical and ultrastructure immunocytochemical techniques, along with investigation of cytoskeletal and membrane proteins, growth factors, oncogenes and tumor growth dynamics have lead to better understanding of tumor histogenesis.

Thirty years ago neuroradiologic diagnosis of brain tumors consisted of standard radiographs and invasive techniques, such as cerebral angiography and pneumoencephalography (PEG).

Standard radiographs (special views, tomography) can reveal cranial bone lesions, enlargement of physiologic cranial foramina, pathological endocranial calcifications, pineal gland dislocation if it is calcified, etc. When any of the above mentioned abnormalities is found, invasive diagnostic techniques are justified.

Angiographic radiographs were used to prove vascular pathology. There are several indirect signs seen in angiography which can arouse suspicion of endocranial tumor, such as: different forms of pathologic vascularization, avascular areas, compressed or dislocated blood vessels, etc. It is of utmost importance to display blood vessels and their relationship to the tumor for preoperative planning. In order to obtain best possible diagnosis all three phases (arterial, parenchymal and venous) in latero-lateral (LL), antero-posterior (AP) and semioblique projections should be recorded. Apart from complicated and partly risky invasive technique, interpretation of the angiography findings require a skilled and experienced radiologist.

In smaller hospitals without CT equipment, angiography is still used for emergencies such as intracerebral and particularly extracerebral hemorrhage. Intracranial hematomas can mimic tumors and it is necessary to differentiate between them. Emergency surgery for extracerebral hemorrhage is necessary to save a patients life.

Pneumoencephalography (PEG) is nowadays used only for double contrast CT examination. It is useful for the diagnosis of minor tumors of cerebellopontine angle or *empty sella syndrome,* using negative air contrast to fill cerebellopontine cistern.

CT examination was the first ever to enable direct visualization of tumor. When Dr. James Ambrosse, neuroradiologist in London on October 1st 1971 made a CT scan of a 41 year old female with suspected brain tumor and displayed a tumor and edema as well, it started a new era in neuroradiology (9).

MR is complementary technique for the brain tumor diagnosis (21). CT scan should be followed by MR imaging when it is necessary:

to get better multiplanar view (supra- or infratentorial) of the tumor and its relationship to the normal brain structures and ventricular system;

to differentiate between low grade astrocytoma and ischemic or infarction zones;

to make diagnosis of oligodendroglioma without calcification;

to differentiate between involved brain structures, tumor and edema or necrosis and hemorrhage inside the tumor which is essential for planning the surgery;

to make diagnosis of the cranial base tumor (to avoid artifacts arising from massive bones overlapping the tumor in CT scan);

to make MR angiography of the main head and neck vessels

to discover early or multiple metastasis in different cases when required.

MR imaging is indicated if the information about tumor obtained by CT is insufficient, if the tumor is blurred by other brain pathology, when there is diagnostic confusion or dilemma between surgery and conservative treatment (23).

Numerous problems can arise about CT, so that the indications to MR have been considerably widened according to the clinical appearance of the patient (8).

Clinical signs of the brain tumor can be caused by a direct compression of different brain structures by a tumor or general signs caused by elevation of the intracranial pressure induced by space occupying lesion. Progressive focal lesion is due to the first cause. Malignant potential of the tumor and the way of spread determine the development of such a lesion. Benign or infiltrative tumors can grow "silently" for years without causing neurologic deficit because of the neural tissue adaptation. Rapidly growing tumors will cause progressive neurologic deficit in the early phase. Regressive lesions, such as necrosis and hemorrhage can cause sudden onset of neurologic signs like in apoplexy.

Epileptic fit could be the first sign of a tumor, especially in tumors arising from highly epileptogenic areas, such as central sulcus, cortex and temporal lobe. Focal signs can differ depending on tumor location.

General signs of brain tumors are caused by elevated intracranial pressure. *Stagnant papilla*, headache, vomiting, bradycardia and blurred vision (obscuration).

All the tumors reported in this book were diagnosed in the Clinical center of Serbia.

1. Tumors of neuroepithelial origin

Neuroepithelial tumors are astrocytal, oligodendroglial, ependymal, mixed, chaired plexus tumors, neuroepithelial tumors of unknown origin, neuronal and mixed neuronal-glial, pineal and embryonic.

MR imaging enables multiplanar localization of the expansive lesion as well as destroyed or jeopardized normal brain structures and prediction of the direction of the tumor spread. It is of utmost importance to differentiate between tumor and edema, to reveal hemorrhage, necrosis or calcification inside the tumor and assess tumor tissue qualities.

MR imaging of a tumor should be done in axial, coronal and sagittal planes. Slice thickness should be 3-5-10 mm spaced by 0.1-2 mm with whole endocranium to C2-C3 encompassed. Slice thickness could be reduced in order to reveal minor lesion with finer resolution. In that case the field gets narrow, but the summation or overlapping of the pathologic and normal lesions is avoided. Such technique is useful for discovering the Silvius aqueduct obstruction or sellar tumors, etc.

Spin Echo and Gradient Echo sequences are used along with special rapid sequences to reveal calcification, blood collections, changed blood vessels, etc.

Enhanced MR with paramagnetic contrast is useful for better demarcation between tumor and edema or improved display of the tumor, especially meningioma or glioma. Paramagnetic contrast helps to make differential diagnosis between tumor and other lesions. Clinical practice acquires new applications of the paramagnetic contrast in the diagnosis of the CNS tumors and other lesions daily.

a) Astrocytic tumors

According to the dominant changed astrocytic cells there are following types of astrocytic tumors: astrocytoma, astroblastoma, pilocytic astrocytoma, etc. Regarding modified WHO classification astrocytic tumors in adults are: astrocytomas, anaplastic - malignant astrocytoma, glioblastoma, pilocytic astrocytoma, pleomorphic xanthoastrocytoma, subependymal giant-cell astrocytoma (in tuberous sclerosis). Neuroepithelial tumors are histologically divided in four grades (I-IV). Ratio of supratentorial and infratentorial tumor is 4:1, while neuroepithelial tumors of different grades represent $^3/_4$ three quarters of all malignant supratentorial tumors.

a-1 Astrocytoma

In the above mentioned study 2/3 of all supratentorial gliomas are astrocytoma of a varying degree of malignancy. There are several different pathological forms of astrocytoma: fibrillar, protoplasmic, gemistocytic and mixed, belonging to grade II astrocytoma.

Pilocytic astrocytoma, characterized by multiple tiny cysts and occasional hemorrhage and necrosis, because of its benign clinical course is classified as grade I, as well as subependymal giant-cell astrocytoma.

Grade I and II astrocytoma belong to the benign, slowly growing group, also called *low grade astrocytoma*.

Anaplastic astrocytoma and glioblastoma belong to grade III or IV category.

Low grade astrocytoma present typically as cerebellar childhood astrocytoma, brainstem astrocytoma or cerebral astrocytoma.

Cerebellar childhood astrocytoma is a big, cystic, slowly growing tumor, causing hydrocephalus and brainstem compression. Complete microsurgical excision of the tumor is a method of choice leading to complete cure.

Brainstem astrocytoma are usually seen in children and adolescents. They pose a problem to neurosurgeon because of the infiltrative type of spread and eventual malignant alteration and their prognosis is generally poor (15-18).

Unlike anaplastic astrocytoma, low grade cerebral astrocytoma is usually found in younger patients (second, third or fourth decade). While low grade cerebellar astrocytoma is seen in children, cerebral astrocytoma is frequently found in young adults and it is seldom cystic. Prolonged clinical course with slowly progressive symptoms and long standing epilepsy is usually seen. Their growth is diffuse and infiltrative, without considerable dislocation of surrounding structures. Typical locations of cerebral astrocytoma are frontal, fronto-precentral, fronto-temporal, temporal and temporo-parietal.

Pilocytic cerebellar astrocytoma has typical CT image of a cystic hypodense tumor usually surrounded by an edge of solid tissue enhanced by an intravenous application of iodine contrast. Neuroimage of supratentorial variety is quite the same, but it is rarely found.

Low grade brainstem astrocytoma is seen in CT scan like homogenous hypodense expansive formation, but they can be non-homogenous, with cysts and necrosis as well.

Supratentorial slowly growing astrocytoma are seen in CT scan without contrast application like homogenous, well defined low density areas. There is no noticeable enhancement after the intravenous administration of iodine contrast. Therefore astrocytoma can pose a problem to differentiate between infarction, edema or demyelination zone.

MR tomographs in T-1W sequence shows astrocytoma as lower signal intensity zone, while in T-2W sequence it is shown as a mixed zone of higher signal intensities. Cysts and necrosis has high signal intensities (37).

Intratumoral hemorrhage has usual signal properties regarding to the sequence applied (Figg. 106, 107).

The following lesions can be considered in differential diagnosis: oligodendroglioma without calcification, solitary metastasis, recent infarction, local brain edema, intracerebral hematoma in resorption phase, phlegmonous encephalitis, focus of multiple sclerosis, etc.

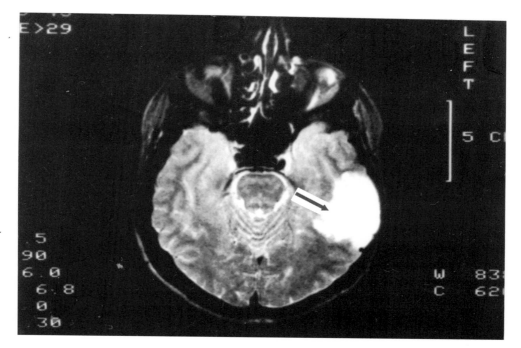

Figure 106. Axial image (SE 4000/90)- Patient T.D. with left temporal grade II astrocytoma (postoperatively histologically proven) with high signal intensity - arrow. No differentiation between tumor and edema is possible.

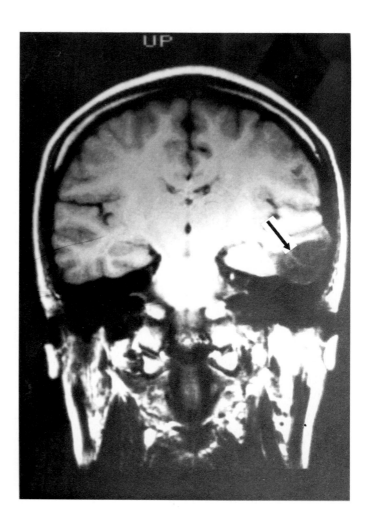

Figure 107. Coronal image (SE 500/15). Same patient (T.D.) with left temporal grade II astrocytoma shown in lower signal intensities - arrow.

a-2 Glioma of the optic nerve and glioma of the optic chiasm

Glioma of the optic nerve and chiasm, as well as hypothalamic-chiasmatic glioma should be mentioned separately because they combine low grade malignancy with extremely unfavorable location where radical surgery is impossible. Glioma of the optic nerve can be either intraorbital, intracanalicular or combined.

Glioma of the optic nerve are frequently seen intraorbitally in children suffering from type 1 neurofibromatosis; its incidence being 15%.

Clinical signs are progressive proptosis and vision problems. It has been discussed over the years whether they belong to hamartomas or tumors.

When hypothalamus is involved by glioma, the hypothalamic syndrome with endocrine disorders, such as pubertas praecox, insipid diabetes, hyperactivity, sleep and feeding disorder, etc., arises.

Pontine and cerebellar glioma belonging to the low grade glioma class will be discussed further in the text.

Computer tomography was considered sufficient for the diagnosis of those tumors before the MR era (13).

However, MR imaging is a method of choice for multiplanar visualization of tumors and delineation of tumor from the normal anatomy structures, being of utmost importance for delicate surgery planning (Figg. 108-110).

Surgical treatment should be perfectly timed considering that the vision is usually preserved for quite a long time and possible tumor spread towards chiasm and contralaterally. In chiasmal glioma removal of the cyst and tumor reduction is considered the best possible treatment (12).

Treatment of the low grade cerebral astrocytoma is still controversial in neurosurgery regarding the feasibility, timing and the extent of the resection, especially for tumors located in the vicinity of the vital functional zones. The hazards of the slowly growing tumor should be carefully compared to a postoperative morbidity risk.

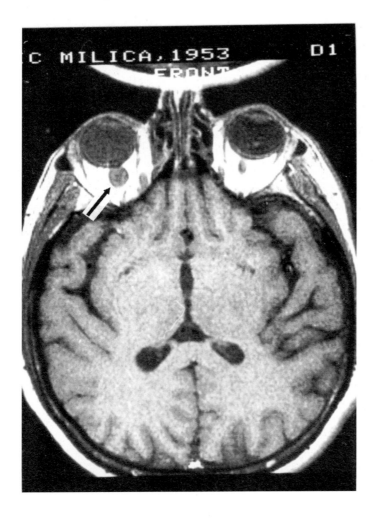

Figure 108. Axial image (SE 500/15). Glioma of the optic nerve in the right orbit - arrow.

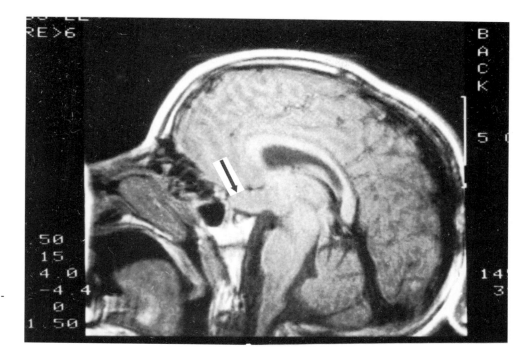

Figure 109. Sagittal image (SE 500/15). Glioma of the optic chiasm in patient M.M. - arrow.

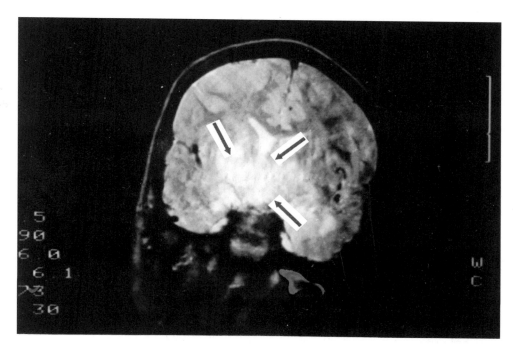

Figure 110. Coronal image (SE 2500/90). Glioma of the optic chiasm in the same patient (M.M.). Glioma is surrounded by ample perifocal suprasellar and bilateral temporal edema - arrows.

Postoperative radiotherapy after partial resection of a tumor, even for grade I astrocytoma, is advocated by a majority of Authors, although there is histological evidence that in 2/3 recurrent tumors higher grade astrocytoma was found. It could be attributed to postoperative radiotherapy as well.

It has been generally accepted that radiotherapy can postpone the tumor recurrence considerably. According to Laws and col. in 1984, younger age at the time of surgery is a significant factor of favorable prognosis (16).

There are still a lot of controversies concerning radiotherapy effectiveness for tumors with delicate localization, because of diversifying clinical course and relatively passive tumors.

b) Oligodendroglial tumors

Mixed tumors, oligodendroglioma and anaplastic tumors belong to a group of oligodendroglial tumors.

b-1 Oligodendroglioma

Tumors originating from the myelin sheath cells in the white matter of the brain are usually supratentorially located. Younger males, aged 35 to 55, are most frequently affected. Biologically similar to astrocytoma, they have some specific features, such as frontal localization, major compression effect despite slight surrounding edema, etc. Intraventricular location is rarely seen, when the tumor of subependymal origin tend to spread into the ventricular system.

Tumor tissue, usually well delineated from surrounding tissue, is of pinkish-grey color, uneven consistency, with mucoid zones, necrosis, cystic degeneration, hemorrhage and typical calcification. Oligodendroglioma is histologically recognized by small round or polygonal cells with big nuclei. Pathologic blood vessels has thin walls with endothelial swelling and proliferation seen under the microscope. Perivascular calcification is a typical feature of oligodendroglioma. Irregular calcifications are usually seen in peripheral zones of the tumor.

Oligodendroglioma are graded regarding malignancy as well as astrocytoma, but patients with grade III and IV oligodendroglioma survive longer than patients with respective grade astrocytoma.

Epileptic seizures and stagnant papilla seen in more than 50% of patients represent the characteristic features of oligodendroglioma, while hemiparesis is found in about one third of patients, especially with frontoparietal tumors.

Neuroradiology is quite successful in preoperative diagnosis of oligodendroglioma.

Pathologic calcification can be confirmed by plane skull radiography.

CT scan without iodine contrast injection shows oligodendroglioma as an irregular area of lower and mixed density, with characteristic hyperdense zones of calcium deposits. Contrast application enhance tumor density only in grade III oligodendroglioma and makes no substantial difference for other forms. Tumor density can be quite uneven. Low density perifocal edema is occasionally seen.

MR image in T-2W shows tumor with high signal intensity and intratumoral calcifications with maximally high signal intensity. Tumor is well defined, but not clearly delineated from perifocal edema (4).

Administration of paramagnetic contrast enhance signal intensity in grade III oligodendroglioma and not in other tumor forms. Islands of uneven signal intensities can be seen inside the expansive lesions (Figg. 111, 112).

It is important to differentiate oligodendroglioma from calcified meningioma and angioma, ependymoma, tuberculoma, tuberous sclerosis, etc. (18, 29). If there is no calcification inside oligodendroglioma, MR image could resemble astrocytoma or gangliocytoma (30).

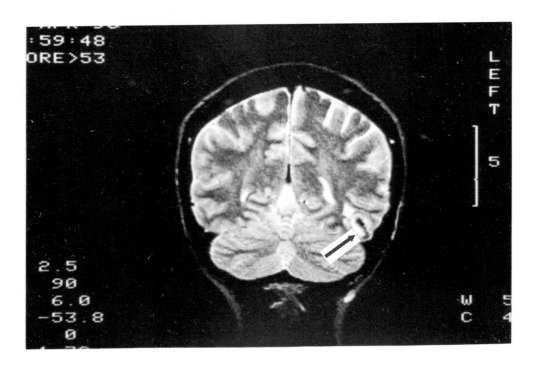

Figure 111. Coronal image (SE 2500/90). Calcified oligodendroglioma of high signal intensity, surrounded by discrete edema, is seen in left temporobasal region - arrow.

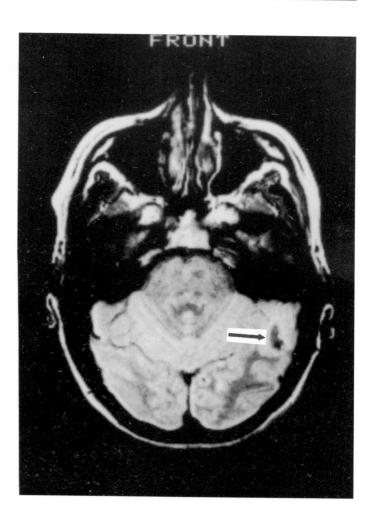

Figure 112. Axial image (SE 2500/15). It is practically impossible to delineate left temporobasal calcified oligo-dendroglioma from edema. Arrow pointing at central cal-cification inside the tumor.

Of all neuroepithelial tumors, oligodendroglioma is the most suitable for the radical surgical excision. Postoperative radiotherapy should be administered in higher grade tumors, regarding the radicality of the excision. Radical excision, frontal localization, calcification and cysts inside the tumor, along with middle aged patient, according to the clinical experience, provide for the favorable prognosis.

c) Poorly differentiated and embryonic tumors

Glioblastoma and medulloblastoma are the most frequent among poorly differentiated and embryonic tumors. According to the latest modification of WHO, classification glioblastoma are included in astrocytoma group and medulloblastoma in embryonic tumors, subclass PNET (primitive neuroectodermal tumors of multipotent differentiation).

c-1 Glioblastoma

According to the WHO classification glioblastoma correlates to grade IV astrocytoma. In patients operated for glioma in the Institute of neurosurgery in Belgrade more than 50% were anaplastic astrocytoma. Grade IV tumors were found in 15% of cases (astrocytoma, glioblastoma, multiform glioblastoma), while grade III astrocytoma were the most frequent in this group. According to the literature data male patients in their fifties are usually affected.

Glioblastoma is usually located in the frontal or temporal lobe of the brain. Histopathology of glioblastoma is characteristic for hemorrhage, a-v shunts, cysts, necrosis, being a sign of higher grade of malignancy.

Glioblastoma has infiltrative growth with rapid onset of neurologic deficit and general signs of increased intracranial pressure.

In CT scan without contrast administration glioblastoma is either isodense or hypodense with occasional hyperdense zones of hemorrhage. Compression effect and surrounding edema are noticed.

After contrast injection tumor becomes clearly delineated or blurred hyperdense formation with central hypodense zones of cysts and necrosis. Extendeed hypodense zone of perifocal edema is present as well (34).

MR image in T-2W sequence shows glioblastoma with mixed signal intensities, while central area of cysts and necrosis has high signal intensity. Irregular, narrow sheath of higher signal intensity and perifocal edema with high signal intensity are seen. In T-1W sequence, glioblastoma shows faint signal intensities with lower signal intensities of necrosis and cysts. Intratumoral hemorrhage are seen as islets of high signal intensities (10, 20).

Application of paramagnetic contrast enhances signal intensities in certain parts of tumor, while central zone of necrosis and cysts remains of low signal intensity (Figg. 113, 114).

Treatment of those malignancies is surgery followed by radiotherapy and occasional chemotherapy. Best results are achieved in tumor located in silent areas of the brain when complete resection of the neoplasm is possible, so that the best survival rates were recorded for frontal and temporal localization in non-dominant cerebral hemisphere. However, no matter haw radical the surgery has been, local recurrence will show soon because of the infiltrative nature of the tumor.

In grade III astrocytoma 24 month survival rate is 16%, while in grade V 15 month survival rate is 8%.

Local radiotherapy and chemotherapy improves the survival span, especially if cytostatic drug is administered intraarterially, increasing the concentration and efficacy of drug in the tumor and diminishing general toxic effects.

Development of new drugs and new techniques of its application in chemotherapy could improve the therapeutic results more than advances in surgical technique, but genetic engineering of the growth and aggression factors in tumor will probably be the future technique to solve the problem.

c-2 PNET - Medulloblastoma
[see chapter: Posterior fossa tumors (9)]

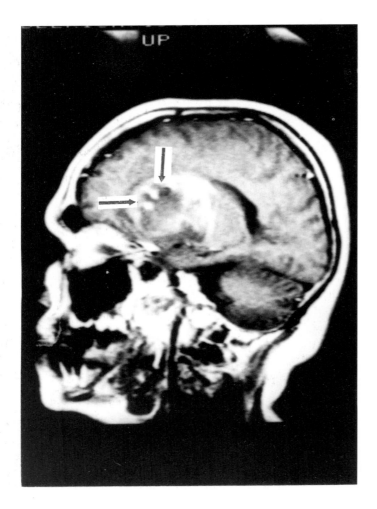

Figure 113. Sagittal image (SE 200/15). Patient V. J. with right frontotemporal glioblastoma of mixed signal intensity with islets of hemorrhage and cysts - arrows.

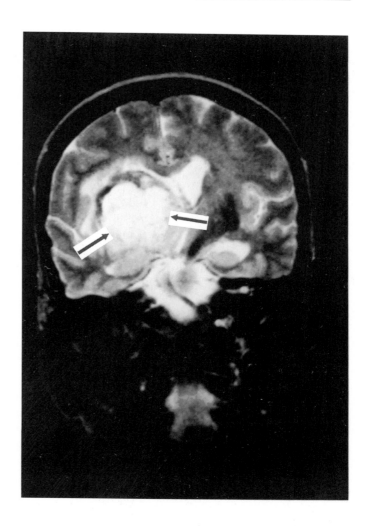

Figure 114. Coronal image (SE 2500/90). Same patient (V.J.) with right frontotemporal glioblastoma of high signal intensities, with third and both lateral ventricles compression and dislocation to the left - arrows.

d) Ependymal tumors

Ependymal tumors are: ependymoma, anaplastic ependymoma, mixopapillar and subependymoma.

d-1 Ependymoma

Ependymomas make 6.2% of all cerebral tumors in the series from Institute of neurosurgery in Belgrade. According to the literature data supratentorial ependymoma are more frequent.

These gliomas of ependymal origin have variable prognosis depending on histopathology, localization, age of patient, adjuvant radiotherapy, etc.

Ependymomas are found in children and adolescents. They make 10% of all brain tumors in children under 16. In our series of patients both genders were equally affected, with 2/3 of the patients aged between 21 and 50.

Most Authors have found that supratentorial ependymomas affect elder patients than infratentorial ones. In Belgrade series ratio between paraventricular and intraventricular ependymomas is 3:2, with supratentorial localization in 55% of cases.

Pathohistologically, ependymoma is red in color, nodular or lobular, clearly delineated from surrounding tissue with occasional cysts filled with xanthochromatous contents. Ependymomas could be classified regarding their form, cellular arrangement or type of stroma, and graded like astrocytoma in four malignancy grades (I-IV).

Arising from ependymal and lower glial layer surrounding brain ventricles, usually from posterior parts of the lateral ventricles, ependymoma follows ventricular morphology. They can be found in third and fourth ventricle as well, exceptionally in pontocerebellar angle. Tumor spread by cerebrospinal liquor is possible.

Clinical features depend on localization, with preoperative duration of symptoms being relevant to prognosis. Increased intracranial pressure causes main symptoms, and epileptic seizures (grand mal) are occasionally seen.

CT scan show hyperdense area of tumor with calcium encrustation of maximal density. Some of cerebral ependymoma are seen as hypodense lesions because of cysts. Administration of intravenous contrast enhances the tumor density, while calcification remain extremely hyperdense and cysts hypodense.

MR tomographs in T-1W sequence shows ependymoma as low intensity signal lesion and in T-2W high intensity one. Calcifications have low signal intensity in both sequences. Cysts have high signal intensity in T-2W and low in T-1W sequence (30, 36).

MR image after paramagnetic contrast application in T-1W sequence enhances the signal of ependymoma solid tissue, while cysts and calcification remain unchanged (Fig. 115).

MR and CT scans of medulloblastoma and chorioidal plexus papilloma can resemble ependymoma.

Prognosis of ependymoma depends on localization and malignancy grade. There is substantial difference regarding prognosis between paraventricular, suitable for resection and intraventricular ependymomas, inserted in the vicinity of basal ganglia, which can not be completely removed.

Postoperative radiotherapy for malignant ependymoma can improve survival rates, but there are still controversies on radiotherapy doses to prevent liquor spread. Irradiation of the complete neuroaxis for posterior fossa malignant ependymoma and complete brain for the benign type is acceptable.

e) Chorioid plexus tumors

Chorioid plexus tumors are: papilloma and carcinoma.

e-1 Chorioid plexus papilloma

Tumors arising from chaired plexus epithelium, *plexus papilloma*, are rarely seen (1%), affecting younger patients (1.5-3.9% in children), most of them in the first two years of age (65%).

Plexus papilloma in children arise from the lateral ventricles, while in adult patients they are found exclusively in the fourth ventricle (79%) and cerebellopontine angle. Exceptionally they could be found

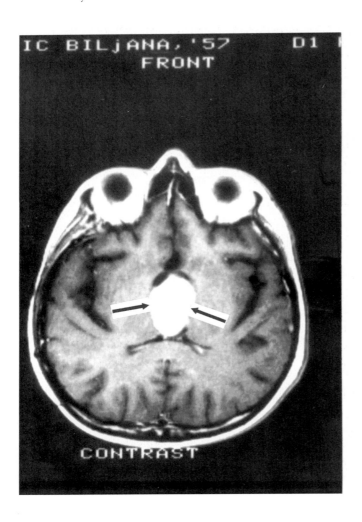

Figure 115. Axial image (SE 500/15) after gadolinium - DTPA administration. Ependymoma with mixed signal intensity in the third brain ventricle - arrows.

in the third ventricle. Cubical cells upon the rare fibrous stroma are seen, making this benign tumor hard to differ from normal chaired plexus tissue.

Malignant form of plexus papilloma is not infrequent (10-35% of all plexus tumors).

Clinical features are caused by increased intracranial pressure. Main symptoms are nausea, vomiting, restlessness, visual impairment, ataxia, meningismus (in children) or headache accompanied by cranial nerve disorders.

In children aged 2-4 craniomegaly caused by hydrocephalus is frequently found, followed by stagnant papilla, cranial nerve disorders and ataxia. Hydrocephalus in this case is caused by hyperproduction and obstruction to the liquor circulation.

CT scan shows chaired plexus papilloma as a smooth or lobulated, slightly hyperdense tumor with hyperdense calcifications (24-80%), without signs of local invasion. Intravenous administration of iodine contrast enhances the tumor density. If a calcified intraventricular tumor accompanied by hydrocephalus is found in childhood, it is most probably a plexus papilloma.

MR image in T-1W sequence shows *plexus papilloma* with low signal intensities, while in T-2W sequence it has higher signal intensities and clearly defined edge, with tortuous low intensity bands corresponding to the blood vessels. If a low intensity zone is not homogenous, but diffuse, calcification or hemorrhage should be considered, and CT scan is required to prove them (35). Administration of paramagnetic contrast enhances signal intensity of the tumor in MR (Figg. 116, 117).

Finest morphology details and relationships can be assessed by MR image, but calcifications and hemorrhage are better displayed in CT scan. It should be kept in mind that the patients are usually children under 2, in whom general anesthesia for CT and MR examination is necessary, so that each case should be treated individually. Useful information can be obtained through angiography because of the abundant vascularization of tumor.

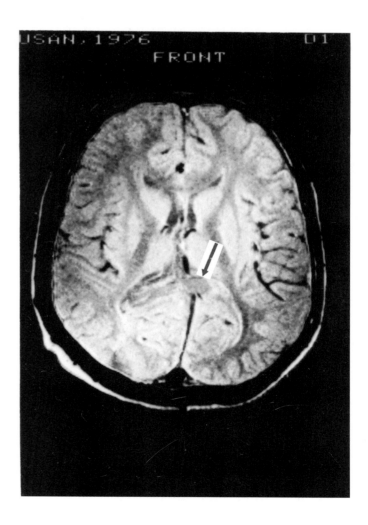

Figure 116. Axial image (SE 2500/15). Left parasagittal plexus papilloma of the left lateral ventricle, with mixed signal intensities - arrow.

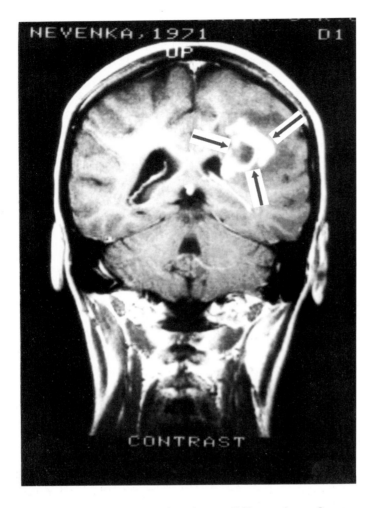

Figure 117. Coronal image (SE 500/15) after gadolinium-DTPA administration. Plexus papilloma in the left lateral ventricle trigonum - arrows.

Plexus papilloma is hard to differentiate from ventricular meningioma, ependymoma or solid angioblastoma.

Surgical treatment for those tumors begins with external drainage of the hydrocephalus. Radical excision of the papilloma is sufficient for the complete cure, whereas carcinoma has poor prognosis (3).

Most of the Authors suggest *"en bloc"*, resection of the tumor with complete control of the afferent blood vessels to prevent uncontrolled bleeding, but bigger tumors sometimes require staged surgery. Transcortical-transventricular or transcallous access is advised for supratentorial, whereas suboccipital access is the best for infratentorial tumors.

Radiotherapy is still controversial, while chemotherapy should be administered in chaired plexus carcinoma, especially in children under 3 years of age.

f) Pineal cell tumor

Pineal cell tumors are: pineocytoma, pineoblastoma and mixed tumors (pineocytoma/pineoblastoma), while germinomas in this area, which do not arise from pineal parenchyma, belong to the germinal cell tumors.

f-1 Pinealoma

Pinealoma (pinealocytoma, pineocytoma) is rare, representing only 0.5% of all tumors, usually found in younger patients. Its structure resembles that of a pineal gland. It is located in the area of quadrigeminal lamina and pineal gland. Its histological structure shows typical cellular extensions towards vascular stroma. Ectopic pinealoma can be found in the fourth ventricle or in the hypophyseal stalk (infundibulum).

Pinealoma is graded in three malignancy grades (I-III). They are well defined without local invasion signs.

Pineoblastoma is an extremely malignant tumor, similar to medulloblastoma in its biological nature, highly invasive, infiltrative and extremely radiosensitive. Invasion of the surrounding structure helps to determine the degree of malignancy, considering the fact that neuroradiologic imaging could not differentiate between benign and malignant formations.

Clinical features are mainly due to the increased intracranial pressure, with upward glance paresis, insufficient pupil accommodation, and occasional cerebellar signs. Pinealoma is displayed in CT scan as an isodense spherical formation with hyperdense calcifications. Tumor density is substantially enhanced by iodine contrast injection. MR image of pinealoma in T-1W sequence shows pinealoma with signal intensities similar to those of the pineal gland (Fig. 118). Pinealoma in T-2W sequence has high signal intensity with islets of the lower signal intensity corresponding to calcifications (36). Administration of paramagnetic contrast helps to define the tumor optimally by high signal intensities (Fig. 119). Pinealoma should be differentiated from ependymoma, pilocytic astrocytoma and suprasellar craniopharyngeoma in MR tomographs. It is particularly hard to differ pinealoma from hyperplasia of the pineal gland parenchyma.

Most of the Authors suggest to commence the therapy with liquor drainage and to determine the radiosensitivity of tumor by tumor markers in order to plan further therapy. Exploration surgery is advisable for radioresistant tumors, whereas for radiosensitive tumors, such as germinoma, excellent results could be achieved by radiotherapy. Feasibility for resection could be decided upon neuroradiology findings (26). For example, if the thalamus is infiltrated surgery is not recommended.

Surgery should be staged in two acts, first to cure hydrocephalus by liquor drainage, and second act of direct exploration. The most convenient access is suboccipital-transtentorial, transcallous, transcortical-transventricular, as well as infratentorial-supracerebellar.

For malignant types, especially for germinoma, radiotherapy is effective, whereas chemotherapy is useful in treatment of germinal tumors, recurrent or metastatic tumors. Radiotherapy should be administered in invasive or insufficiently resected pineocytoma.

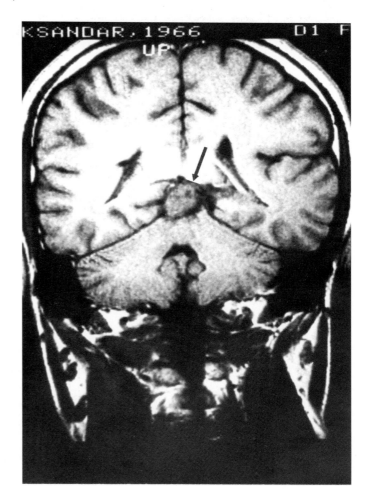

Figure 118. Coronal image (SE 500/15). Mediosagittally, in the projection of a pineal gland, pinealoma with mixed lower signal intensities is shown - arrow.

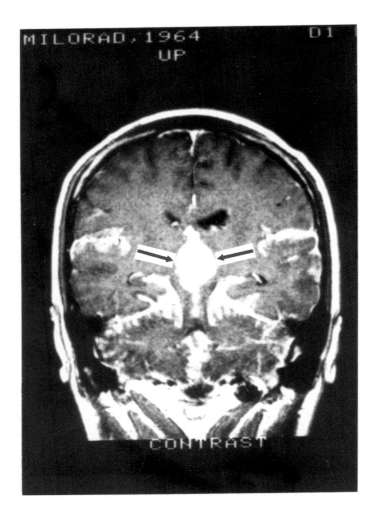

Figure 119. Coronal image (SE 500/15) after gadolinium-DTPA administration. Mediosagittally, in the projection of a pineal gland, pinealoma with high signal intensity is shown- arrows.

f-2 Other tumors of the pineal region

Other tumors arising from the pineal region could be divided upon cytogenetic principles in three groups: tumors of the pineal parenchyma origin, of the germinal cell origin, glioma and miscellaneous extraventricular tumors in the pineal area.

Germinal cell tumors are the most frequent tumors of this region making 70%, especially germinomas representing one half of the neoplasms in the pineal area (See: Germinal cell tumors).

Multiplanar MR image provides for the perfect display of germinoma. Gadolinium contrast is used to help delineate the tumor boundaries (Fig. 120).

Teratoma is infrequently seen, especially in male children, being well defined, sometimes cystic and radioresistant. (See: Germinal cell tumors).

Pineal glioma are usually astrocytomas of varying degrees of malignancy.

Neuronal tumors

Neuronal tumors, are: gangliocytoma, arising from neurons; and ganglioglioma, arising from both neurons and glia. There are different types according to the maturity of cells and ratio of neuronal and glial elements.

Neuronal tumors could be classified as gangliocytoma, dysplastic cerebellar gangliocytoma, desmoplastic infantile ganglioglioma, dysembryoplastic neuroepithelial tumors, ganglioglioma, anaplastic ganglioglioma, central neurocytoma, olfactory neuroblastoma. They are either solid, well defined, gray in color, with eventual calcifications, or cystic with a solid mural portion. There is typical lymphocyte infiltration around blood vessels.

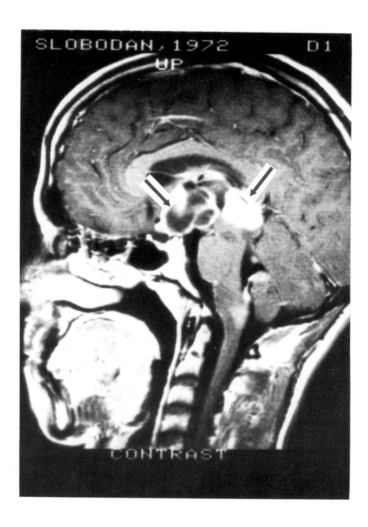

Figure 120. Sagittal image (SE 500/15) after gadolinium-DTPA administration. Arrows pointing at germinoma in pineal and suprasellar region. Suprasellar portion of a tumor is cystic with septa, while the pineal portion is solid.

Neuronal tumors are slowly growing, benign lesions, suitable for radical excision.

Ganglioma and gangliocytoma represent less than 1% of all neuroepithelial brain tumors in adults. Supratentorial localization is frequent, especially in brain hemispheres or third ventricle floor. They are usually seen in younger patients.

Gangliocytoma (ganglioneuroma) is a rare tumor, affecting both genders equally, usually in the third decade of life.

Central neurocytoma is a separate entity, with lateral ventricles being the site of predilection. Recurrences after surgery are extremely rare and the prognosis is generally favorable.

Clinical features depend on localization, but all of these tumors are slowly growing. The diagnosis of neurocytoma could not be made only upon CT scan finding, showing well defined mass inside the dilated ventricle, with occasional calcifications.

Features of the tissue signal intensities of neuronal tumors and neurinoma in MR tomographs are practically identical, in both T-1W and T-2W sequences. Paramagnetic contrast enhances the signal intensities of all neuronal tumors alike. MRI improves the definition of surrounding structure. Typical intraventricular localization, well defined boundaries and relationship with septum pellucid implies possible diagnosis of central neurocytoma (30).

Generally speaking, neuronal tumors grow slowly and are benign in nature, so that they can be radically resected. Although they are radiosensitive, they should never be treated by radiotherapy unless there is an anaplastic variety.

2. Tumors of nerve sheath origin

According to the latest WHO classification following tumors are included in this group: a) schwannoma (neurilemmoma, neurinoma), b) neurofibroma and c) MPNST (malignant peripheral nerve sheath tumor).

The most frequent among them are acoustic nerve neurinoma, making 6-8% of all primary intracranial tumors and 80% of cerebellopontine angle tumors, according to the literature data (they will be discussed later on in the text).

Neurinoma

a-1 Supratentorial neurinoma

Tumors of the nerve sheath origin can be found supratentorially in cranial nerve root area (optic nerve, oculomotor nerve, trochlear nerve, trigeminal nerve, abducent and, occasionally, facial nerve).

Clinical features depends on the certain nerve disorder and lesions of the surrounding structures. It is impossible to tell the origin of tumor sometimes, when the tumor encompasses the whole cavernous sinus compromising all the local cranial nerves. It makes the clinical appearance diversified. Usually, if the oculomotors are impaired, diplopia is the first symptom to be noticed.

CT scan, even with contrast application, is insufficient to make conclusions about tumor nature and localization. Neurinoma of the cavernous sinus in its early stage is hard to tell from normal variety of hyperplastic cavernous sinus.

CT provides insufficient information on tumor relationship to the major blood vessels in the parasellar region.

Multiplanar MR image in T-2W, and particularly in T-1W sequence with intravenous administration of paramagnetic contrast, clearly delineates the tumor by signal enhancement. MR angiography defines precisely major blood vessels of parasellar region and tumor (Fig. 121).

MR is a keystone for diagnosis of the cranial nerve tumors, especially in the parasellar, i.e. cavernous sinus area (32).

Treatment for those slowly growing tumors is surgery. Complete excision is usually impossible. Radiotherapy has no effect.

a-2 Infratentorial neurinoma (5)

Acoustic nerve neurinoma - vestibular schwannoma

(see chapter on posterior fossa tumors)

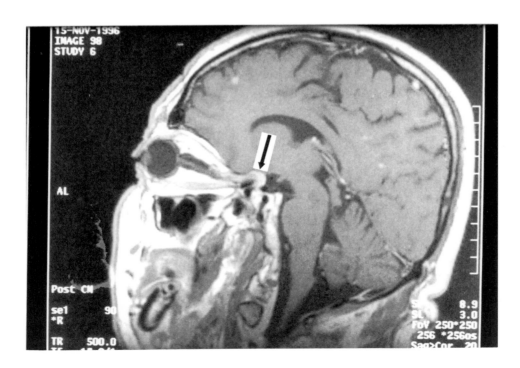

Figure 121. Sagittal image (SE 500/15) after gadolinium-DTPA administration. Arrow pointing at left optic nerve neurinoma (right in front of the optic nerve canal).

3. Meningeal tumors

Benign meningioma is the most frequent meningeal tumor, whereas meningosarcoma or melanocytic tumors are rarely found.

a) Meningioma

According to the WHO classification meningeal tumors are divided as follows:
a-1 Meningioma (including subtypes)
meningothelial
transitional
fibrous
psamomatous
angiomatous
microcystic
secretory
clear cell
chaired
reach in lympho-plasmocytes
metaplastic (xanthomatous, mixoid, osseous, cartilaginous)
a-2 Atypical meningioma
a-3 Anaplastic - malignant meningioma

a-1 Meningioma

Meningioma arises from the cell on top of the arachnoidal villi, in the vicinity of dural venous sinuses, dural foramina for cranial nerves, cribrous lamina and middle fossa scull base.

Meningothelial cells, found in chaired plexus, tela chorioidea, arachnoid extensions engulfing spinal nerve roots, are supposed to be responsible for the genesis of intraventricular, pineal and spinal meningiomas.

Meningioma are typical intracranial tumors of extracerebral origin, making 20% of all intracranial tumors. Patients in their fourth or fifth decade of life are usually affected; women predominate, whereas in children those tumors are exceptionally rare. Latest genetic studies have shown monosomy of 22 chromosome or deletion of the long limb of one of those chromosomes in 70% of patients affected by meningioma. Increased incidence is found in patients with type 2 neurofibromatosis; familial susceptibility is frequent.

Topographical by meningioma can be:
supratentorial - in the convexity (parasagittal, in the falx, or strictly in the convexity), basal (of the anterior base - olfactory, parasellar, sphenoid, of the middle cranial base) and
posterior fossa (convexity, tentorial, posterior pyramidal, clival, of foramen magnum).

Otherwise, they could be topographically classified as convexity, parasagittal, falx, intraventricular, basal (olfactory, suprasellar, sphenoidal, temporal fossa, pyramidal, clival, posterior fossa), tentorial (anterior, posterior, falcotentorial) (2).

Meningioma of the convexity: parasagittal meningioma arise from Pacchioni's granulation inserted along sagittal sinus, have long and slow evolution, with postponed onset of increased intracranial pressure and long-standing epilepsy or psychological alteration or contralateral hemiparesis, depending on tumor location. Incidence of the meningioma of the falx is five times smaller than of parasagittal ones. They are situated in the midline, between the hemispheres. Meningiomas of the convexity could be inserted practically anywhere on the dura out of the midline or sagittal sinus.

Basal meningioma of the anterior cranial fossa inserted on the cribrous bone dura (olfactory) can grow enormously without causing any neurologic deficit, save for the anosmia and psychological alteration. Parasellar meningioma, inserted either on planum, jugulum, tuberculum or dura of the sellar diaphragm, causing major vision impairment due to the compression of optic nerve and chiasm, could be difficult to differentiate from optic neuritis. They are small, solid, well vascularized, and often asymmetric.

Meningioma inserted on the small wings of the sphenoid bone has the highest incidence among extracerebral tumors of the scull base. Sphenoid meningioma could be either of pteryon, alar or clinoid type. In the middle cranial fossa meningioma is most often inserted on a pyramid.

Within posterior fossa it could be inserted either on convexity, tentorium cerebelli, nearby internal acoustic meatus, superior petrous sinus or clivus.

Clinical features of meningioma, including headache, hemiparesis, epileptic fits, pshological alteration, visual impairment, etc., depend on the tumor location. Headache and hemiparesis are found in one third of the patients with meningioma of different location.

There are a few locations with typical presentation, such as olfactory meningioma (anosmia, Foster-Kennedy-s syndrome), tuberculum meningioma (chiasmal syndrome), cavernous sinus meningioma (ptosis, diplopia, bulbomotor impairment) or foramen magnum meningioma (nuchal or suboccipital pain, progressive neurologic deficit).

Meningioma in children is extremely rare presented by the signs of intracranial hypertension and no focal signs whatsoever.

Hyperostosis, enhanced impressions digitate or occasional calcifications could be seen in native radiographs. Most of the hyperostoses are caused by meningioma (38-61%). Bone alterations are relevant if found in the sphenoid bone, clinoid or tuberculum. Calcifications are found in 3-18% of those tumors.

CT scan is reliable in establishing the diagnosis of meningioma. Intravenous administration of iodine contrast displays the hyperdense tumor optimally, defining tumor boundaries from surrounding edema. Some meningiomas (15%) shows typical appearance in CT with alternating hypo- and hyperdense zones and uneven binding of the iodine contrast.

Conventional or digital subtraction angiography was mandatory in the past. MR angiography have diminished the significance of those methods for the diagnosis, but they are still used occasionally to display abundant tumor vascularization or enable preoperative embolization (35).

MR is suitable for multiplanar display and delineation of meningioma from normal structures in hard to access locations, such as infratentorial area, cranial base, cavernous sinus and falx cerebri (tumor relationship to venous sinuses), etc.

Meningioma is isodense, compared to the gray matter, in 60-90% and slightly hypodense in 10-30%, as seen in MR image in T-1W sequence, whereas in T-2W sequence tumor shows slightly elevated signal intensity and perifocal edema higher signal intensity (Fig. 122). After the paramagnetic contrast has been administered, MR image in T-1W sequence shows meningioma with high signal intensity, clearly defined from perifocal edema (20). Inside bigger meningiomas occasional zones of lower signal intensities (necrosis) or mixed signal intensities (hemorrhage) could be seen (Figg. 123, 124).

In the recent time histologic type of meningioma could be assumed on the basis of MRI findings (in T-2W sequence). Meningothelial and angioblastic meningioma have higher signal intensities in T-2W sequence, due to hypervascularity, than fibroblastic or transitional ones. Perifocal edema is more pronounced in meningothelial or angioblastic variety.

MR tomographs of meningioma could resemble those of neurinoma, metastasis, malignant lymphoma, anaplastic astrocytoma, internal carotid artery aneurysm, chondroma, *glomus jugulare* tumors, etc. (37).

Radical surgical excision with extraarachnoidal cleavage is a method of choice for meningioma treatment. In spite of the careful microsurgical excision, early recurrence could occur due to the unpredictable nature of those tumors.

If the local aggression signs are seen during the surgery the above mentioned possibility could be assumed. Radiotherapy should be administered either for incompletely resected tumors, for benign tumors of the cavernous sinus region or particularly for the control of atypical or malignant varieties.

MR is inexpendable for the detection of residual or recurrent tumors.

a-2 Atypical meningioma
Histology of atypical meningioma shows signs of local aggression and tendency towards recurrent growth (irregular architectonics, hypercellularity, increased mitosis index, necrosis, pronounced nucleoli, nuclear polymorphism, hypervascularity and hemosiderin deposits)(22) (Fig. 125).

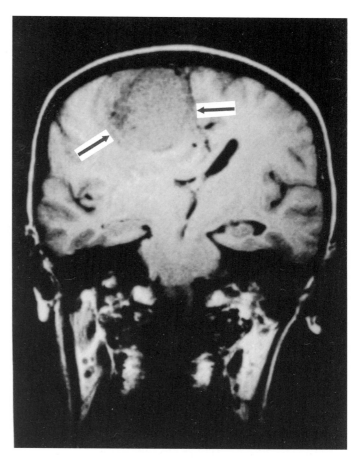

Figure 122. Coronal image (SE 500/15). Right frontoparietal meningioma with moderately high signal intensity - white arrows. Perifocal edema has low signal intensity - black arrows. Falx cerebri is shifted to the left.

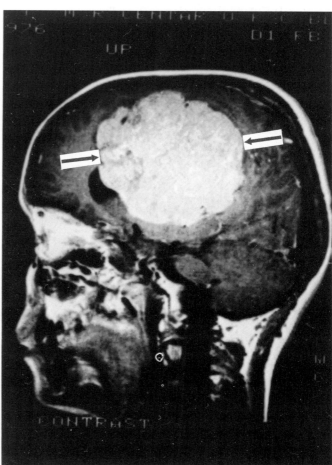

Figure 123. Sagittal image (SE 500/15) after gadolinium-DTPA administration. Arrows pointing at a huge falx meningioma.

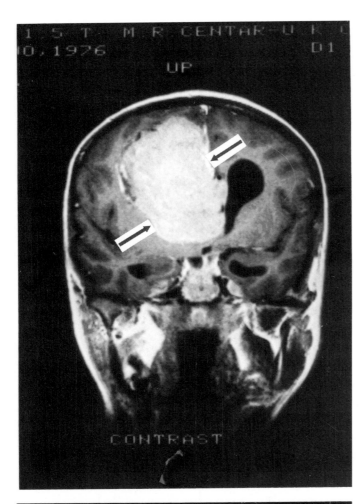

Figure 124. Coronal image (SE 500/15) after gadolinium-DTPA administration. Arrows pointing at a huge falx meningioma.

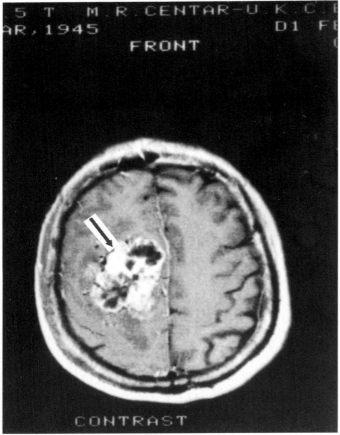

Figure 125. Axial image (SE 500/15) after gadolinium-DTPA administration. Arrow pointing at a huge, well defined meningioma, of mixed and high signal intensities, located high in right parietal region.

Adjuvant radiotherapy should follow surgery for the atypical variety.

a-3 Malignant meningioma

Diagnosis of a rare variety of malignant meningioma needs histologic confirmation or existence of the distant metastasis.

Papillary malignant meningioma, usually seen in children or young adults, is unpredictable, aggressive, with exceptional distant metastases and big, vesicular, partly atypical, hyperchromatous cellular nuclei. Pathologic mitoses are hard to differentiate.

Prognosis in malignant meningioma is based upon histology and intraoperatively found signs of local aggression towards brain, dura, venous sinuses and bone. Bromodeoxyuridine index exceeding 1 is considered a sign of atypical meningioma and tendency to recur. According to our studies, the average PCNU/cyclin index being 0.25 makes it not so significant for the recurrence prediction as much as the synergetic action of N-myc and pan-ras oncogenes (22).

Malignant meningioma, found in 10% of cases (22), has blurred edges and fungiform peripheral growth.

Calcifications, necrosis and compression effects of malignant meningioma are superbly displayed in CT scan. Iodine contrast administration enhances the tumor density.

MR image in T-1W sequence after Magnevist administration shows maximally enhanced signal intensity of the tumor. Excellent delineation between tumor and edema is obtained (37). Lower signal intensity zones inside the tumor are caused by calcium deposits, necrosis, hemorrhage, etc. (Fig. 126).

Malignant meningioma with high signal intensities is shown in the left temporo-occipital region. Demarcation between tumor and edema is good (Fig. 126). Treatment for meningioma is surgery, with access and extent of the resection being adjusted to the tumor location.

Simpson in 1957 stated that the recurrence risk depends on the degree of surgical radicality (28).

I degree of radicality means complete excision of the tumor, dura and involved bone (recurrence risk - 9%).

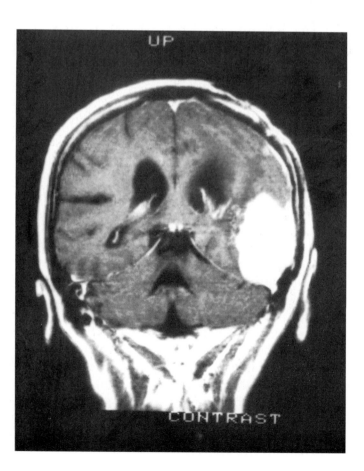

Figure 126. Coronal image (SE 500/15) after gadolinium-DTPA administration. Malignant meningioma with high signal intensities-left temporooccipital region.

II degree of radicality means complete excision of the tumor and coagulation of dural insertion (recurrence risk - 19%).

III degree of radicality means complete excision without dural coagulation, because of the sinus or bone involvement (recurrence risk - 29%).

IV degree of radicality means reduction of a tumor mass (recurrence risk - 44%).

V degree means only biopsy or decompression.

This classification is clinically significant even nowadays.

Postoperative radiotherapy should be applied for anaplastic and atypical forms.

4. Tumors of vascular origin

Tumors of vascular origin represent 1-2% of all central nervous system tumors. They could be located practically anywhere, but most often they are situated in the posterior cranial fossa. According to the present WHO classification they are included in the group of meningeal tumors subclass of non-meningothelial origin, while in children they represent a separate category of vascular origin.

Typical tumors of vascular origin are: a) hemangioblastoma and b) hemangiopericytoma.

a) Hemangioblastoma

Hemangioblastoma has a lot of blood vessels, particularly thin walled capillaries with swollen endothelium. There are polymorph, big, ovoid cells in between blood vessels. Hemangioblastoma is benign tumor of vascular origin, usually arising in cerebellum, making 2.5% of all intracranial tumors (38).

When they are a feature of von Hippel-Lindau-s disease, developing between 15 and 20 years of age, accompanied by retinal angioma, kidney carcinoma, pancreatic cysts, pheochromocytoma and polycytaemia, the prognosis is really bad. Retinal angioma is seen in 10-40% of patients affected by von Hippel-Lindau disease. They are usually small and asymptomatic, but they could b multiple and bilateral as well (35).

Headache, internal hydrocephalus and ataxia are the clinical features of hemangioblastoma.

CT scan with iodine contrast administration shows hyperdense tumors of vascular origin. Hemangioblastoma is shown either as hypodense cyst with hyperdense mural knot or as a solid vascular mass. Sometimes is hard to display a solid mass by contrast CT examination, so that angiography or MR is needed to prove it.

MR tomographs with paramagnetic contrast administration in T-1W sequence displays high signal intensity of hemangioblastoma or hemangiopericytoma. In T-1W sequence hemangioblastoma has slightly lower signal in intensities and tumor could be suspected only upon the disturbed morphology of the cerebral parenchyma. In T-2W sequence the tumor has slightly elevated signal intensity (11). Surgery is a treatment of choice for hemangioblastoma and prognosis is good unless other malignancies are present.

b) Hemangiopericytoma

Hemangiopericytoma is malignant tumor of vascular origin, usually affecting adult males, typically situated on meninges (1-7% of meningeal tumors, classified as angioblastic meningioma), extremely aggressive and recurrence prone. They could be found in the spinal canal occasionally.

Both dural or soft tissue hemangiopericytoma shows similar features of high cellularity and typical radial proliferation of endothelial cells. This tumor is hard to differentiate from angioblastic meningioma upon histologic features, but recent cytogenetic studies have shown substantial difference.

Clinical features can be variable depending on the localization.

CT scan of hemangiopericytoma shows a hyperdense, well vascularized expansive lesion.

MRI defines the tumor as low signal intensity zone in T-1W sequence and as slightly elevated signal intensity zone in T-2W sequence (30). Angiography is very useful for the diagnosis of those lesions (Fig. 127).

Considering the high recurrence risk, one stage radical surgical excision is a method of choice. According to the literature data it could be achieved in 50-70% of patients. Postoperative radiotherapy

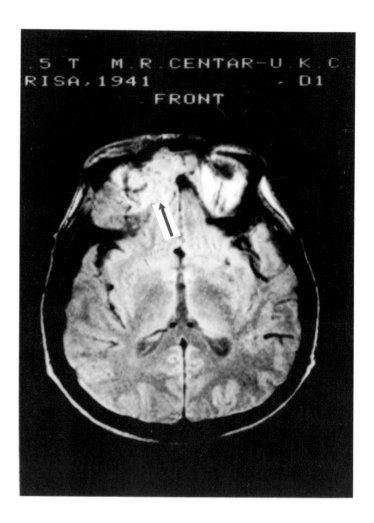

Figure 127. Axial image (SE 2500/15). Bilateral fronto-basal hemangiopericytoma with mixed higher signal intensity. Tumor is poorly delineated from perifocal edema-arrow.

is administered. Preoperative radiotherapy, advocated in the past, is nowadays abandoned because of the problems when dissecting tumor from the healthy tissue. Preoperative embolization is necessary in cases with abundant vascularization (30).

5. Germinal cell tumors

According to the WHO classification germinal cell tumors are: germinoma, embryonic carcinoma, endodermal sinus tumors, choriocarcinoma, teratoma (mature, immature and malignant) and mixed germinal cell tumors.

As stated in the literature, they make 0.4-3.4% of all intracranial tumors. Germinoma is the most frequent, being 40-65% of all germinal cell tumors, followed by teratoma (18-20%), endodermal sinus tumor (4-6%), embryonic cell tumor (3-5%), and choriocarcinoma (3-5%). They develop in the first two decades of life, with different symptomatology depending on the region involved (6).

Preoperative detection of tumor markers is extremely important if germinal cell tumor is suspected (alpha feto protein, beta HCG). Positive results of marker tests induces the choice of radiotherapy for those tumors that are highly radiosensitive (see chapter on pineal tumors).

a) Germinoma

Germinoma is malignant, extremely radiosensitive tumor, arising extracranially anywhere along the midline or intracranially in the pineal and/or sellar region. The tumor usually destroys the pineal gland, involving third ventricle wall and mesencephalon. Liquor dissemination and even extracranial metastases are occasionally seen.

Histology of the tumor is identical to the testicular seminoma or ovarial dysgerminoma, consisting of the two types of cells: big, primitive germinal cells (oblong, polynuclear, gigantic) and lymphocytes. Fibrous-vascular stroma contains specific tiny cells. Calcifications are often seen inside germinoma.

Suprasellar germinoma can cause insipid diabetes, visual field deficits, as well as other hypothalamo - hypophyseal disorders, including hypopituitarism, praecox puberty, growth and sexual maturation delay, seldom behavior disorders, obesity or anorexia. Pineal germinoma causes intracranial hypertension due to hydrocephalus and bulbomotor disorders.

Neuroradiology imaging in germinoma is diversified, making preoperative differential diagnosis very complicated.

Calcifications inside germinoma are best displayed by CT scan. Administration of the iodine contrast tumor is clearly seen in CT scan because of the enhanced density.

MRI in T-1W sequence shows germinoma as a low and lower signal intensity lesion (35). In T-2W sequence germinoma has higher signal intensities. Germinoma is best displayed in T-1W after paramagnetic contrast administration, showing high signal intensities save for intratumoral calcifications retaining extremely low signal intensities (Fig. 128).

Germinoma with high signal intensities, shown mediosagittally, suprasellary in the III ventricle projection - arrow.

Surgery consist merely of biopsy or tumor reduction, to confirm diagnosis (31).

Radiosensitivity is the main feature of this tumor (1). Preoperative determination of tumor markers is essential for the choice between surgery and radiotherapy. Alpha-feto-protein, beta choriogonadotropin (sub-unit beta), as well as placental alkalic phosphatase are well known.

Germinoma is extremely radiosensitive and it could be cured by radiotherapy alone, save for the recurrent or multiple tumors when adjuvant chemotherapy is necessary.

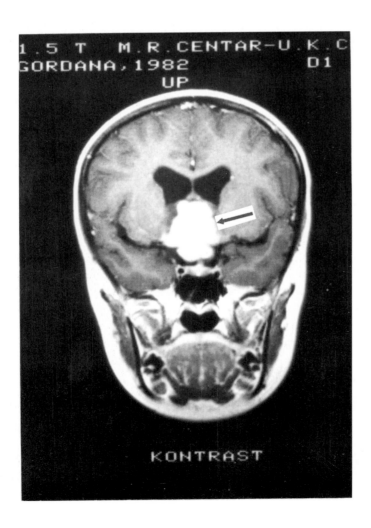

Figure 128. Coronal image (500/15) after gadolinium-DTPA administration. Germinoma-arrow.

b) Teratoma

Teratoma is a rare tumor of the younger population between 20-40 years of age, located in the pineal region, III or lateral ventricles. They could be either ectodermal, mesodermal or endodermal, usually a combination of two or all three germinal layers, resulting in the diversity of the tumor. Beside squamous cell epithelial islets, teratoma contains epidermoid and dermoid cysts, glandular elements resembling bronchial or intestinal epithelium, etc. Smooth muscle, cartilage and bone elements can be found as well. Neural tissue elements or parts of other organs are also seen. Teratoma can contain embryonic tissues and organs, such as denticles, medullar epithelium, etc.

Clinical symptoms are similar to those of germinoma.

Heterogeneous histology of teratoma is responsible for its neuroradiologic diversity. CT scan of germinoma shows multiple, variable, irregular pathologic area with uneven iodine contrast binding. CT scan reveals areas of the density of fat, soft tissues, calcification or liquid. Malignant teratoma tend to invade surrounding tissue.

Teratoma is well defined in CT scan, unlike the other tumors of the pineal region. Hypodense zones are due to the fat. Tissue imbibition after intravenous administration of iodine contrast is quite irregular.

MR in T-1W sequence shows teratoma with higher signal intensities with low signal intensity zones of calcification (30, 35). Variable signal intensities are due to the compound teratoma structure. In MR tomographs teratoma could resemble lipoma (Fig. 129).

Surgery is particularly useful in the treatment for benign teratoma, whereas adjuvant therapy for the malignant teratoma is required.

6. Malformation and miscellaneous tumors

Craniopharyngioma, colloid cyst, lipoma, epidermoid and dermoid cysts belong to a group of malformation and miscellaneous tumors.

a) Craniopharyngioma

Craniopharyngioma is usually of suprasellar location, affecting all ages, with a peak incidence between 5 and 14 years of age. Craniopharyngioma makes 2.5-4% of all intracranial tumors; incidence in children being 6-7% and 1% in adults (32).

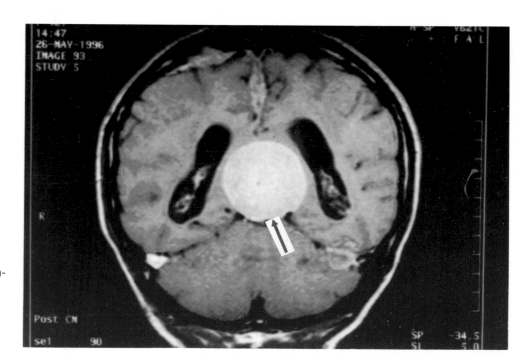

Figure 129. Coronal image (SE 570/15) after gadolinium-DTPA administration. Arrow pointing at a huge teratoma in the pineal region.

Intrasellar and parasellar extension are frequently seen.

Considering the fact that craniopharyngioma origin are the embryonic remnants of the Rathkes pouch, it could be found anywhere along the embryonic path of those cells incorporated later on in adenohypophysis and inferior portion of the stalk.

Konovalov (36) had divided those tumors in three basic types: extraventricular, intra-extraventricular and intraventricular or ectopic, completely situated in the III ventricle (infrequent).

Craniopharyngioma is built of squamous epithelial cells, with peripheral layer of cylindrical cells in the fibrous stroma. Cystic degeneration of cells leads to cavity formation, whereas keratinized epithelial cells acquire calcium deposits. Calcium deposits are found in stroma as well. Calcification and cystic degeneration are typical features of craniopharyngioma (more than 75%). Hemorrhage with hemosiderin deposits and necrotic zones are seen in bigger tumors. Cholesterol deposits, xanthochromatous cells and lymphocytes can be found as well. Banna M. (5) recognizes two histological subtypes with substantially different prognosis: adamantinous and papillary (seen exclusively in adults, has favorable prognosis).

Symptoms can be divided in three groups: chiasmal visual impairment, endocrine disorders (hypogonadism in adults or growth and maturational delay in children) as well as neurologic deficit. Hydrocephalus is due to compression at the III ventricle level.

Plane x-rays show disorders in 55-68% of patients (adults-children) (18).

Craniopharyngioma is seen in CT scan as a solid isodense zone with hyperdense calcification or hypodense cysts occasionally found inside the tumor. Solid part of the tumor gains density after i.v. administration of the iodine contrast which makes tumor easily visible among normal anatomy structures (7). Calcifications are found in 60-96% of patients (adults-children) and cystic degeneration of tumor in 87-99% (adults - children). Gigantic tumors, exceeding 6 cm in diameter, being the real surgical problem, are 6 times as frequent in children than in adults. One third of children, surgically treated for craniopharyngioma in the Institute of neurosurgery in Belgrade, have had a tumor exceeding 6 cm.

MR tomographs in T-1W sequence shows solid portion of a tumor in middle and low signal intensities, with fat collection in high signal intensities and extremely low signal intensities of the calcifications (Figg. 130, 131). In T-2W sequence the signal intensities of the fat and calcium remains unchanged. Solid portion of the tumor has mixed lower signal intensities. After paramagnetic contrast administration solid tumor shows high signal intensities. Calcifications, cysts and necrosis have low signal intensities (Fig. 132).

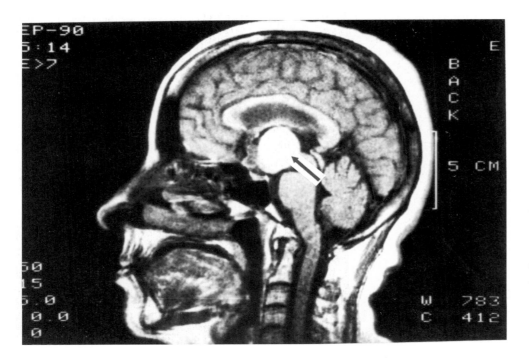

Figure 130. Sagittal image (SE 500/15). Cystic, well defined craniopharyngioma in suprasellar region - arrow. Cyst containing cholesterol has high signal intensity. In front of the cyst, above the clinoidal process, a small solid portion of a tumor with lower signal intensity is shown.

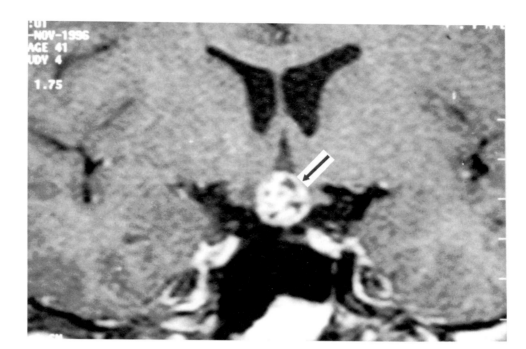

Figure 131. Coronal image (SE 500/15). Well defined craniopharyngioma of suprasellar region - arrow.

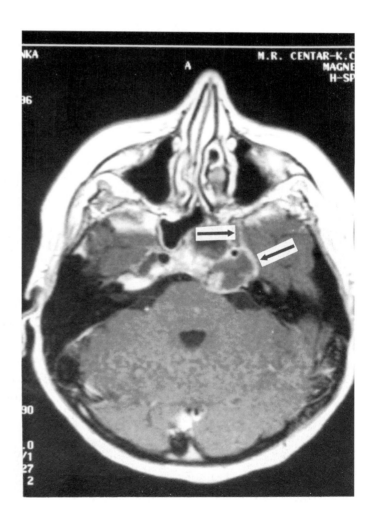

Figure 132. Axial image (500/15) after gadolinium-DTPA administration. Arrows pointing at a huge residual/recurrent cystic craniopharyngioma of a sellar region.

MR is of utmost importance for a precise location of craniopharyngioma and definition of its relationship to normal intrasellar, parasellar and suprasellar structures (Fig. 95), although calcifications are poorly displayed. MR is important for the diagnosis of huge, intraventricular, atypical or recurrent tumors.

Differential diagnosis of craniopharyngioma is made in cases of hypophyseal adenoma, meningioma or internal carotid artery aneurysms.

In spite of its benign character, craniopharyngioma has unpredictable behavior and marked tendency towards recurrence, so that radical one stage surgical excision is a method of choice in the therapy (Fig. 132). Radiotherapy is needed for the rest of the patients in order to postpone, if not prevent the recurrence, for the majority of the cases.

The most suitable surgical access is subfrontal or pteryonal, translaminar terminalis or transcallous, as well as combined pteryonal-transcallous or bifrontal for intraventricular tumors. Suboccipital approach is suitable for the rare posterior fossa tumors. Transsphenoidal approach is used for a rare intrasellar craniopharyngioma. Choice of the access depends on the tumor size and location, as well as on the experience of the surgeon. Extensive basal calcifications or tumor adherent to the chiasm, hypothalamus or major blood vessels pose a problem to an attempted radical excision (34).

Some Authors advocate postoperative radiotherapy after a radical excision as well, because of the theory of multicentric tumor origin as a reason for recurrent disease. Pathologists have found peripheral finger-like extensions as a sign of tumor aggression, although there is still a layer of gliosis enabling successful resection.

Adequately treated patients with craniopharyngioma can survive quite a long period of time, with fifteen year survival rate being 29% in children and 65% in adults in the series of patients in our Institute.

Histologic subtype of craniopharyngioma could affect the prognosis tremendously. For example, adamantinous type found in children has poor prognosis with frequent and early recurrence.

One stage radical surgery provides for the best survival rates, quality of life and preservation of sight. Preoperative adjustment, as well as postoperative monitoring and intensive care, have prevented severe hormonal and electrolyte disorders and improved surgical results.

Surgical mortality rate is however still high, being 2-20%. Yasargil have stated 16% mortality in 144 patients with radical resection (13, 24). We have had quite similar experiences in 126 patients (17% up to 30 days), mortality rate depending on the tumor size (less than 2 cm - 0% and bigger than 6 cm - 35%).

Radiotherapy can control the tumor growth and postpone the recurrence, with an average time span of the recurrence being 75 months after the radiotherapy, and 43 months without it, for a 10 year follow-up.

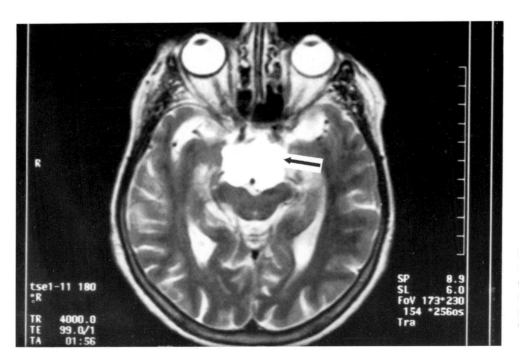

Figure 133. Axial image (TSE 4000/99). Colloidal cyst of high signal intensity is shown in the third ventricle projection, centrally and bilaterally paracentrally.

Radical surgery for a recurrence is seldom possible, so that sometimes tumor reduction or aspiration of a cyst is the only available solution. Omaya reservoir implantation to evacuate the cyst or administer cytostatic (Bleomycin), as well as instillation of radioactive materials (Au, P, Y) directly into the cyst, with varying success, have been described (17).

b) Colloidal cyst

Colloidal cyst (neuroepithelial cyst or paraphyseal cyst) is a congenital cavity built of primitive neuroepithelium in the third ventricle roof with well vascularized fibrous collagenous wall. Inside of a cyst is lined with cubic or cylindrical epithelial hair cells. Cyst contains colloid. This is an infrequent, slowly growing expansion with occasional long-standing stationary cysts.

Colloidal cyst is a pretty rare entity (less than 2% of the brain tumors), interesting for the benign nature and resectability, but on the other hand if untreated they could cause sudden neurologic deficit and occasionally sudden death of the patient. Found exclusively in the anterior part of the third ventricle with insertion right behind Monroes foramina, they are the most frequent pathologic condition in this area.

Colloidal cyst affects all ages and both genders as well, frequently being asymptomatic.

Classic definition of clinical features consists of headache and sudden drop without unconsciousness, following head tilt, because of the peduncular movement of the cyst within the ventricle, thus obstructing Monroes or Silvius foramina. This explanation seems to be inadequate, for only a few cysts have such symptomatology nowadays. Long-standing headache, accompanied by intracranial hypertension and occasional progressive dementia, similar to one seen in normotensive hydrocephalus.

CT scan of colloidal cyst shows hypodense formation which could be hard to differentiate from basal cisterns. According to the series of 144 patients, in 70% of cases cyst can be hyperdense even before the contrast administration. Density corresponds the variable viscosity of the contents of the cyst. Application of the iodine contrast could possibly enhance the density of the cysts wall, depending on vascularization.

MR tomographs in T-1W sequence shows cyst in low signal intensities, unless there is blood or cholesterol inside the cyst, when they show typical high signal intensities (Fig. 134). MR image can differentiate between the colloidal cyst and basilar artery aneurysm or basal cisterns. MRI is not as significant for deduction on the cyst contents density as the CT examination (32). Colloidal cyst is treated either by stereotactic aspiration or by a direct open access through transcallous and occasionally transcortical route. Nowadays, endoscopy is considered superb technique for the treatment of this lesion. Recurrence is extremely rare (35).

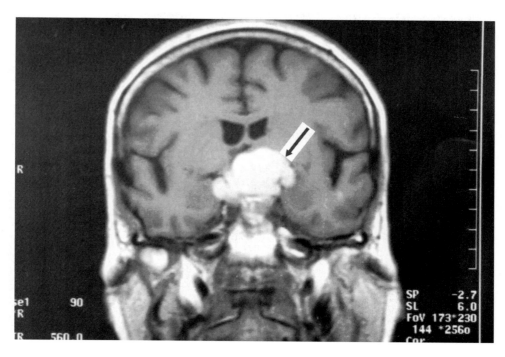

Figure 134. Coronal image (SE 500/15) Colloidal cyst of high signal intensity is shown in the third ventricle projection, centrally and bilaterally paracentrally - arrow.

c) Lipoma

Lipoma is a rare tumor, containing fat and scarce collagenous fibrous tissue. They are slowly growing, benign lesions. Occasional calcifications and even ossification are found in lipoma.

Glial, ganglional, smooth or striped muscle fibers in the lipoma are due to the disturbed development.

Intracranial lipoma is extremely rare, always in the sagittal plane in the corpus callosum area.

Lipoma is usually asymptomatic and therefore found accidentally by the neuroradiologist.

CT examination, with or without iodine contrast, shows lipoma in low signal intensities. Smaller or calcified lipoma could cause confusion because of their resemblance to a cyst, teratoma, etc.

MR tomographs in T-1W and T-2W sequence show lipoma in high signal intensities of the fat (24) (Fig. 135).

d) Dermoid, epidermoid and neuroenteric cysts

Dermoid and epidermoid cysts make 0.2-1.8% of all intracranial tumors, according to the literature data. Previous attitude that dermoids affect mainly children and epidermoid adults is abandoned nowadays, because recent data have shown equal distribution in all ages and both sexes for both entities.

d-1 Dermoid cyst

They are sites of predilection for a dermoid cyst: along the midline, vermis, orbit, paranasal sinuses and scalp. Suboccipital cyst can be connected to a dermal sinus and complicated by meningitis.

Dermoid cysts are well defined, multilobular, adherent to the surrounding brain tissue, with viscous, fat, xanthomatous because of desquamation and secretion, with occasional hair or rudimentary teeth. Histologically they are made of simple squamous epithelium with dermal elements.

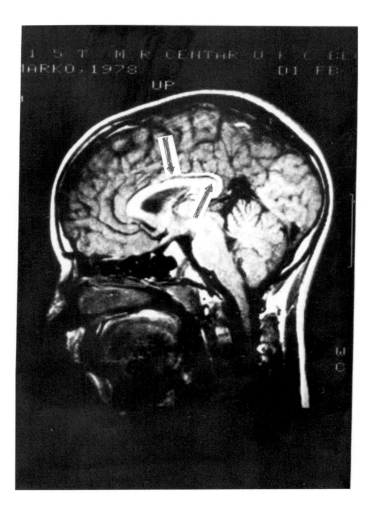

Figure 135. Sagittal image (500/15). Vermicular lipoma with high signal intensities, surrounding the body and splenium of the corpus callosum - arrows.

d-2 Epidermoids

Epidermoids are located laterally, usually in the cerebellopontine angle (37%), parasellar area (31%), in the diploe (16%), in the rhomboid fossa (11%) or in the spinal channel (5%). They spread along the ventricular system with occasional ventricular rupture.

Epidermoid (cholesteatoma, pearl tumor) has shiny, nodular, pearly, well defined and scarcely adherent capsule and uniform shiny contents with a lot of cholesterol crystals and layers of squamous epithelium.

d-3 Neuroenteric cysts

Neuroenteric cysts are found extremely rare, usually in cervicodorsal region, but a few intracranial or craniocervical junction cysts have been reported as well. They are usually located anteriorly to the neuroaxis, and the communication with posterior mediastinal cyst through a bony structure is possible. They are congenital, slowly growing, silent lesions. They adjust to the shape of the existing cavities, so that they are usually discovered when they reach enormous size. Endocranially, they usually grow inside the basal cisterns.

Neuroenteric cysts, causing compressive syndrome of the cervical spine, are usually accompanied by incomplete closure or scoliosis seen in native radiographs.

Neuroenteric cyst is smooth, translucent, filled with clear, xanthochromatic or dark fluid. Epithelium is usually cylindrical with hairs.

Symptoms are usually present for 7-8 years before the diagnosis is established. The most frequent symptoms being epilepsy (53%), headache (47%), hemiparesis, cranial nerve deficits. In posterior fossa cysts cerebellar signs (42%) and cranial nerve deficit (27-50%) are seen.

There are five typical intracranial locations for those cysts: suprasellar-chiasmal (chiasmal and hypothalamic syndrome accompanied by endocrine disorders), parasellar (epilepsy, vision deficit), retrosellar (trigeminal neuralgia or hemifacial spasm, ataxia, nystagmus, hemiparesis), basilar region (deficit of the lower cranial nerve group) and intraventricular (psychological alteration). Caudal, extramedullar location is the most frequent among the spinal ones.

CT scan show these lesions as a hypodense zone. Dermoids are usually calcified. There is no hydrocephalus or brain edema, because of the slow growth of the lesion.

MRI is valuable to display the relationships, especially for the posterior fossa cysts. Epidermoid has low signal intensity in T-1W and high ones in T-2W sequence. Signal intensity varies dependent on the lipid contents (18, 20, 35).

Surgery consists of the radical resection and capsule removal, whenever possible. Subtotal, intracapsular resection is satisfactory as well, because of the slow growth and benign nature of the lesion.

7. Primary malignant lymphoma

Central nervous system lymphoma make 3% of all intracranial tumors, with primary malignant lymphoma representing one half, or 0.85-1.5% of all IC tumors. Dramatic increase in the incidence of intracranial lymphoma have been observed lately (8% of all IC tumors in 1992), because of the increased number of the AIDS patients and extensive use of the immunosuppressive therapy, but a substantial increase have been recorded in immunocompetent patients of both sexes as well (6).

This infrequent expansive lesion is usually located in the brain hemispheres or basal ganglia, affecting primarily the patients in the fifth and sixth decade of life.

According to the classification in use cerebral lymphoma can be either non-Hodgkin or Hodgkin type, primary or secondary, affecting immunocompetent or immunodeficient patients.

Non-Hodgkin lymphoma:

primary cerebral lymphoma in immunocompetent or immunodeficient patients - AIDS, following organ transplantation, congenital or therapeutic.

Secondary cerebral lymphoma

Hodgkin's disease:

-primary

-secondary cerebral Hodgkin's disease
Ocular lymphoma
Mycosis fungoides
Lymphomatoid granulomatosis
Malignant endotheliosis

Cerebral lymphoma encompasses a lot of tumors previously described as reticular or adventitial cell sarcoma, microgliomatosis, perivascular sarcoma, perithelial sarcoma, plasmacytoma, Morbus Hodgkin, histiocytosis, etc. They are homogenous tumors without marked compression effect.

Introduction of radiotherapy and chemotherapy for lymphoma have improved prognosis and remission duration tremendously, which used to have rapid lethal outcome in the past. Considering the excellent therapeutic response to radio- and chemotherapy, it has become important to know the type of tumor without biopsy. Careful examination of the cerebrospinal liquor could be sufficient for the diagnosis of cerebral lymphoma. Diagnosis of lymphoma is confirmed if the abnormal monomorph population of lymphocytes, typical for medium and high grade lymphoma, is found after cytocentrifugation of the liquor (increasing the cellularity up to 60 times) and immunohistochemically proven as monoclonal, combined with elevated protein level, reduced glucose level and pleocytosis. According to the literature data, 10% of patients have had positive findings in liquor at a moment of initial presentation of the disease, but the diagnosis was seldom based on the liquor findings before CT or MR confirmation (30).

CT scan of malignant lymphoma shows hypo- or isodense lesion with mild to moderate edema. After the administration of iodine contrast hyperdense tumor is clearly delineated from a hypodense perifocal edema. Multifocal lesions are seen in 30-45% of cases. Malignant lymphoma is similar to meningioma, astrocytoma, metastasis, recent focus of MS, leukemic infiltration, etc., so that differential diagnosis is required.

MRI of malignant lymphoma in T-1W sequence shows weak signal intensity, whilst in T-2W sequence the strong one. Perifocal edema and tumor could not be defined in T-2W. Intravenously administered paramagnetic contrast in T-1W enhances malignant lymphoma by a high signal intensity, separating it from the perifocal edema with unchanged low signal intensity. MR with application of the paramagnetic contrast has no substantial advantage over CT examination with iodine contrast, except for a few cases of subarachnoidal or spinal localization (Fig. 136).

Before commencement of the treatment for malignant lymphoma it is necessary to assess the systemic spread of the disease, including examination of the liquor and ophthalmologic one. Natural history of malignant lymphoma is rapid death. Therapeutic options are surgery, corticosteroids, radiotherapy and

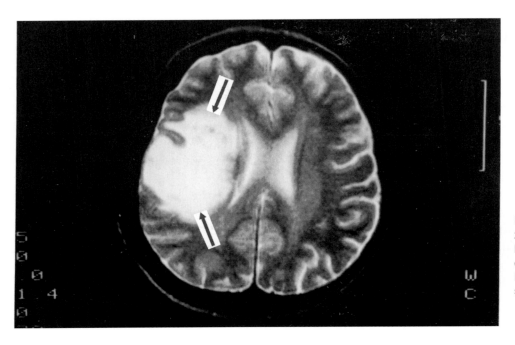

Figure 136. Axial image (SE 2500/90). Primary malignant lymphoma in the right parietal region shown as irregular area of high signal intensity - arrows.

chemotherapy. Surgery in malignant lymphoma should provide tissue specimen for the histology without the peril for the patient (stereotactic biopsy). Tumor is highly radiosensitive, so that radiotherapy significantly improves the survival span. If radiotherapy alone is used, one year survival rate is 66% and five year survival 7%. Results are even better if chemotherapy is administered, but the optimal combination of drugs is still to be found. Literature data are still diversified.

CT and MRI help to evaluate and notice considerable tumor reduction following radiotherapy, even before the clinical signs of recovery are noticed.

8. Metastases

Solitary or multiple brain metastases are usually due to the hematogenous dissemination of carcinoma. Besides the bronchogenic carcinoma, carcinoma of the kidney, breast, prostate, colon, etc. could give metastases to the brain. Malignant melanoma and testicular seminoma are prone to hematogenous dissemination. Some of the tumor, such as medulloblastoma, can disseminate by a liquor.

According to the literature data incidence of the brain metastases is 10/100000 inhabitants of North America. Older males are usually affected. In a cohort of patients under 35 incidence is 1/100000, whereas in patient over 60 years of age it is 30/100000. Metastases of the lung tumors are the most frequent in overall population and breast cancer metastases in women. They are usually supratentorial (80-85%), located in the temporo-parieto-occipital junction in the vicinity of the terminal branches of the medial cerebral artery.

Incidence of the solitary or multiple metastases depends on the primary tumor. Multiple metastases are seen in melanoma and occasionally in lung and breast cancer. Carcinoma of the colon usually has multiple metastases (50%), whereas the kidney cancer is prone to solitary metastasis. Autopsy data have shown that 60-85% of patients with malignancies die of multiple brain metastases (27).

Metastases are a segment of the systemic malignant disease and therefore they could not be treated separately. According to the literature reviews and our own experience, the average survival span for the patients with solitary metastases has been 9-12 months, and with multiple ones 4-6 months. Survival is influenced by a patients general condition, age, control of a primary malignancy and the absence of the extracranial metastases.

Clinical appearance and known primary tumor are important for the MR confirmation of the metastatic tumors. Symptoms of the metastases are occasionally present even before the primary has been discovered. Onset of the symptoms could be sudden, mimicking apoplexy through an epileptic seizure or hemiplegia, or gradual in a form of progressive focal deficit, psychoorganic or intracranial hypertension syndrome.

CT examination with contrast application is usually sufficient for the majority of metastases. In the early phase of the secondary deficit formation CT could be negative or inconclusive especially in the cranial base or posterior fossa. Although CT examination have revealed 37-50% of patients with solitary metastasis, additional MRI have found multiple metastases in one fifth of those patients (27).

MR imaging, especially with paramagnetic contrast administration, is capable to detect majority of the solitary or multiple metastases in the earliest possible stage and delineate secondary deposit from perifocal edema precisely (20). Magnetic resonance could sometimes suggest a histological type of the deposit and possible location of the primary. However, MRI appearance of the metastases is not specific (Figg. 137, 138).

It is essential to differentiate metastases from multiple abscess, meningioma, lymphoma, glioblastoma and tuberculoma in the MR tomographs. Solitary or multiple metastases of the malignant melanoma to the brain or meninges are typical.

Malignant melanoma is built of fusiform and polygonal cells with granulated protoplasm with melanin deposits. Metastasis could contain giant cells as well. Afore mentioned cells have pathologic mitoses, more or less. Inside malignant melanoma hemorrhage or even bigger hematoma could be found.

Specific structure of melanocytes is shown in the magnetic field by unusually high signal intensities, similar to those of the lipid collections or hematoma, in all sequences. Metastases of malignant

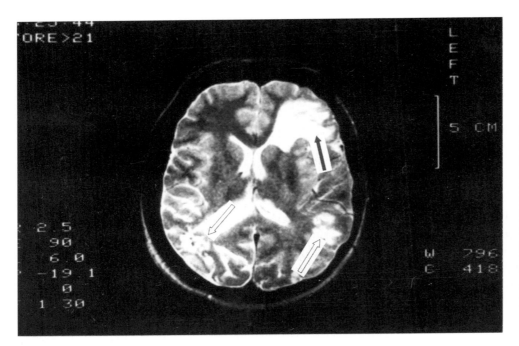

Figure 137. Axial image (SE 500/15). Bilateral multiple metastases. Cystic degeneration of the metastasis with marked irregular edema in the left frontoparietal region-black arrow. Several smaller metastases shown in the left parieto-occipital region - white arrows. Metastases in the right parieto-occipital region as well. Primary tumor is unknown.

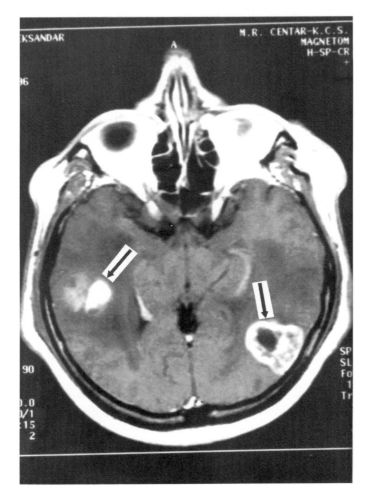

Figure 138. Axial image (SE 500/15) after gadolinium-DTPA administration. Multiple metastases with high signal intensities shown in the right and left temporo-occipital region - black arrows. Primary tumor is unknown.

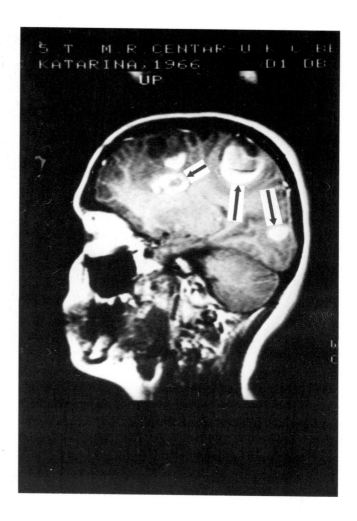

Figure 139. Sagittal image (SE 200/15). Multiple metastases of the malignant melanoma are seen in the right fronto-parieto-occipital area. Secondary deposits are of high, mixed and lower signal intensities-arrows.

melanoma could be easily recognized in MR tomographs for their bizarre features, multiplicity, well defined boundaries and perifocal edema.

Secondary deposits of the malignant melanoma vary in shape and size, but they are generally well defined from surrounding edema (17). It should be emphasized that beside the metastases with high signal intensities, low and mixed signal intensity varieties could be seen as well (Fig. 139). Blood collections are shown in typical signal intensities, depending on the sequence applied.

Carcinomatosis represent a special type of metastases. It is usually seen in breast and lung cancer, etc. MRI with intravenous application of paramagnetic contrast is a method of choice for differentiation between carcinomatosis and extracerebral hematoma or empyema (Fig. 140).

Considering the fact that secondary deposits are treated by palliative therapy it is hard to assess value of certain therapeutic modalities.

Neurosurgical resection of the solitary metastasis with or without postoperative radiotherapy is much cheaper than non-invasive stereotactic radiosurgery, whereas the results are practically equal.

Chemotherapy has more favorable results for sensitive tumors, than for brain metastases acquired in the later stages of malignant disease, when the chemotherapy effects are already exhausted.

Chemotherapy alternatives are investigated. Improved selectivity, opening of the blood-brain barrier and combination of the immunologic and genetic therapy are searched for.

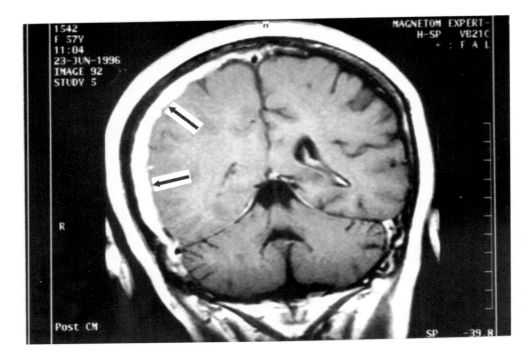

Figure 140. Coronal image (500/15) after gadolinium-DTPA administration. Meningeal carcinomatosis in the right fronto-temporo-parietal region (secondary deposit of the lung cancer)-arrows.

REFERENCES

1. Allen JC., Kim JH., Packer RJ.: Neoadjuvant chemotherapy for newly diagnosed germ cell tumors of the central nervous system. J. Neurosurg., 67: 65-70, 1987.
2. Al-Mefty O.: Meningiomas. Raven Press. New York, 1991.
3. Apuzzo M., Litofsky S.: Surgery in and around the anterior third ventricle. In Apuzzo M. (ed.): Brain surgery, complication avoidance and management. Churchill Livingstone. New York, Edinburgh, London, Melbourne, Tokyo, 1993.
4. Araki T., Inouye T., Suzuki H., Mashida T., Iio M.: Magnetic resonance imaging of brain tumors: Measurement of T-1. Radiology, 150: 95-98, 1984.
5. Banna M.: Craniopharyngeoma based on 160 cases. Br. J. Radiol., 49: 206-223, 1976.
6. Brant-Zawadzki M., Kelly W.: Brain tumors. In Brant-Zawadzki M., Norman D. (eds): Magnetic resonance imaging of the central nervous system. Raven Press, New York, 151-186. 1986.
7. Fitz CR., et al.: Computed tomography in craniopharyngeomas. Radiology, 127: 687-691, 1978.
8. Gademann G.: NMR-Tomography of the Normal Brain. Springer-Verlag. Berlin, Heidelberg, New York, Tokyo, 1988.
9. Gerhardt P., Fromhold W.: Atlas of Anatomic Correlations in CT and MRI. Thieme. New York, Tokyo, Heidelberg, 1988.
10. Halbsgut A, Lechner B: Magnetresonanz-Tomographie (NMR). Springer-Verlag. Frankfurt, 1986.
11. Huk WJ., Gademann G., Friedman G.: Magnetic Resonance Imaging of Central Nervous System Diseases. Springer-Verlag. Berlin, New York, Heidelberg, Tokyo, Paris, London, 1989.
12. Humpreys R.: Optic gliomas. In Apuzzo M. (ed.): Brain surgery, complication avoidance and management. Vol. 1, 643-688, Churchill Livingstone. New York, Edinburgh, London, Melbourne, Tokyo, 1993.
13. Kazner E., Wende S., Grumme Th.: Computer und Kernspin-Tomographie intrakranialler Tumoren aus klinischen Sicht. Springer Verlag. Berlin, Heidelberg, New York, London, Paris, Tokyo, 1989.
14. Konovalov AN.: Technique and strategies in direct surgical management of craniopharyngiomas. In Apuzzo M. (ed): Surgery of third ventricle. Churchill Livingstone. New York, Edinburgh, London, Melbourne, Tokyo, Vol. 1, 542-553, 1987.
15. Kovacs K., Miller M.: Intracranial Tumors of Infants and Children. Georg Thieme Verlag. Stuttgart, 213-220. 1971.
16. Laws ER. Jr., et al: Neurosurgical management of low grade astrocytoma of cerebral hemispheres. J. Neurosurg., 61: 665-673, 1984.
17. Licter AS., et al.: The treatment craniopharingeomas. J. Radiat. Oncol. Biol. Phys., 2: 675-683, 1977.
18. Liessner J., Seider M.: Klinische Kernspintomographie. Enke. Stuttgart, 1987.
19. Litofsky S., Levy M., Apuzzo M.: Craniopharyngioma. In Apuzzo M. (ed.): Brain surgery, complication avoidance and management. Churchill Livingstone. New York, Edinburgh, London, Melbourne, Tokyo, Vol. 1, 313-318, 1993.
20. Pomeranz JS.: Craniospinal Magnetic Resonance Imaging. WB Saunders Company. Philadelphia, London, Toronto, Sydney, Tokyo, 1989.

21. Pykett IL.: NMR imaging in medicine. Sci. American., 246: 78- 88, 1982.
22. Rakic M., et al.: The expression of N-myc and pan-ras oncogenes in intracranial meningiomas. J. of Neurooncol., 30/2: 24-29, 1996.
23. Ramm B., Semmler W., Laniado M.: Einfuerung in der MR-Tomographie. Enke Verlag. Stuttgart, 1986.
24. Reiser M., et al.: Magnet-rezonanz-Tomographie. Springer Verlag. Berlin, Heidelberg, New York, Paris, London, Tokyo, Hong Kong, 1989.
25. Russel D., Rubinstein L.: Pathology of Tumors of the Nervous System. Edward Arnold. London, 1977.
26. Sano K.: Pineal region masses. In Apuzzo M. (ed.): Brain surgery, complication avoidance and management. *Churchill* Livingstone. New York, Edinburgh, London, Melbourne, Tokyo, Vol. 1, 463-473, 1993.
27. Schoerner W.: Kontrastmittel in der Kernspintomographie. Deutsche Arzte Verlag. Berlin, 1988.
28. Simpson D.: The recurrence of intracranial meningiomas after surgical treatment. J. Neurol., Neurosurg. and Psychiatr., 20: 22-39, 1957.
29. Spagnoli MV., Gorssman RI., Packer RJ., Hackney DB., Goldberg HI., Zimmerman RA., Bilaniuk LT.: Magnetic resonance imaging determination of gliomatosis cerebri. Neuroradiology, 29: 15-18, 1987.
30. Stark D., Bradley GWJR.: Magnetic Resonance Imaging. The CV Mosby Company. St. Louis, Washington D.C., Toronto. 1988.
31. Takeuchi J., Hanada H., Nagata I.: Suprasellar germinoma. J. Neurosurg., 49: 41-48, 1978.
32. Van M. Runge: Enhanced Magnetic Resonance Imaging. The C.V. Mosby Company. St. Louis, Baltimore, Toronto, 1989.
33. Venes J., Brunberg J.: Cysts. In Apuzzo M. (ed.): Brain surgery, complication avoidance and management. Churchill Livingstone. New York, Edinburgh, London, Melbourne, Tokyo, Vol. 1, 313-318, 1993.
34. Yasargil MG., et al.: Total removal of craniopharyngiomas. J. Neurosurg., 73: 3-11, 1990.
35. Zawadcki MB., Norman D.: Magnetic Resonance Imaging of the Central Nervous System. Raven Press. New York, 1987.
36. Zeitler E.: Kernspintomographie. Deutsche Artze, Verlag, Koeln, 1984.
37. Zimmerman RA., Bilaniuk LT., Grossman RI., Goldberg HI., Edelstein HI., Bottomley P., Redington RW.: Cerebral NMR: Diagnostic evaluation of brain tumors by partial saturation technique with resistive NMR. Neuroradiology, 27: 9-15. 1985.
38. Zulch KJ.: Brain tumors: Their biology and pathology, 3rd ed., Springer, New York, 1986.

VII. TUMORS OF THE POSTERIOR CRANIAL FOSSA

Vaso Antunović, Gradimir Dragutinović, Miodrag Rakić

There are numerous classifications of the expansive lesions in the posterior cranial fossa. One of them classify tumors according to their location either as intraaxial or extraaxial, with brainstem tumors as a separate entity.

1. Intraaxial tumors are: medulloblastoma, cerebellar astrocytoma, ependymoma, plexus chorioideus papilloma, etc.
2. Extraaxial tumors are: meningioma, neurinoma, epidermoid, dermoid, lipoma, paraganglioma, arachnoidal cyst, glomus jugulare tumor, chordoma, etc.
3. Tumors of cerebellar hemispheres are: astrocytoma, hemangioblastoma, metastases.
4. Primary tumors of the brainstem are usually low grade glioma, being malignant for their malignant location and inability of surgical resection (8).

Clinical appearance could be completely asymptomatic, and neuroimaging could accidentally reveal the tumor. Polymorph clinical picture is however found in the majority of cases, including cerebellar symptomatology, cranial nerve impairment, ataxia, etc. Intracranial hypertension, due to compromised liquor circulation, could often be the first sign.

Standard radiographs are insignificant for the modern diagnosis of the posterior fossa tumors.

Posterior fossa is not easily accessible for CT examination. Massive bone structures, such as occipital bone, clivus, sellar dorsum and especially pyramids and mastoids, can cause a lot of artifacts in computer tomography.

Bone structures could be precisely differentiated if the extended scale of CT examination is used, whilst the morphology of rombencephalic soft tissue is poorly displayed by this method. Relationship between gray and white matter or eventual pathology could not be clearly seen.

Intravenous administration of iodine contrast could enhance most of the posterior fossa tumors in CT scan.

Triplanar MR examination enables detailed visualization of posterior fossa brain structures, eliminating the artifact completely.

Tumors, both supra- and infratentorial, have identical signal intensities in MR tomographs. Differential diagnosis of posterior fossa tumors, that could extend supratentorially, have been discussed in the previous chapter.

MR diagnostic of the expansive lesions in posterior fossa or craniocervical junction requires multiplanar approach in sequences used also for other brain tumors. Special sequences and paramagnetic contrast Gd-DTPA are chosen according to the pathoanatomic features of the tumor.

Slice thickness is 3-5 with distance of 0.1-0.2.

1. Intraaxial posterior fossa tumors

a) Medulloblastoma

Medulloblastoma belongs to a group of embryonal tumors, subgroup PNET and, according to WHO classification a group of primitive neuroepithelial tumors (gr. IV). Medulloblastoma is a rapidly growing malignancy. It makes 25% of all intracranial tumors in childhood and 2/3 of all posterior fossa tumors.

According to the Authors from Institue of Neurosurgery in Belgrade, medulloblastoma is quite frequent in childhood, so that one half of the children operated on for posterior fossa tumor or 1/3 of those operated children for any intracranial tumor, have had medulloblastoma (9).

Medulloblastoma is a frequent lesion in patients in the first two decades of life, located in the posterior fossa, usually in cerebellar vermis, but the cerebellar hemisphere could be affected, especially in adults, as well. Cerebrum is exceptionally involved and that could be due to dissemination of primary medulloblastoma located practically anywhere in the posterior fossa, nearby liquor cavities. Systemic metastases have been reported in 5-15% of cases.

Posterior fossa PNET is rarely found in adults. Those tumors have higher incidence than astrocytoma and lower than cerebellar metastases (2).

Pathologically, medulloblastoma is a pinkish-gray tumor with enhanced blood vessels in the capsule.

Pathohistologically, medulloblastoma has a lot of non-differentiated, i.e. immature cells, tightly packed, small, with scarce cytoplasm, eventual pseudorosettes, with poor fibrous stroma and few blood vessels. Having a lot in common with astrocytic, neuronal and ependymal tumors, medulloblastoma have been classified as primitive neuroectodermal tumor, with or without differentiation (2).

Medulloblastoma arises from the roof of the IV ventricle, invading it, thus causing the obstruction to liquor circulation and internal hydrocephalus. Morning vomiting and headache could be the first signs of increased intracranial pressure. Neurologic examination reveals cerebellar symptomatology such as: gait on a wider base, falling backwards, asynergism, dysmetry. Fundus examination confirms stagnant papilla of even 10 dioptries. Brainstem disorders could be found in the later phase.

In CT scan, medulloblastoma is seen as iso- or hypodense lesion in the IV ventricle, and its density could be enhanced by a contrast injection. Hypodense perifocal edema is poorly differentiated. Typical CT scan of medulloblastoma shows uniform or heterogenous imbibed mass in the IV ventricle, after iodine contrast administration.

MR image in T-1W sequence displays medulloblastoma in equal or low signal intensities (Fig. 141).

In T-2W sequence tumor is shown in equal to higher signal intensities, with clear demarcation of edema with high signal intensity from a solid tumor tissue (Fig. 142).

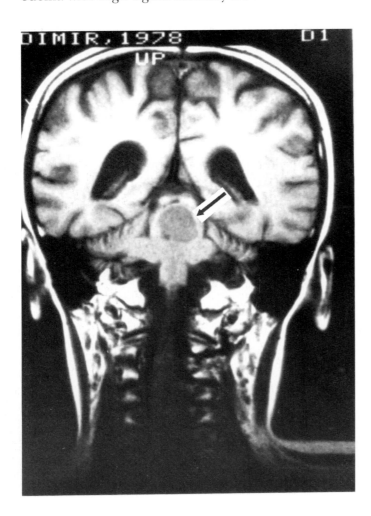

Figure 141. Coronal image (SE 500/15). Well defined medulloblastoma of low signal intensities is shown in the IV ventricle projection - arrow.

After paramagnetic contrast administration, MR image in T-1W sequence shows signal enhancement of a tumor, whereas edema retains low signal intensities (2) (Fig 143). CT and MR features of supra- and infratentorial medulloblastoma are identical. Differential diagnosis should rule out ependymoma or, rarely, pylocytic astrocytoma, cerebellar angioma, etc. (11).

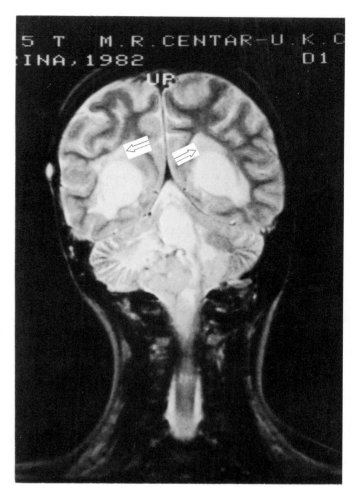

Figure 142. Coronal image (SE 2500/90). Medulloblastoma in the projection of the inferior pole of the right cerebellar hemisphere, compressing medulla and causing obstruction hydrocephalus and dilation of IV, III and both lateral ventricles. Tumor of isointensive signal is well delineated, surrounded by a slight perifocal edema - arrows.

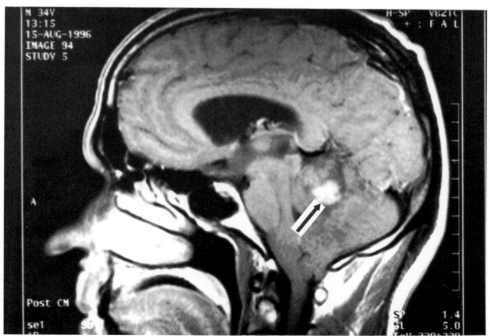

Figure 143. Sagittal image (SE 500/15) after gadolinium-DTPA administration. Medulloblastoma has high signal intensities - arrow, with perifocal edema with low signal intensities.

Surgical objectives are radical resection of medulloblastoma and restitution of liquor circulation. According to the literature data, the degree of the surgical radicality is proportional to the survival span.

Considering exceptional radiosensitivity of those tumors, the WHO protocole includes postoperative radiotherapy of the whole neuroaxis in order to control, the local growth and liquor dissemination of the tumor.

Chemotherapy is mostly used for recurrent medulloblastoma or systemic metastases.

Therapy results have been improved a great deal recently, so that, according to the literature data, expected survival span for children operated on for medulloblastoma and treated according to WHO protocole, is 8 years after the surgery and 50-70% patients have no evidence of recurrence after 5 years (9).

b) Ependymoma

Ependymoma, making 5% of all brain tumors, are usually situated in the fourth ventricle, but could be found in the lateral recesse of the IV ventricle and extend through to Luschkas foramen as well.

Histology and biology of ependymoma is similar to the supratentorial ependymomas described in a previous chapter. Posterior fossa ependymomas may have a variable degree of malignancy, but their prognosis is generally worse as compared to suprasellar ones, because of their origin in the floor of the fourth ventricle.

Clinical course of ependymoma depends on this location. Dominant symptoms are due to the increased intracranial pressure caused by IV ventricle obstruction (internal hydrocephalus), such as: ataxia, vision impairment, hemiparesis, pain in the neck caused by compression of the anatomic structures in the posterior fossa, etc.

Lobulated, well delineated mass protruding into fourth ventricle, usually hyperdense with occasional calcifications, is shown by a CT scan.

Ependymoma has high signal intensity and precise demarcation in T-1W sequence after contrast administration (19). Internal hydrocephalus is frequently associated (Figg. 144, 145).

Surgery, including radical tumor resection and restitution of liquor circulation, is the most effective treatment. Tumor can be easily dissected from the top or lateral walls of the fourth ventricle, but if the floor of the IV ventricle is involved, tumor can not be completely removed because of the high surgical risk. Microsurgical resection, CUSA and laser have reduced operative mortality to the smallest possible extent (8%), as compared to 17-50% mortality rate in pre-microscopic era (20).

Microsurgical resection can be followed by radiotherapy.

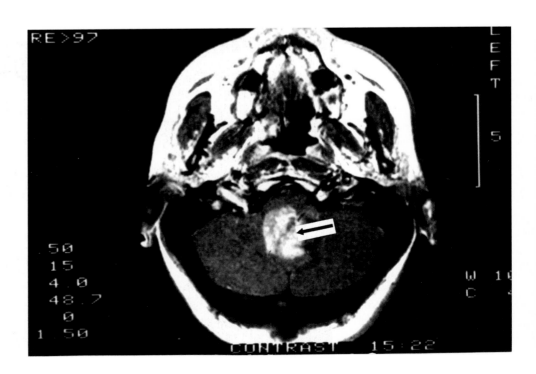

Figure 144. Axial image (SE 500/15) after gadolinium-DTPA administration. Ependymoma of high signal intensities involving the major part of the fourth ventricle with subsequent obstructive internal hydrocephalus. Arrow pointing at the tumor.

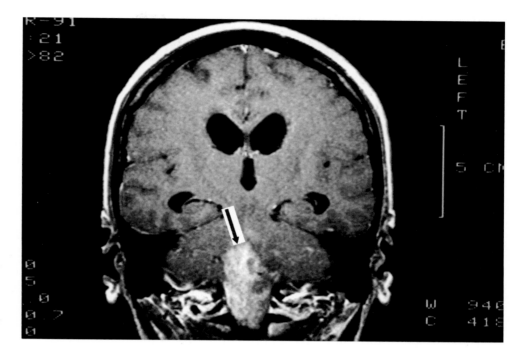

Figure 145. Coronal image (SE 500/15) after gadolinium-DTPA administration. Ependymoma of high signal intensities shown in a projection of the IV ventricle - arrow pointing at the tumor.

c) Papilloma of the chorioid plexus

Plexus papillomas in adults are usually situated in the IV ventricle (79%) (20), whereas in children they are almost exclusively supratentorial.

Origin of those tumors is still unclear, but there is a possibility that they arise from chorioid plexus and extend towards cerebellopontine angle or through Luschkas foramen.

Clinical course depends on the internal hydrocephalus evolution (see previous chapter).

CT and MR features of both supratentorial and infratentorial plexus papilloma are the same (4).

Plexus papilloma in MR image in T-1W after paramagnetic contrast administration is shown with heterogenous high signal intensities (19). These tumors often compromise liquor circulation, thus causing obstructive internal hydrocephalus (Fig. 146).

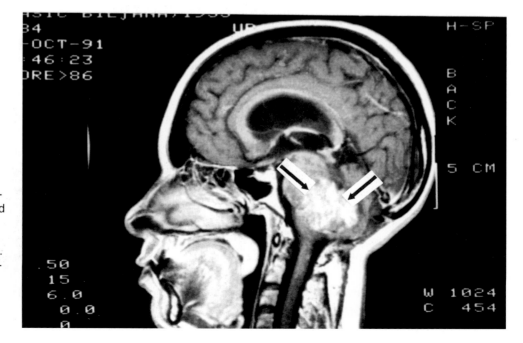

Figure 146. Sagittal image (SE 500/15) after gadolinium-DTPA administration. Chorioid plexus papilloma with high signal intensities is shown in the fourth ventricle projection. Tumor fills the ventricle, compress cerebellum, pons and medulla oblongata causing obstructive internal hydrocephalus - arrows.

Surgical treatment should provide for radical resection of a tumor and restitution of liquor circulation. Recurrence is rare after the radical surgery, so that those tumors should be considered surgically curable. Radiotherapy and chemotherapy could be administered in case of malignant variety (plexus carcinoma) or an incompletely removed tumor with controversial results.

2. Extraaxial posterior fossa tumors

Extraaxial tumors originate from neural sheaths, meninges or non-brain structures. They induce compression of the soft tissues in the posterior cranial fossa. Extraaxial tumors can cause destruction of pyramid, mastoid or cranial base bones, depending on the location, size and pathohistology.

The most frequent extracranial tumor in the cerebellopontine angle is acoustic neurinoma.

a) Neurinoma of the acoustic nerve

Acoustic neurinoma is the most frequent tumor of neural sheath origin, making 8% of all intracranial tumors and 80% of tumors in the cerebellopontine angle. They could be bilateral in 4-5% of cases Neurofibromatosis type 2.

Neurinoma and meningioma make 96% of all benign tumors in the cerebellopontine angle. Neurinoma is ten times more frequent than meningioma.

Natural history of neurinoma is quite variable, but it could be generally said that this is a slow growing tumor, with an annual increase of less than 2 mm, in the majority of patients (9).

They affect middle aged patients, usually in fifth and sixth decade (50%), where as patients with neurofibromatosis are generally younger, under 30 years of age. The incidence in females is slightly higher. It could be sporadic or hereditary. Unilateral, sporadic acoustic neurinoma is found in 96% of cases. Hereditary type is bilateral, seen in type 2 neurofibromatosis, caused by gene deletion in the long arm of the chromosome 22.

Hystopathologic features of neurinoma include two types of Schwann cells (Antony type A and B) with cystic and mucous degeneration. Fibrous tissue inside the tumor is variable, but there is fibrous capsule on the surface. Blood vessels are grouped. Lymphocyte infiltrations, as well as hemosiderin deposits and xanthochromatous cells are found. Malignant variety is exceptionally rare.

Progressive unilateral hearing loss and tinnitus remains the only symptom for quite a long time. Lesion of the trigeminal nerve (V1) manifested by ipsilateral corneal hypoaesthesia (decreased or absent corneal reflex) is the first neurologic sign. Vertigo with nistagmus and dysbalance is seen in the later phase. Tumor growth inflicts further symptomatology due to impairment of other nerves in posterior cranial fossa, first of all trigeminal and facial nerves, as well as homolateral cerebellar hemisphere and ipsilateral ataxia. Brainstem compression can cause impairment of the long sensitive and motor pathways and contralateral hemiparesis. Tumor usually has slow evolution with late onset of decompensation, massive symptomatology and increased intracranial pressure.

Special and tomography views of pyramids enable visualization of the bony structures such as *porus and meatus acousticus internus*. Increased diameter of *porus acousticus internus* over 7 mm (normal value 5-7 mm) suggest suspected expansion in the cerebellopontine angle.

CT examination is indicated upon the otological findings. Auditory evoked potentials should be done always, as well as the laboratory findings.

There is a special technique of CT examination required for the diagnosis of microtumors (diameter range 5-10 mm): 5 ml of air is injected intrathecally and led to the cerebellopontine cistern by a special head positioning (mini gas-cisternography). Iodine contrast injected intravenously enhances the density of neurinoma or meningioma a great deal. The idea is to surround a tumor, imbibed by iodine contrast, with air which helps the demarcation of the smallest lesions. Targeted axial view with slice thickness of 2-3 mm and reconstruction is used in order to obtain best possible visualization of *meatus acousticus internus*. Double contrast CT examination can reveal the small cerebellopontine angle tumors with high certainty.

The first double contrast CT examination was performed in Belgrade by Dragutinović G. and coll. in the Institute of Radiology in 1983. The tumor of 3 x 3 x 3 mm in diameter was diagnosed and subsequently operated on.

MR imaging is a non-invasive method of choice for the diagnosis of cerebellopontine and other extraaxial tumors. Standard sequences, multiplanar views and slice thickness of 5 mm are used. Paramagnetic contrast should always be used if neurinoma, meningioma or other tumors with signal enhancement are suspected (5).

Neurinoma and meningioma are alike in MR tomographs in all sequences, even after contrast administration (Figg. 147, 148).

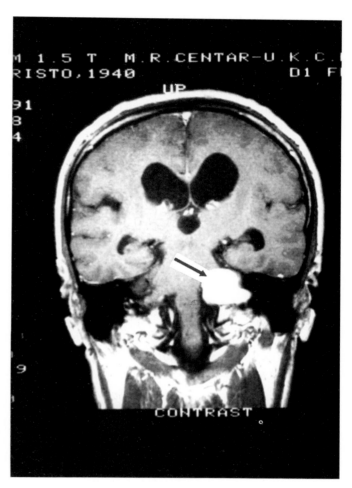

Figure 147. Coronal image (SE 500/15) after gadolinium-DTPA administration. Well demarcated neurinoma with high signal intensities is shown in the left cerebellopontine angle of the patient P.R. - arrow. Tumor fills meatus acousticus internus and cerebellopontine cistern, causing lateral compression of the pons.

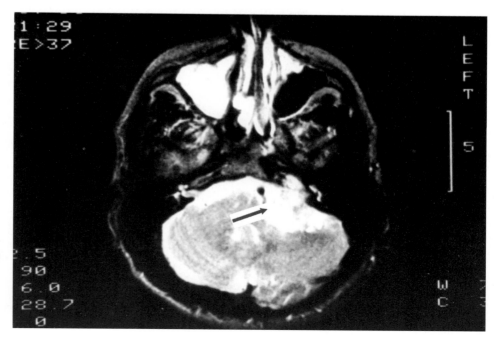

Figure 148. Axial image (SE 2500/90). Same patient with poorly defined expansive lesion in the left cerebellopontine angle-arrow. Comparison to **Figure 147.** Justifies administration of paramagnetic contrast.

MR imaging have replaced double contrast CT examination, except in those centers where MR is not available (7, 12).

b) Neurofibroma

Benign neurofibroma consists of Schwanns cells, fibroblasts, myelinated and non-myelinated nerve fibers, diffuse collagen and fibrous tissue with hyalin degeneration (Fig. 149).

Increased cellularity, giantic cells, atypia and hyperchromia of nuclei, as well as pathological mitoses are found in malignant neurofibroma (see chapter on malformations) (17).

Surgery for neurinoma or neurofibroma is identical; translabyrinthine, suboccipital- retromastoid, middle cranial fossa or combined approach is used. Advantages of certain aproach have been discussed, but the choice depends on tumor size, hearing threshold on the tumor side and contralaterally, as well as on the surgeons experience. Translabyrinthine approach enables better identification of the facial nerve, but the results are as good in suboccipital approach for the experienced surgeon (19).

Hearing preservation has become surgical objective recently, following improved results in preservation of the facial nerve and decreased mortality. In case of the facial nerve lesion direct repair, graft or hypoglosso-facial anastomosis are used successfully, especially in younger patients.

c) Meningioma

Location of meningioma in the posterior fossa (1):
in the convexity (medial, lateral, superior)
posterior pyramidal
clival and petroclival
craniocervical junction
the fourth ventricle

Clinical course of meningioma is slowly progressive, similar to neurinoma. Neurologic deficit depends on the location of tumor.

CT scan with iodine contrast administration enables good visualization of the posterior fossa meningiomas.

Extraaxial meningioma could be shown in multiplanar MR tomographs in T-1W sequence with paramagnetic contrast administration. Contrast helps delineate the tumor from edema. Tumor has high signal intensities (3). The examination technique for extraaxial neurinoma is quite the same. Those two types of tumor could not be differed in MR images (Figg. 150, 151).

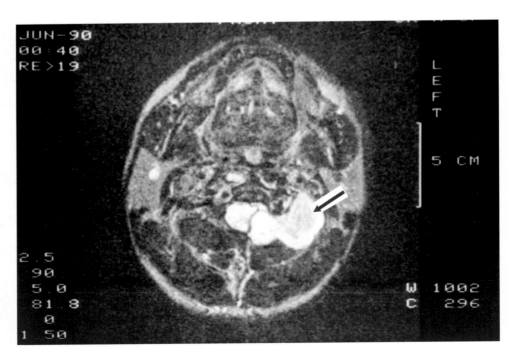

Figure 149. Axial image (SE 2500/90). Neurofibromatosis - tumefact in the level of craniocerebral junction, compressing medulla oblongata and beginning of medulla spinalis - arrow.

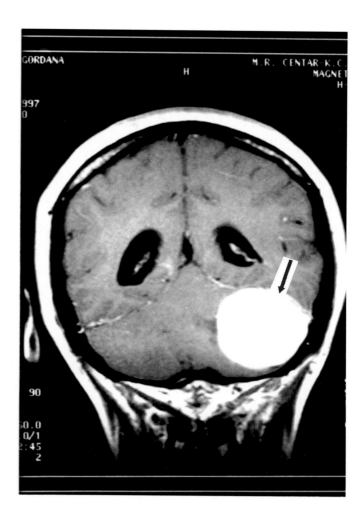

Figure 150. Coronal image (SE 500/15) after gadolinium-DTPA administration. Huge meningioma, with high signal intensity, is shown infratentorially in the convexity - arrow.

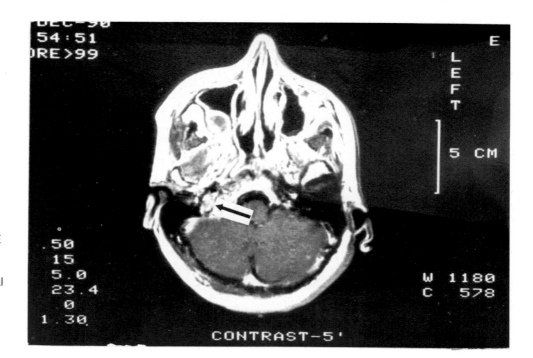

Figure 151. Axial image (SE 500/15) after gadolinium-DTPA administration. Meningioma, with high signal intensities, is shown in the right cerebellopontine angle with considerable caudal propagation - arrow.

Indirect signs, seen in MR tomographs, could not determine the histologic nature of the tumor for sure (tumor insertion dimensions or location, degree of hyperostosis, etc.) (14).

Meningiomas of the frontal and parietal falx, and left cerebellopontine angle have been diagnosed in the same patient, P.M. (Figg. 152-154).

Surgical treatment depends on precise tumor location. Meningioma of the convexity in the posterior cranial fossa could be easily excised. Meningioma inserted in the posterior wall of the pyramid could interfere with lower group of cranial nerves, which should be preserved during tumor dissection. Medial or lateral suboccipital approach issued (1).

Clival and petroclival meningiomas pose a problem in neurosurgery, for they arise in the vicinity of the brainstem and could be adherent to a basilar artery or cranial nerves, and have a high perioperative mortality rate during microsurgical resection. Several approaches for those tumors have been described: fronto-temporal, occipito-transtentorial, suboccipital, combined subtemporal-translabyrinthine and transtemporal. Medial suboccipital access is used for a extremely rare meningiomas of the fourth ventricle.

d) Epidermoid

Cholesteatoma is a developmental tumor (see: epidermoid cysts), which tend to grow laterally inside endocranium. They are usually located in cerebellopontine angle (37%), parasellary (31%), diploic (16%), fossa rhomboidea (11%), spinal canal (5%). If they are located in the petrous bone progressive hearing impairment and facial paralysis can occur (19).

Acquired inflammatory cholesteatoma is a separate entity. It is based on the fat degeneration of the middle ear granulations. It involves temporal bone, and exceptionally occipital, frontal or cranial base bones.

Histopathology has been described before.

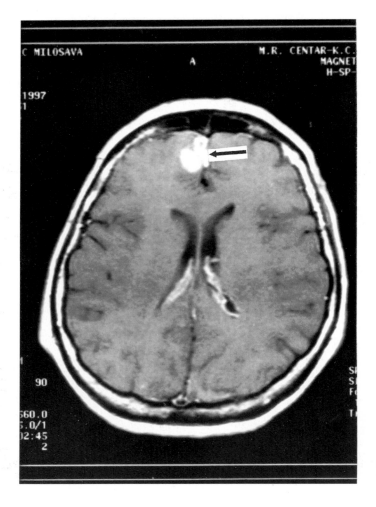

Figure 152. Axial image (SE 500/15) after gadolinium-DTPA administration. Frontal falx meningioma - arrow.

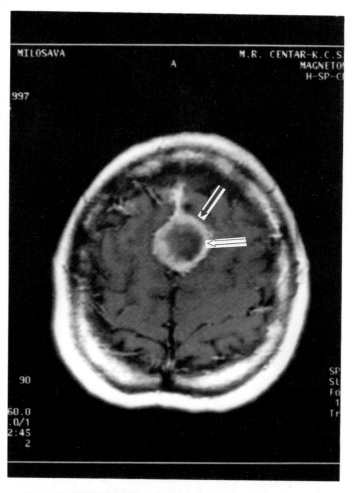

Figure 153. Axial image (SE 500/15) after gadolinium-DTPA administration. Parietal falx meningioma high under the calotte - arrows.

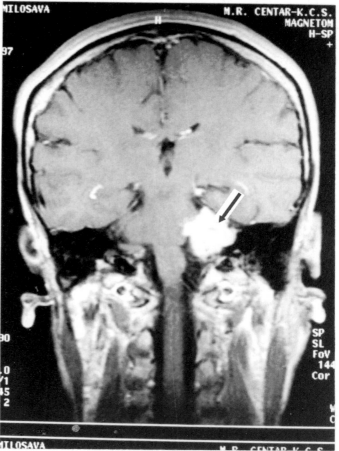

Figure 154. Coronal image (SE 500/15) after gadolinium-DTPA administration. Meningioma of the left cerebellopontine angle - arrow.

Epidermoid compress brain structures of the posterior fossa and depending on the size can cause obstructive internal hydrocephalus.

CT scan shows epidermoid as well defined, hypodense and partly isodense expansion, without marked alteration after contrast application.

MR tomographs in T-1W sequence show epidermoid as demarcated heterogenous mass of low signal intensity; if there are fat collections they are shown as high signal intensity zones inside a tumor (Figg. 155, 156).

In T-2W sequence the tumor has non-homogenous signal intensities. Signal intensities of epidermoid are not altered by paramagnetic contrast application (6).

Regarding slow evolution, extent of the tumor at the time of diagnosis and benign nature of the tumor, the surgical treatment should be rationally radical (2).

e) Chordoma

Chordoma is a slow growing tumor, usually found in middle aged males, originating from embryonal remnants of the dorsal cord.

Macroscopically, chordoma is nodular, red, gelatinous or solid. Big, polyedric cells are sorted in lobules or beams and divided by slender fibrous septa. Pathological mitoses are seen in rapidly growing chordoma. Malignant alteration of particularly invasive chordoma is rare. They are soft and gelatinous, and inside the tumor, which could grow enormously, hemorrhage, cysts and necrosis could be found.

Chordoma is rare, making 2% of all intracranial tumors; 40% of chordoma being primary intracranial, located in clivus, sella, parasellary, nasopharynx or craniocervically. Local invasion and position makes radical excision problematic, so that it should be considered malignant. Chordoma could have spinal, sacral or spheno-occipital location (9).

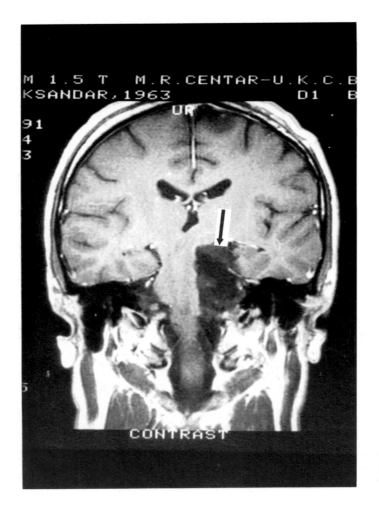

Figure 155. Coronal image (SE 500/15) after gadolinium-DTPA administration. Parasagittally left, infratentorial epidermoid with lower signal intensities - arrow. Paramagnetic contrast did not enhanced signal intensities in the tumor.

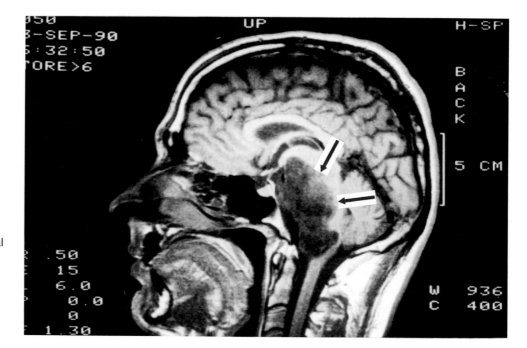

Figure 156. Sagittal image (SE 500/15). Left parasagittal epidermoid with low signal intensities, compromising cerebellar hemisphere, pons and medulla oblongata. Liquor circulation is not critically jeopardized.

Headache and cranial nerve impairment are the most frequent symptoms, especially VI nerve palsy (50-90%) with subsequent diplopia.

Chordoma is shown in CT scan as well defined hypodense or isodense tumor, without density alteration after iodine contrast administration. Eventual cysts, hemorrhage and necrosis density could influence homogenity of the tumor structure.

MR tomographs inT-1W sequence show chordoma as well defined tumor mass with signal intensities similar to a nomal brain tissue. Cysts and necrosis inside the tumor have extremely low signal intensity, and the hemorrhage higher signal intensity (Fig. 157). In T-2W sequence chordoma has slightly higher and mixed signal intensities, whereas cysts and necrosis are shown in high signal intensities (20).

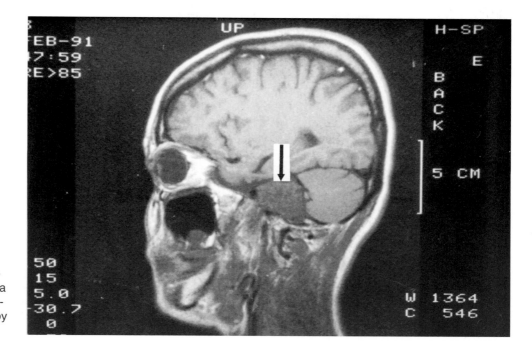

Figure 157. Sagittal image (SE 500/15). Well defined chordoma of homogenous low signal intensities is shown in the right cerebellopontine angle and the tip of a pyramid. Parasagittally, compression of the cerebellum by a tumor is seen - arrow.

Radical surgical excision, sometimes staged or achieved through extensive combined approach, provides for the best results. If it is not possible, reduction surgery followed by postoperative radiotherapy is applied (9).

f) Glomus jugulare tumor

Glomus jugulare tumor belong to the group of neuroendocrine tumors or paragangliomas. Middle aged females are frequently affected. Tumor can be bilateral in 1-2 % and in that case, they are hereditary.

Glomus jugulare tumor has no capsule and it is made of neurovascular tissue with consistent cells and abundant vascular stroma. Tumor celles nests are perfectly seen when reticulin fibres are dyed by silver.

Invasive growth of glomus jugulare tumor destructs cranial base bone, pyramid, mastoid, etc. and compress structures in posterior cranial fossa, infiltrating nerves and venous sinuses.

Glomus jugulare tumor is located in the vicinity of the jugular bulb and could be classified, according to precise location, extension and propagation, in several ways: grade 0, when tumor is confined to the middle ear cavity, up to grade 4, when several cranial nerves are involved; Glomus tympanicus type I-IV; Glomus jugular type I-IV (21). Those are extracranial tumors with intracranial propagation.

CT scan can provide a lot of useful and precise information on bone destruction in cranial base and pyramid. Glomus jugulare is well displayed in CT scan.

Malignant or benign variety of glomus jugulare, dependent on pathological vascularization, is shown in MR tomographs in T-1W sequence after i.v. injection of paramagnetic contrast, as a zone of mixed and higher signal intensities (13). In T-2W sequence those tumors have mixed lower signal intensities (Figg. 158, 159).

Optimal therapeutic modality is still searched for, with radiotherapy, gamma-knife or surgery being currently used. Multidisciplinary team approach will be used in the future.

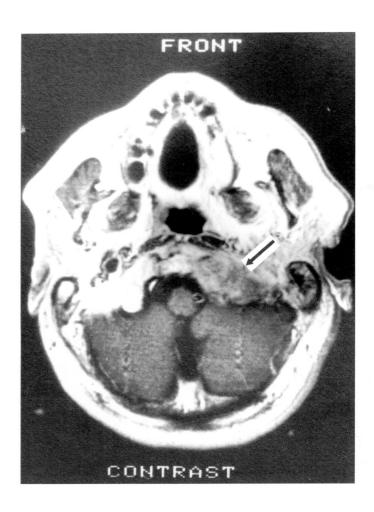

Figure 158. Axial image (SE 500/15) after gadolinium-DTPA administration. Glomus jugulare tumor with mixed higher signal intensities is shown in the cranial base, in jugular foramen projection, in patient D.P. - arrow.
Tumor is well delineated from slightly compressed cerebellar structures.

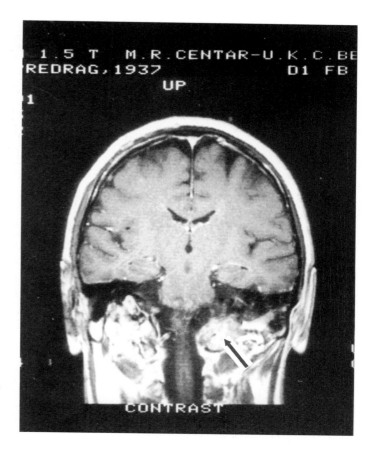

Figure 159. Coronal image (SE 500/15) after gadolinium-DTPA administration. Same patient (D.P.) with glomus jugulare tumor shown in mixed higher signal intensities, located in cranial base, nearby foramen jugulare - arrow.

3. Tumors of the cerebellar hemispheres

Astrocytoma, causing homologous ataxia, is the most frequent tumor of the cerebellar hemisphere. Pylocytic astrocytoma (WHO Gr. I), mentioned earlier in the text, has the highest incidence, but could be cured by surgery. Glioma of higher degree of malignancy could be found in brainstem or cerebellar hemispheres, although infrequently.

a) Astrocytoma

Intraaxial astrocytoma of the posterior cranial fossa have identical features in CT scan as supratentorial ones (Fig. 160).

Pylocytic astrocytoma (Gr. I) seen in children and adolescents is a separate entity. Earlier, this tumor was referred to as polar spongioblastoma or juvenile astrocytoma of the cerebellar hemisphere.

Pylocytic astrocytoma has a cystic portion, filled with yellowish or dark liquid with high protein contents, and solid mural portion. Histology of astrocytoma is confirmed by Rosenthal fibres and granular bodies presence.

Astrocytoma of the posterior cranial fossa has favorable prognosis; when radically resected it does not recur in the majority of cases.

b) Hemangioblastoma

Hemangioblastoma has been described earlier in the text, and most often it affects cerebellar hemispheres. Clinical appearance is manifested by headache, hydrocephalus and ataxia.

Hemangioblastoma in T-2W sequence has high signal intensities and is hard to delineate from the surrounding edema. In T-1W sequence hemangioblastoma have low signal intensities as well as edema (Fig. 161). Therefore it is impossible to define tumor from edema in T-1W or T-2W sequences because of changed anatomy. Paramagnetic contrast application in T-1W sequence enhances signal intensity of hemangioblastoma enabling optimal demarcation from peritumoral edema (18). Fourth ventricle can be compressed or dyslocated depending on tumor size and location.

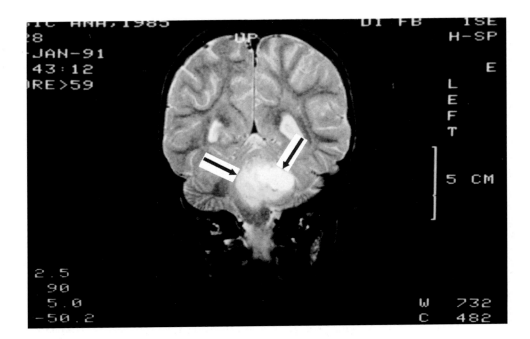

Figure 160. Coronal image (SE 2500/90). Astrocytoma located mediosagittally, centrally in cerebellum and parasagittally bilaterally, predominantly in the left side. Tumor is cystic with higher signal intensities - arrows. Slight perifocal edema has higher signal intensities.

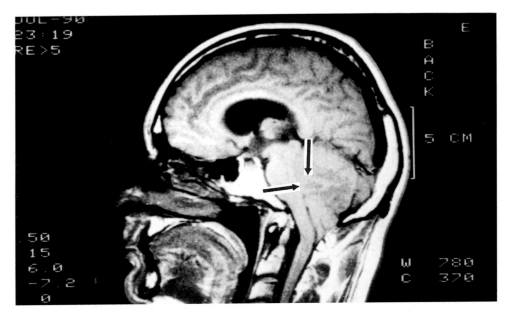

Figure 161. Sagittal image (SE 500/15). Fourth ventricle filled by hemangioblastoma, compressed cerebellum and subsequent obstructive internal hydrocephalus. Tumor has slightly lower signal intensities - arrows.

Surgical treatment provides for radical cure by complete removal of the tumor in majority of the cases.

c) Cavernoma

Cavernoma (described earlier) of the posterior fossa dos not have specific features except the symptomatology induced by precise location of the tumor. Symptomatology is absent or non-specific. Cavernoma can cause obstructive internal hydrocephalus exceptionally and there is no perifocal edema.

Most often cavernomas are accidentally discovered during MR imaging.

Cavernoma can be recognized by intraparenchymatous bleeding, when surgery is indicated even for delicate location. General condition and age of patient, as well as multiplicity of lesions, should be considered.

MR examination is dominant to CT or angiography for the diagnosis of cavernoma. Those occult A-V malformation could be recognized by their prominent features, either in the posterior fossa or supratentorially (Figg. 162, 163).

Cavernoma is treated surgically.

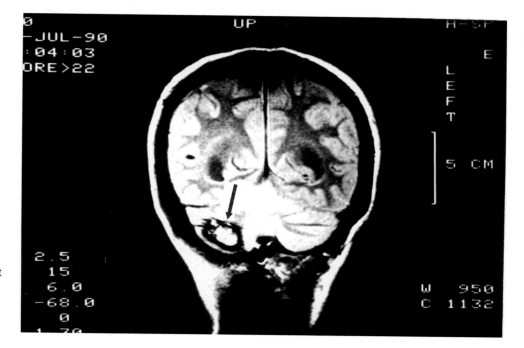

Figure 162. Coronal image (SE 2500/15). Big cavernoma, with prominent hemosiderin edge of low signal intensity, is shown in the right cerebellar hemisphere -black arrow. Smaller cavernoma is seen in periventricular, supratentorial area.

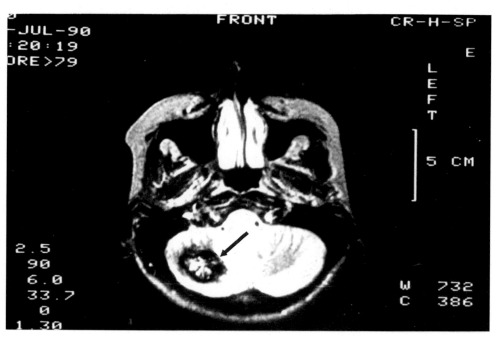

Figure 163. Axial image (SE 2500/90). Cavernoma in the same patient, displayed in Double echo sequence - arrow.

d) Angioma

Smaller angioma, especially in the posterior fossa, are rarely detected by CT examination.

MR imaging can help differentiate the smaller angioma and make the indication for angiography to confirm the diagnosis. Special sequences enable better visualization of angioma, but paramagnetic contrast is occasionally required (8, 15).

Angiomas are shown as various shapes of pathologic blood vessels, with higher signal intensities. Eventual calcifications are shown in all sequences with extremely low signal intensities (Fig. 164).

Surgical principles in the treatment of posterior fossa angiomas are similar to those applied for suprasellar ones (see previous text). Angioma staging after Spetzler is a valuable one, for it considers the size, type of drainage and location for the planning of surgery. Gamma knife is suitable for angiomas less than 3 cm in diameter.

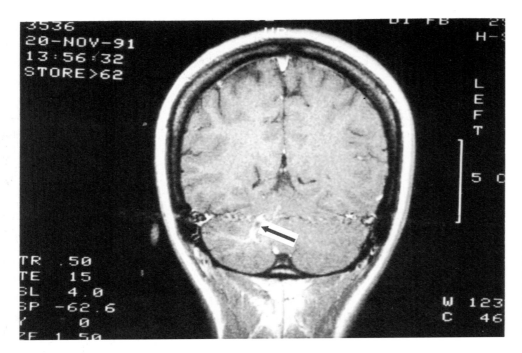

Figure 164. Coronal image (SE 500/15) after gadolinium-DTPA administration. Smaller angioma in a form of irregular, wide blood vessel in the right cerebellar hemisphere - arrow.

e) Metastases

Intracranial metastases are the most frequent tumors of endocranium. They outnumber total of all other intracranial tumors. It has been attributed to the advances in treatment for primary malignancies and extended survival, thus enabling development of intracranial metastase. Intracranial metastases are infratentorial in 10-15% of all intracranial metastases, with brainstem location in 3-5% of cases. Incidence of metastases in those regions is higher than could be expected proportional to the mass or volume. The reason for this has not been explained yet (10).

Multiplicity, marked vasogenous edema and compression effect are basic features of the metastatic growths.

According to our experience, cerebellar metastases are usually of pulmonar origin in males and breast origin in females, but the metastases originating in digestive tract or pelvic organs are seen as well (10).

Clinical manifestations are due to increased intracranial pressure or focal cerebellar deficit.

Metastases could be well shown by CT scan, especially after contrast application.

MR imaging has advantages for posterior fossa metastases. Multiple lesions, overlooked by CT, could often be proved by MR examination. This could alter therapeutic approach considerably.

Multiple metastatic deposits have identical MR features both supratentorially and infratentorially (Figg. 165, 166).

MR imaging with contrast application helps confirm or rule out suspected intracranial metastases and define their precise number and location (20).

Therapeutic approach considers surgery, radiotherapy and chemotherapy, regarding the number, location and type of secondary deposits.

4. Primary tumors of the brainstem

Tumors of the brainstem are divided into several groups by Konovalov (18).

Tumors of the mesencephalon (small thecal focal tumors, lateral tumors of mesencephalon, exophytic tumors propagating towards upper vermis and posterior portion of the third ventricle) (Fig. 167).

Tumors of the pons - diffuse and focal, exophytic propagating dorsally - into fourth ventricle, laterally - to cerebellopontine cistern and ventrally - to parapontine cistern (Figg. 168-170),

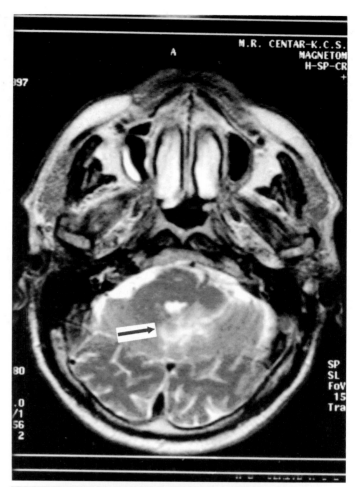

Figure 165. Axial image (SE 4000/99). Poorly defined metastasis of bronchus carcinoma in the left cerebellar hemisphere, in patient G.I. - arrow.

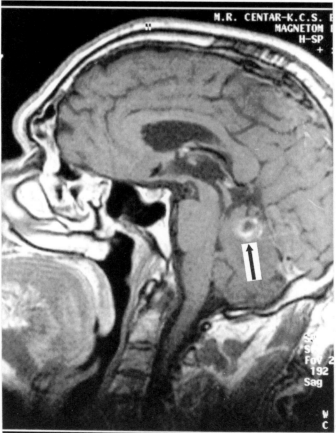

Figure 166. Sagittal image (SE 500/15) after gadolinium-DTPA administration. Clearly demarcated metastasis of bronchus carcinoma and perifocal edema in the same patient (G.I.) - arrow.

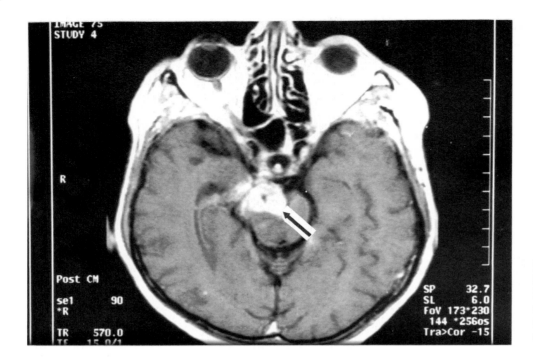

Figure 167. Axial image (SE 570/15) after gadolinium-DTPA administration. Tumor of the mesencephalon is clearly demarcated after contrast application - arrow.

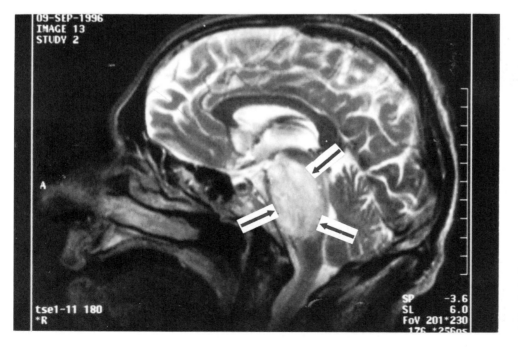

Figure 168. Sagittal image (SE 4000/99). Arrows pointing at infiltrative expansive lesion in pons and mesencephalon. Infiltrative tumor could not be delineated from edema, even in (SE 500/15) after gadolinium-DTPA administration.

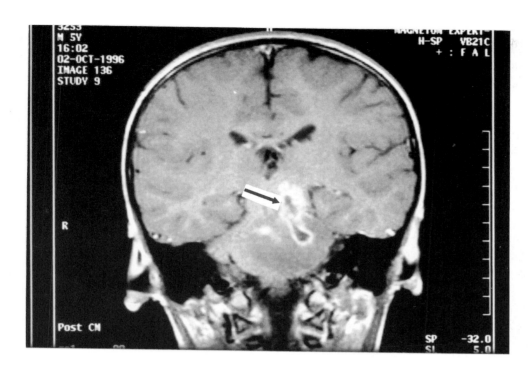

Figure 169. Coronal image (SE 500/15) after gadolinium-DTPA administration. Infiltrative cystic-necrotic tumor of the pons and mesencephalon with marginal enhancement of signal intensities - arrow.

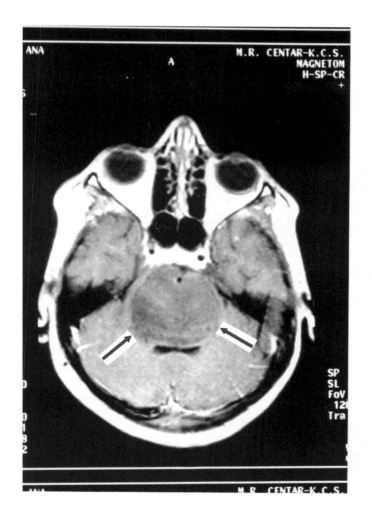

Figure 170. Axial image (SE 560/15) after gadolinium-DTPA administration. Tumor of the pons is inseparable from surrounding edema and does not change signal intensity in (SE 560/15) after gadolinium-DTPA administration.

Tumors of the medulla oblongata - diffuse midline, propagating rostrally towards pons and/or caudally towards medulla spinalis, and focal, being solid or cystic (Fig. 171).

Cervicomedullar tumors - with caudal or rostral propagation (Fig. 172).

Other pathologic lesions, such as metastases, hematoma, cavernoma, etc. could be found in the brainstem as well.

Brainstem tumors induce progressive cranial nerve impairment, as well as long motor and sensory pathways disorders, thus causing various altern syndromes. Headache, vomiting, fainting spells and instability are caused by increased intracranial pressure. Patient could be bradypsychic and torpid. Sudden death could arise because of the compression of the vital centres in the brainstem.

CT examination with i.v. application of the iodine contrast enables moderate visualization of the tumor.

Multiplanar MR, particularly in T-1W sequence with paramagnetic contrast administration provides for precise location and demarcation of the tumor from normal anatomy structures and edema. Certain tumors do not enhance after contrast administration. MR features of tumors in this area are similar to the same tumors elsewhere (10).

Clinical studies have justified shunt surgery for tumors of low biological potential. Exophytic, cervicomedullar and focal tumors propagating towards brainstem surface are generally resectable with reasonable operative risk, if microsurgery, cavitron ultrasonic suction and laser are applied, whereas open or stereotaxic biopsy should be used for deep focal or global brainstem tumors.

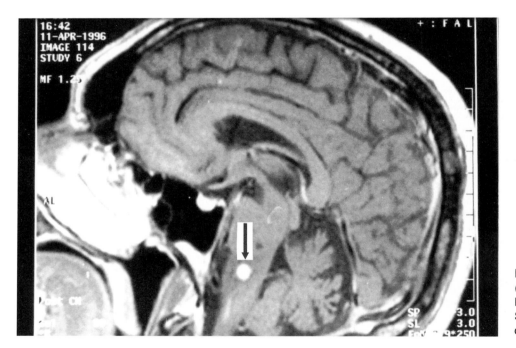

Figure 171. Sagittal image (SE 570/15) after gadolinium-DTPA administration. Small, well demarcated tumor of medullla oblongata - arrow.

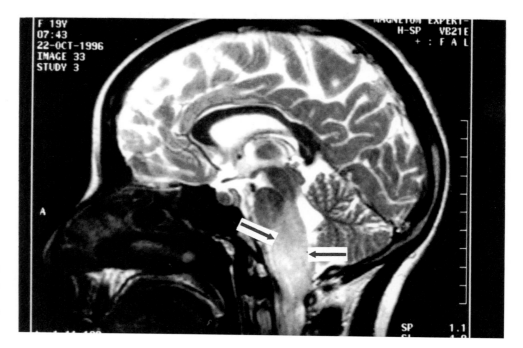

Figure 172. Sagittal image (SE 4000/99). Infiltrative tumor of medulla oblongata and incipient medulla spinalis (craniocervical junction area). Tumor does not change in (SE 560/15) after gadolinium-DTPA administration.

REFERENCES

1. Al-Mefty 0: Meningiomas. Raven Press. New York, 1991.
2. Berger MS., Wilson CB.: Epidermoid cystis of the posterior fossa. J. Neurosurg., 62: 214-219, 1985.
3. Bird CR., Hasso AN., LeBeau DJ.: Meningiomas and skull base neoplasms. Magn. Reson. Imag., 1: 52-62, 1989.
4. Coates TL., et al.: Pediatric choroid plexus neoplasms: MR, CT and pathologic correlation. Radiology, 173: 81-88, 1989.
5. Curati WL., Graif M., Kingsley DPE., Niendorf HP., Young IR.: Acoustic neuromas: Gd-DTPA enhancement in MR imaging. Radiology, 158: 447-451, 1986.
6. Halbsgut A., Lechner B.: Magnetresonanz-Tomographie (NMR). Springer-Verlag. Frankfurt, 1986.
7. Hasso AN., Kwon TS.: Infratentorial and cerebellopontine angle tumors: MRI strategies. MRI Decisions, 4: 2-6, 1990.
8. Huk WJ., Gademann G., Friedman G.: Magnetic Resonance Imaging of Central Nervous System Diseases. Springer Verlag. Berlin, New York, Heidelberg, Tokyo, Paris, London, 1989.
9. Liessner J., Seider M.: Klinische Kernspintomographie. Enke. Stuttgart, 1987.
10. Packer RJ., et al.: Magnetic resonance imaging of lesions of the posterior fossa and upper cervical cord in childhood. Pediatrics, 76: 84-92, 1985.
11. Pomeranz JS.: Craniospinal Magnetic Resonance Imaging. W.B. Saunders Company. Philadelphia, London, Toronto, Sydney, Tokyo, 1989.
12. Press GA., Hesselink JR.: MR imaging of cerebellopontine angle and internal auditory canal lesions at 1,5T. Am. J. Neuroradiol., 9: 241-247, 1988.
13. Randell CP., Collins AG., Young IR., Haywood R., Thomas DJ., Mcn Donnell MJ., Orr JS., Bydder GM., Steiner RE.: Nuclear magnetic resonance imaging of posterior fossa tumors. AJNR, 4: 1027-1034, 1983.
14. Reiser M., et al.: Magnet-rezonanz-Tomographie. Springer-Verlag. Berlin, Heidelberg, New York, Paris, London, Tokyo, Hong Kong, 1989.
15. Spetzler RF., et al.: A proposed grading system for arteriovenous malformations. J. Neurosurg., 65: 476-483, 1986.
16. Spoto GP., et al.: Intracranial ependymoma and subependymoma: MR manifestations. AJR, 154: 837-843, 1990.
17. Stark D., Bradley GWJR.: Magnetic Resonance Imaging. The C.V. Mosby Company. St. Louis, Washington D.C., Toronto, 1988.
18. Vignaud J., et al.: NMR imaging of intraaxial tumours of the posterior fossa. J. Neuroradiol., 11: 249-257, 1984.
19. Zawadcki MB., Norman D.: Magnetic Resonance Imaging of the Central Nervous System. Raven Press. New York, 1987.
20. Zeitler E.: Kernspintomographie. Deutsche Artze Verlag. Koeln, 1984.

VIII. TUMORS OF THE CRANIOCERVICAL JUNCTION

Gradimir Dragutinović, Miodrag Rakić, Ljiljana Djordjić

Both intraaxial and extraaxial expansive processes belong to this group of tumors.

Neurinoma, meningioma, ependymoma, chordoma, A-V malformations, metastases, etc. are usually seen in craniocervical junction area (17).

There are several options: the tumor either propagates from posterior fossa to the cervical region, or invades endocranium from a cervical area, or arises primarily in the craniocervical junction.

Tumors of the craniocervical junction are hard to recognize because of atypical symptomatology. Progressive quadriparesis in the beginning is usually attributed to multiple sclerosis, especially if accompanied by the sensitive symptoms or nystagmus due to spinocerebellar lesion. Invasion of the posterior fossa is followed by cerebellar signs and impairment of inferior cranial nerves (12).

Sensibility level is hard to determine and should be searched for carefully in the neck region. Sphincter disorders are usually absent.

Queckenstedts test is not always positive and there is no hyperproteinorachia in CFS.

Neuroradiology is not sufficiently precise in showing detailed anatomy, particularly the soft tissues of the craniocervical junction.

Classic, special and polytomographic radiographs could suggest bone destruction.

CT scan might display soft tissue pathology, but artifacts caused by bone structures could interfere with reliable diagnosis. Reconstruction planes do not provide for precise spatial location of the tumor (1, 15).

MR examination is a method of choice for investigation of craniocervical junction pathology and tumors in particular (5).

MR image can reveal neurinoma, meningioma, ependymoma, chrodoma, A-V malformations, metastases, etc. located in craniocervical junction area (13).

Slice thickness should be 3-4 mm and distance 0.1-2 for MR tomographs in sagittal, coronal or axial view. Classic sequences are used normally, but special sequences and intravenous administration of paramagnetic contrast may be required for certain tumors (2, 3).

a) Neurinoma

Neurinoma and meningioma of the craniocervical junction are similar, often atypical in their clinical appearance, and could be misjudged for a progressive degenerative disease or MS.

It is hard to determine the type of tumor upon MRI, except for the fact that meningiomas are usually located ventrally and neurinomas laterally.

Neurinoma is best shown by multiplanar MRI in T-1W sequence after intravenous administration of paramagnetic contrast (4, 10). Paramagnetic contrast helps to assess the tumor volume precisely, which is important for surgery planning (Figg. 173, 174).

b) Meningioma mixtus

Meningioma mixtus is a combination of meningoendothelial and fibroblastic meningioma. Vascular stroma is poorly developed as compared to fibrous septa and tissues.

Mixed neurinoma and mixed meningioma of the craniocervical junction have similar signal intensities in MR tomographs. Intravenous injection of paramagnetic contrast does not change the signal inten-

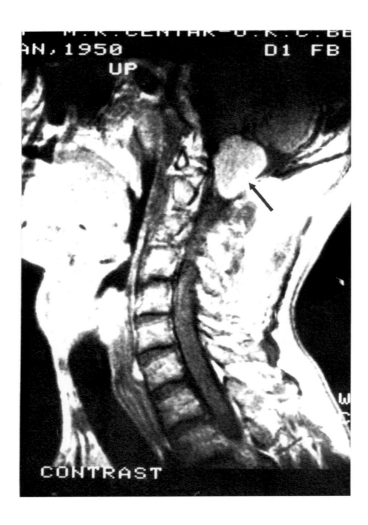

Figure 173. Sagittal image (SE 500/15). Well defined extramedullar neurinoma with high signal intensities is shown in the craniocervical junction area - arrow.

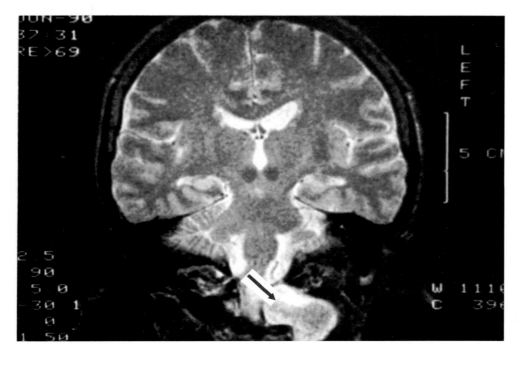

Figure 174. Coronal image (SE 2500/90). Neurofibroma in the craniocervical junction area (white arrows), causing myelomalacia of the medullae spinalis - black arrow.

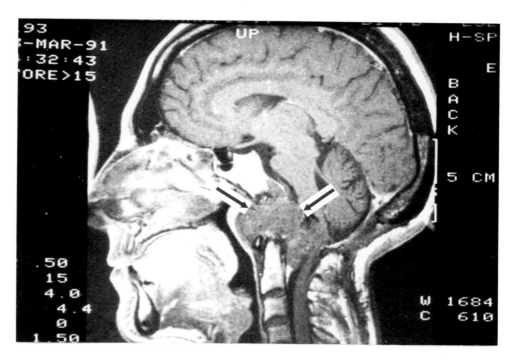

Figure 175. - Sagittal image (SE 500/15) after gadolinium-DTPA administration. Patient J.S. Mixed neurinoma of the craniocervical junction compresses medulla oblongata and incipient medulla spinalis - arrows. Mixed neurinoma has destroyed clivus and reached nasopharynx through endocranial route. Contrast application did not change signal intensities of the tumor. Operative finding: pathohistologically proven mixed neurinoma.

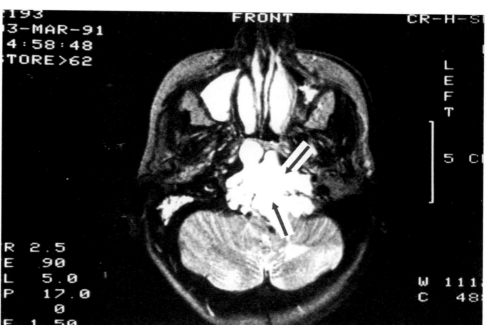

Figure 176. Axial image (SE 2500/90). Mixed neurinoma in the same patient (J.S.) - arrows.

sities substantially (6, 7). Sometimes, it is hard to tell mixed neurinoma or meningioma from a chordoma (Figg. 175, 176).

c) Meningioma

Signal intensities of meningioma in MRI in T-1W sequence are quite different form a normal brain parenchyma, so that paramagnetic contrast is not necessary (Figg. 177, 178). Paramagnetic contrast enhances signal intensities of the tumor and could be used if precise volume assessment or demarcation from surrounding edema is required (8, 13).

Meningiomas and neurinomas are treated surgically, using modern techniques, through posterior or postero-lateral approach or anterior access for the ventral tumors.

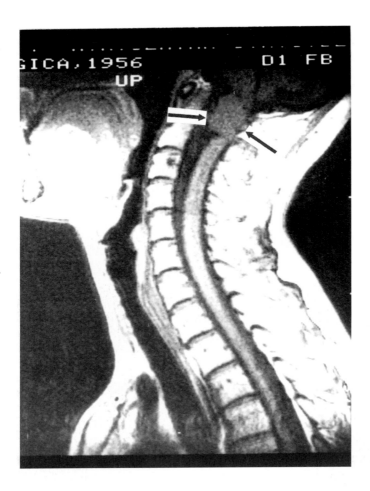

Figure 177. Sagittal image (SE 500/15). Ventral extradural meningioma in the craniocervical junction, causes the compression of the incipient medulla spinalis - arrows.

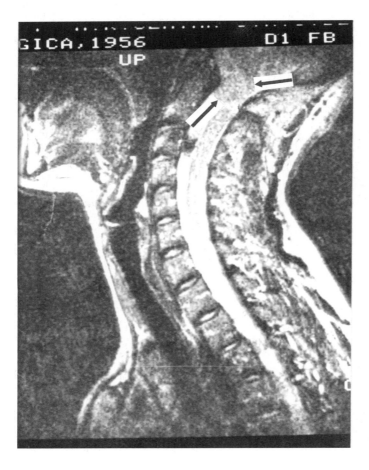

Figure 178. Sagittal image (SE 2000/90). Ventral extradural meningioma in the craniocervical junction, causes the compression of the incipient medulla spinalis - arrows.

d) A-V malformation

A-V malformation is well differentiated in MR imaging. FLASH sequences for slow and rapid blood flow are used (9, 11, 16). Standard sequences help the differential diagnosis (Figg. 179, 180). MR angiography has been used recently.

Indications for surgical treatment of A-V malformations vary depending on location, size and total vascularization of the lesion.

e) Ependymoma

Big ependymomas could propagate towards craniocervical junction and involve incipient medulla spinalis. Ependymoma is shown with high signal intensities in T-1W sequence after contrast administration (9, 14, 17) (Fig. 181).

Ependymoma should be treated by a radical surgery and eventual restoration of compromised liquor circulation (drainage).

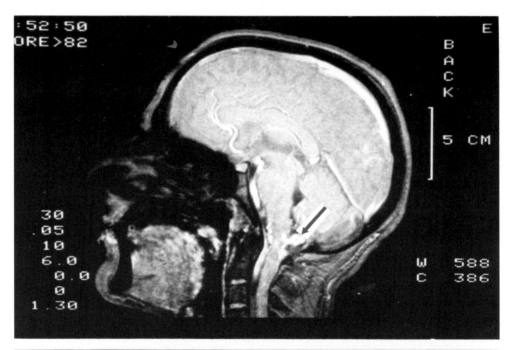

Figure 179. Sagittal image (SE FL 30 TR 50 TE 10) A-V malformation with high signal intensities is shown in the region of craniocervical junction on the dorsal medulla oblongata and medulla spinalis - arrow.

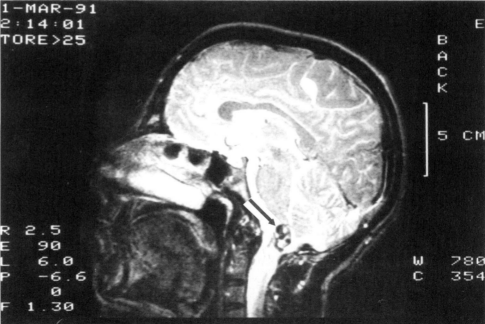

Figure 180. Sagittal image (SE 2500/90). A-V malformation is shown in dorsal medulla oblongata and medulla spinalis in craniocervical junction area, as a band of low signal intensities.

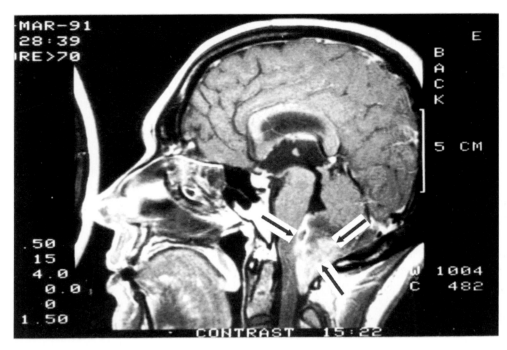

Figure 181. Sagittal image (SE 500/15) after gadolinium-DTPA administration. Ependymoma with high signal intensities shown in craniocervical junction - arrows pointing at a tumor.

REFERENCES

1. Bories J.: Computerized Axial Tomography. Springer-Verlag. Berlin, Heidelberg, New York, 1978.
2. Daniels D., Haughton V., Naidich T.: Cranial and Spinal Magnetic Resonance Imaging-An Atlas and Guide. Raven Press. New York, 1987.
3. Gademann G.: NMR-Tomography of the Normal Brain. Springer-Verlag. Berlin, Heidelberg, New York, Tokyo, 1988.
4. Halbsgut A., Lechner B.: Magnetresonanz-Tomographie (NMR). Springer-Verlag. Frankfurt, 1986.
5. Holland GN., Hawkes RC., Moore WS.: Nuclear Magnetic Resonance (NMR) tomography of the brain: Coronal and sagittal section. J. Comput. Tomogr., 4: 429-433, 1980.
6. Huk WJ., Gademann G., Friedman G.: Magnetic Resonance Imaging of Central Nervous System Diseases. Springer-Verlag. Berlin, New York, Heidelberg, Tokyo, Paris, London, 1989.
7. Kazner E., Wende S., Grumme Th.: Computer und Kernspin-Tomographie intrakranialler Tumoren aus klinischen Sicht. Springer-Verlag. Berlin, Heidelberg, New York, London, Paris, Tokyo, 1989.
8. Kovacs K., Miller M.: Intracranial Tumors of Infants and Children. Georg Thieme Verlag. Stuttgart, pp. 213-220, 1971.
9. Liessner J., Seider M.: Klinische Kernspintomographie. Enke. Stuttgart, 1987.
10. Pomeranz JS.: Craniospinal Magnetic Resonance Imaging. W.B. Saunders Company. Philadelphia, London, Toronto, Sydney, Tokyo, 1989.
11. Reiser M., et al.: Magnet-rezonanz-Tomographie. Springer-Verlag. Berlin, Heidelberg, New York, Paris, London, Tokyo, Hong Kong, 1989.
12. Russel D., Rubinstein L.: Pathology of Tumors of the Nervous System. Edward Arnold. London, 1977.
13. Stark D., Bradley GWJR.: Magnetic Resonance Imaging. The C.V. Mosby Company. St. Louis, Washington D.C., Toronto, 1988.
14. Van M. Runge: Enhanced Magnetic Resonance Imaging. The C.V. Mosby Company. St. Louis, Baltimore, Toronto, 1989.
15. Wackenheim A., Jeanmart L., Beart A.: Craniocerebral Computer Tomography. , Berlin, Heidelberg, New York, Vol.1, 1980.
16. Zawadcki MB., Norman D.: Magnetic Resonance Imaging of the Central Nervous System. Raven Press. New York, 1987.
17. Zeitler E.: Kernspintomographie. Deutsche Artze Verlag. Koeln, 1984.

IX. EXTRACRANIAL TUMORS WITH INTRACRANIAL PROPAGATION

Vaso Antunović, Gradimir Dragutinović, Ivan Piščević

This specific group of tumors consists of nasal cavity carcinoma, tumors of paranasal sinuses, adenoid cystic carcinoma, nasopharyngeal tumors, rhabdomyosarcoma, angiofibroma, paraganglioma, optic nerve glioma, etc.

Clinical appearance depends on tumor type and location. Aggressive growth of those neoplasm usually causes non-specific symptoms, unrelated to neurologic symptomatology. Interdisciplinary coordination is required for the assessment and determination of therapy modalities.

Tumors of the cranial base or neigbouring extracranial structures could induce bone destruction and subsequent endocranial propagation.

Standard and special radiographs, as well as polytomographs can reveal lesions that have caused bone destruction in the facial massive, orbit or cranial base. Radiographs should determine bone destruction, foramina enlargement, etc.

Native or contrast CT scan contribute to a diagnosis of soft tissue mass of the neoplasm and its intracranial propagation. CT scan is usually sufficient for the diagnosis and choice of treatment, especially if combined with pathohistology obtained by biopsy of easily accessible tumor.

CT examination has advantage over any other diagnostic method, because it could show bone structures, especially the cranial base, and soft tissue tumor at the same time (1).

MR examination is seldom indicated, if CT scan and radiographies are inconclusive or tumor volume could not be estimated precisely (3, 4).

a) Chordoma

Chordoma (see earlier) is extracranial tumor, which destructs bones of the cranial base, thus invading endocranium. Basic advantage of MR image over CT scan is a multiplanar tumor display with precise definition of a tumor from normal anatomy structures (9) (Fig. 182).

b) Nasopharyngeal adenocarcinoma

Nasopharyngeal adenocarcinoma is malignancy, that propagates to sphenoidal and ethmoidal sinuses, destructs cranial bone and invades endocranium. Tumor propagation to parapharyngeal space and oropharynx should be observed with care.

Origin of extended malignancies of the ethmoid, such as squamous cell carcinoma and adenocarcinoma, is hard to assess.

Tumor biopsy is required for definiton of the tumor type and origin, as well as for determination of further treatment.

Multiplanar MR imaging in classic T-1W and T-2W sequences, enables demarcation of tumor from normal anatomy structures (6, 7, 10).

As compared to normal soft tissues of the nasopharynx, adenocarcinoma has equal or slightly decreased signal intensities in T-1W sequence (Fig. 183). Infiltration and compression of brain parenchyma induced by a tumor is shown in T-2W sequence.

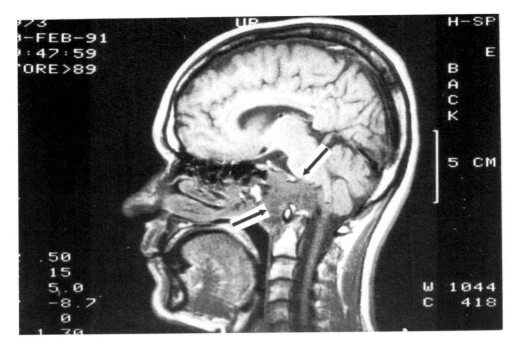

Figure 182. Sagittal image (SE 500/15). Well delineated chordoma with lower signal intensities, in the projection of markedly destroyed clivus. Tumor propagates towards posterior cranial fossa, as well as towards nasopharynx and sphenoidal sinus - arrows.

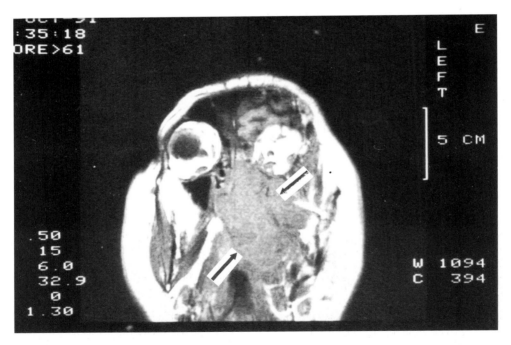

Figure 183. Coronal image (SE 500/15). Huge adenocarcinoma of the nasopharynx, obturates nasal cavity, left maxillary sinus and partly mesopharynx. Tumor infiltrates left orbit, sphenoid and ethmoid and propagates endocranially. Tumor has mixed lower signal intensities - arrows.

c) Squamous cell carcinoma of nasopharynx

Squamous cell carcinoma of nasopharynx invades sphenoid and ethmoid, destructs bones of the cranial base and extends to the anterior, middle and posterior cranial fossa. Paramagnetic contrast in T-1W sequences enhances signal intensities of carcinoma and enables multiplanar assessment of its volume and routes of extension (Fig. 184).

It is important to stress that incipient carcinoma of nasopharynx, ethmoid and sphenoid could not be differentiated from non-specific inflammation, unless bone destruction is present. Tumor biopsy from several locations is a method of choice for the diagnosis of malignant tumors in this region.

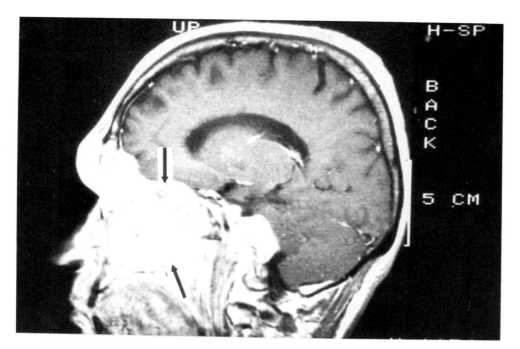

Figure 184. Sagittal image (SE 500/15) after gadolinium-DTPA administration. Enormous squamous cell carcinoma of nasopharynx, with higher signal intensities, fills right nasal cavity, maxillar, ethmoidal, sphenoidal and frontal sinuses and orbit. Tumor propagates intracranially, infiltrating right cavernous sinus, destructing clivus and shifting ventral portion of pons and medulla oblongata - arrows.

d) Squamous cell carcinoma of maxilla and zygomatic bone

Squamous cell carcinoma of maxilla is a neoplasm with invasive growth and destruction of surrounding bones. Maxillar carcinoma has a tendency to invade orbit, nasal cavity, ethmoid and sphenoid, as well as endocranium.

MR tomographs in T-2W sequence shows tumor mass of squamous cell carcinoma in hypo and isointensive signals, whereas a huge edema of temporal regions of the brain, caused by infiltration and compression by carcinoma is hyperintensive (Fig. 185). Paramagnetic contrast application helps to demarcate tumor from edema (8, 11) (Fig. 186).

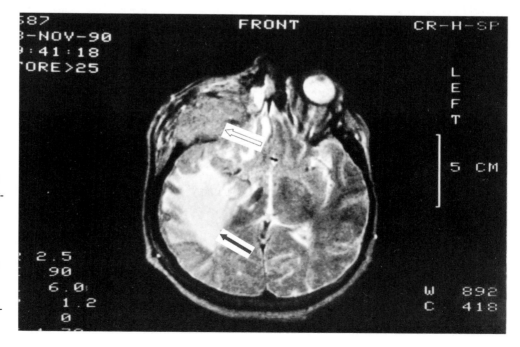

Figure 185. Axial image (SE 2500/90). Squamous cell carcinoma of the right maxilla with right orbit destruction and intracranial extension. Tumor mass in right frontotemporal area is isointensive - white arrow, and surrounded by a huge, irregular edema with high signal intensities - black arrow.

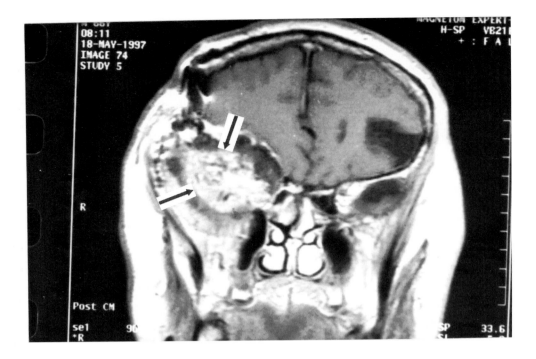

Figure 186. Coronal image (SE 500/15) after gadolinium-DTPA administration. Arrows pointing at mixed hyperintensive carcinoma of the right zygomatic bone with propagation to the maxillar sinus, orbit and endocranium, in the right temporo-basal region.

e) Benign tumor of the pterygoid fossa

Various benign tumors could be found in the pterygoid fossa and parapharyngeal region. Crucial feature of the benign tumors is slow growth and compression of the surrounding structures, which induce symptomatology.

Precise multiplanar display obtained by CT and MR examinations have enabled surgical resection without sequels (2, 5).

MR tomographs in T-1W sequence shows a tumor with non-homogenous high signal intensity in the pterygoid fossa with invasion of the middle cranial fossa. Multiplanar display in T-1W is sufficient to indicate neurosurgical treatment. Tumor is perfectly delineated from normal structures, clearly demarcated and according to tissue characteristics with high lipid contents. Tumor is probaly benign; possibly it is teratoma. Pathohistology is unknown (Fig. 187).

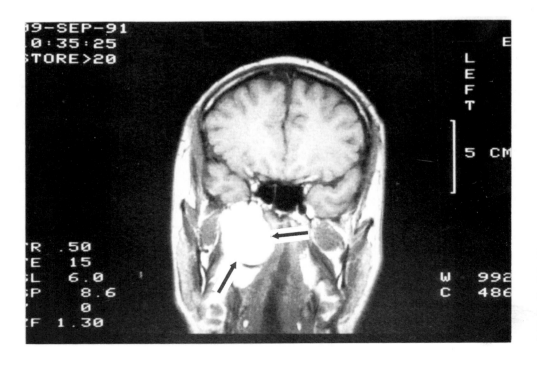

Figure 187. Coronal image (SE 500/15). Benign tumor with non-homogenous high signal intensities in the right pteryngoid fossa, propagating towards endocranium - arrows.

f) Optic nerve glioma

Optic nerve gliomas in children are usually benign, whereas in adults they are often malignant. Few percents of benign optic nerve tumors regard Recklinghausen disease.

Glioma of the optic nerve is hard to dissect from the optic nerve and its growth compromises optic bulb shifting it outwards. Apart from destruction of the normal orbital structures, they tend to invade endocranium and destruct optic nerve canal (6).

MR examination enables multiplanar display of the tumor (Fig. 188). Malignant glioma is hard to tell from the optic nerve, whereas MR image can clearly demarcate tumor from the other anatomic structures of the orbit (10).

Surgical treatment of the tumors of paranasal sinuses and cranial base, with endocranial extension, by the experienced team including head and neck surgeon, ENT surgeon, ophthalmologist surgeon and neurosurgeon, consisting of radical excision of the tumor and cranial base and dural reconstruction, through a combined transcranial-transfacial approach, have achieved favorable results recently. Postoperative radiotherapy, depending on histology, could have positive effects.

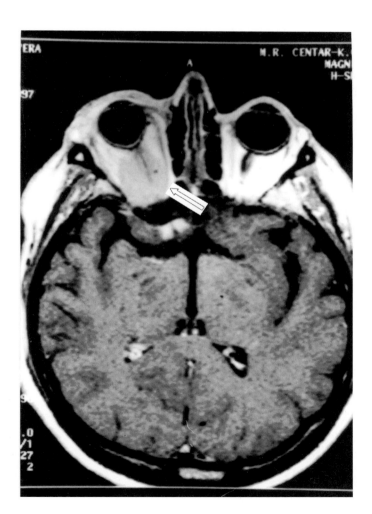

Figure 188. Axial image (SE 500/15) after gadolinium-DTPA administration. Retrobulbar optic nerve tumor invades orbita and tends to propagate endocranially - arrow.

REFERENCES

1. Bories J.: Computerized Axial Tomography. Springer-Verlag. Berlin, Heidelberg, New York, 1978.
2. Curtin HD., Wiliams R., Johnson J.: CT of perineural tumor extension: pterygopalatine fossa. AM J. Neuroradiol., 5: 731-740, 1984.
3. Halbsgut A., Lechner B.: Magnet-resonanz-Tomographie (NMR). Springer-Verlag. Frankfurt, 1986.
4. Huk WJ., Gademann G., Friedman G.: Magnetic Resonance Imaging of Central Nervouss System Diseases. Springer-Verlag. Berlin, New York, Heidelberg, Tokyo, Paris, London, 1989.
5. Laine FJ., et al.: Perineural tumor extension through the foramen ovale: evaluation with MR imaging. Radiology, 174: 65-75, 1990.
6. Liessner J., Seider M.: Klinische Kernspintomographie. Enke. Stuttgart, 1987.
7. Pomeranz JS.: Craniospinal Magnetic Resonance Imaging. W.B. Saunders Company. Philadelphia, London, Toronto, Sydney, Tokyo, 1989.
8. Reiser M., et al.: Magnet-rezonanz-Tomographie. Springer-Verlag. Berlin, Heidelberg, New York, Paris, London, Tokyo, Hong Kong, 1989.
9. Stark D., Bradley GWJR.: Magnetic Resonance Imaging. The C.V. Mosby Company. St. Louis, Washington D.C., Toronto, 1988.
10. Zawadcki MB., Norman D.: Magnetic Resonance Imaging of the Central Nervous System. Raven Press. New York, 1987.
11. Zeitler E.: Kernspintomographie. Deutsche Artze Verlag. Koeln, 1984.

X. TUMORS OF THE HYPOPHYSIS

Gradimir Dragutinović, Vaso Antunović, Miroslav Samardzić

Tumors of the hypophysis are the most important tumors of the sellar region. Extrasellar tumors are rare and induce neurologic disorders.

Hypophyseal tumors are hormone secreting adenomas and other non-secreting tumors.

Regarding the size microtumors or microadenomas are less than 10 mm in diameter and macrotumors or macroadenomas exceed 10 mm.

Intrasellar tumors can propagate parasellary, suprasellary or infrasellary. Enormous tumors can extend retrosellar or even infratentorially to the posterior fossa.

Hormone secreting hypophyseal tumors are:

HGH (human growth hormone) cell adenomas (densely or scarcely granulated)

PRL (prolactine) cell adenomas (densely or scarcely granulated)

HGH and PRL mixed adenomas

"stem" cell acidophylic adenoma

ACTH (corticotropic) cell adenomas (scarcely or densely granulated)

TSH (thyreotropic) cell adenomas (scarcely or densely granulated)

FSH and LH (gonadotropic) cell adenomas (scarcely or densely granulated)

undifferentiated cell adenomas (oncocytic and non-oncocytic).

According to the histological type, hormone secreting tumors can be papillar, sinusoid, diffuse or mixed.

Non-secreting tumors can be either chromofob or chromafine adenoma.

Tumors of neurohypophysis are astrocytoma and pituicytoma.

Tumors of the hypophyseal stalk (*infundibulum*) are primary or secondary. Primary tumors are germinoma, "stem cell" tumor, pituicytoma, granuloma, etc.

Expansive processes in the sellar region, apart from hypophyseal tumors, are craniopharyngioma, meningioma, epidermoid, dermoid, Rathkes cyst, germinoma, etc. (30)

Extrasellar expansive processes are meningioma, chiasmal glioma, suprasellar craniopharyngioma, germinoma, etc.

Pseudotumors include intrasellar aneurysm, intracavernous a-v shunt, infundibular recess dilation and "Empty sella syndrome" as a separate entity.

Neuroradiologic classification of the hypophyseal and all sellar tumors is made according to the local finding and size:

I grade - tumors which do not cause local deformities

II grade - local enlargement of sella without extrasellar propagation

III grade- enlargement of sella with orosion of walls

IV grade- invasion of surrounding structures (33).

Endocrinology examination is crucial for the diagnosis of secretory hypophyseal adenoma. Endocrine disorders caused by hyperproduction or insufficiency of certain hormones are indication for further radiologic examination (14).

The only neurologic symptom of the intrasellar tumor is a headache for quite a long time.

Extrasellar extension of the tumor is followed by the rupture of the sellar diaphragm, cessation of the headache and chiasmal compression with visual field impairment. As the inferior crossed fibers are first to be invaded by the expansive process, bitemporal anopsia in the superior quadrants will show. The further growth of the tumor will destruct all of chiasmal crossed fibres, causing complete bitemporal hemianopsia. The rest of the neurologic symptoms will depend on the tumor propagation. Compression of hypothalamus will induce *diabetes insipidus,* somnolence and hypothermia, and invasion of the temporal lobe will cause epilepsia.

Parasellar propagation can damage bulbomotors, i.e. n III, IV and VI, as well as V-1 and V-2 branches of trigeminal nerve. In huge intra, para and suprasellar tumors optic chiasm could be combined with impairment of parasellar cranial nerves.

Neuro-opthalmologic examination is essential for the early diagnosis of suprasellar extension of the tumor.

Classic radiographs of sella (special profile views, polytomographs, etc.) can help to discover bone pathology of the sella, thus enabling diagnosis of bigger tumors (grades II-IV) (3, 10).

Mini gas cisternography using a small amount of air is the history.

Cerebral angiography is important for extrasellar tumors to display morphology and position of major blood vessels in parasellar and suprasellar region.

Angiography is important for the diagnosis of pseudotumors, i.e. aneurysms, which can simulate tumor.

CT examination is sufficient for the diagnosis of majority of intrasellar microadenoma and particularly macrotumors. Intravenous application of iodine contrast is obligatory. Axial view with reconstruction of coronal and sagittal planes, as well as direct coronal view with reconstruction of the sagittal plane are used in CT examination (7, 8, 15, 26).

Magnetic resonance have some advantages:
- higher resolution and better visualization of tumor
- direct multiplanar display
- no ionizing radiation
- frequent controls, without any harm to the patient, are possible.

Specific MR imaging technique is required for the following reasons:
sellar region is directly visualized in axial, sagittal and coronal views in T-1W sequence;
same views are used following Magnevist administration;
slice thickness is 2-3 mm;
slice distance is 0.1-2.

Duration of the examination could be shorter if only the multiplanar views after contrast administration are used, especially for the MR controls, when signal intensities of the diagnosed tumor are allready known.

MR controls are usually made using the same technique, without reduction of the imaging protocol.

a) HGH-Producing adenomas

Growth disorders are typical for the clinical appearance of the HGH-producing Adenomas. Gigantism in younger patients or acromegaly in adults, apart from subjective symptoms, have gigantic growth and numerous disorders, such as: enlargement of cartilages and visceral organs, hypogonadism, etc. (24, 41).

Neurologic finding in HGH-producing adenoma is negative. Visual deficit (optic chiasm syndroma) is usually present. Parasellar extension can cause compression to III, IV, V1, V2 and VI cranial nerves, depending on the route of extension. In the cavernous sinus region, parasellary, huge HGH- producing macroadenoma can engulf the syphon of the internal carotid artery, thus causing subocclusion symptoms.

Classic radiographs can show stage II-IV of the sellar bone destruction, depending on the size of the tumor.

CT can make the diagnosis of HGH-producing macroadenoma with certainty. In HGH-producing microadenoma CT scan could be inconclusive (15).

MR should follow CT in cases of HGH-producing macroadenoma only if multiplanar view is required for further determination of tumor relationship with cavernous sinus or optic chiasm.

HGH-producing adenoma is shown in MR tomographs after contrast administration with high signal intensities. Mixed higer signal intensities could be seen in mixed or diffuse varieties of tumor. Diffuse type of HGH-producing adenoma could hardly be differentiated from normal hypophyseal parenchyma, thus making the neurosurgical treatment extremely difficult.

MR diagnosis of HGH-producing adenoma is quite sure. It sometimes could be hard to differentiate the tumor from the cavernous sinus (Figg. 189, 190).

Treatment modalities for acromegaly include surgery, radiotherapy and drugs, and all of them have certain advantages and disadvantages. Selective transsphenoidal adenomectomy is a method of choice, successful in 65-75% of patients. If the transsphenoidal approach is not feasible, transcranial subfrontal access should be used. Radiotherapy has delayed effect and could be either primary or postoperative (2).

Higher doses of dopamine agonists (exceeding 20 mg/day) administered as a sole treatment or in combination with other modalities, is effective in 70% of patients. Somatostatin analogue, octreotid, has been used lately with favorable results.

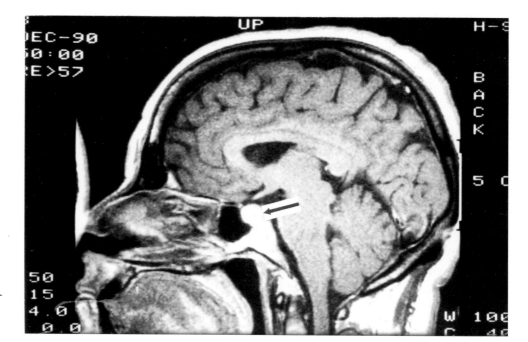

Figure 189. Sagittal image (SE 500/15) after gadolinium-DTPA administration. Patient V.P. HGH-Producing Macroadenoma with high signal intensities, invades sellar fossa and distends sellar diaphragm cranially - arrow.

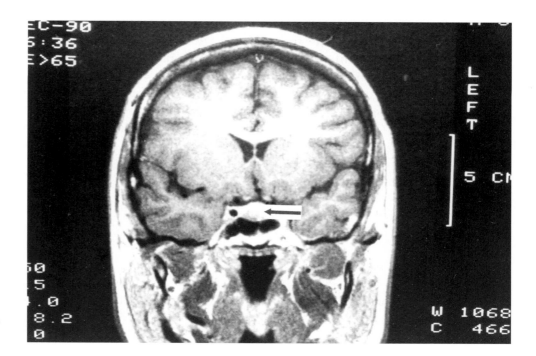

Figure 190. Coronal image (SE 500/15) after gadolinium-DTPA administration. Same patient, V.P. HGH-Producing Macroadenoma , distending sellar diaphragm, shown intrasellary - arrow.

b) Prolactinomas

Prolactinomas are benign, slowly growing, chromofob adenomas of smaller size, whit intense prolactin production.

Women with these tumors usually have amenorrhoea, dysmenorrhoea, galactorrhoea and sterility. Lack of estrogen could cause decreased libido, dyspareunia, osteoporosis, etc.

Endocrine symptoms in men are disorders of potency and libido, sterility, gynecomastia, etc. (3, 39).

If not treated, macroprolactinomas could destroy bony sellar structures, like HGH producing macroadenomas.

Plane X- ray radiographs in microprolactinomas are negative (9, 13).

CT scan of microprolactinoma could be negative or inconclusive. CT scan with intravenous injection of iodine contrast shows prolactinoma in low densities (less than 50 H) (11, 22).

MR image of microprolactinoma is typical for its low signal intensity as compared to normal glandular parenchyma (Fig. 191).

Mixed prolactinomas can have higher signal intensities as well. Extremely low signal intensities in macroprolactinomas are the sign of necrosis, infarction, and cyst (6, 35).

Conservative therapy of prolactinoma by bromocryptine, and recently other dopamin agonists (pergolid, tergurid, cabergolin), was successful in 80% of patients, with tumor diminishing observed in 70% of cases (4, 11, 37, 43).

Surgery for microprolactinoma could be applied in cases of medical therapy resistance or intolerance, in order to normalize hormonal status. Transsphenoidal approach is a method of choice for microprolactinomas. Macroprolactinomas should be approached transcranially (47, 52).

c) ACTH-Producing adenomas

Endocrine disorders in ACTH-producing adenomas cause Cushings syndrome. First group of symptoms is due to hypercortizolemia, such as: arterial hypertension, "buffalo hump", diabetes, hirsutism, acne, pletora of the facial skin, anxiety, depression, etc. Other symptoms are caused by extraadrenal effect of elevated ACTH concentration, so that hyperpygmentation is present (19, 39).

Bone destruction in sellar fossa could be found, depending on the size of ACTH-producing adenoma.

CT scan of ACTH-producing adenoma is inconclusive, because of the variable density of this tumor. Size of tumor is the crucial feature for the diagnosis of ACTH-producing adenoma (36).

ACTH-producing adenomas are shown in MR tomographs by elevated signal intensities and mixed form with variable signal intensities (38, 44). Precise diagnosis depends on the size of tumor, i.e. the diagnosis is certain in voluminous tumors (Fig. 192).

Of all hypersecreting hypophyseal tumors, ACTH-producing adenomas have clearly defined surgical indications, because of the severity of clinical appearance induced by adrenal hypersecretion. Tumors could be very small (2-3 mm), located in the anterior or medial portion of hypophysis, and they are often multicentric. Some Authors advocate hypophysectomy in the first act, to avoid frequent relapses (25%), or adenomectomy with postoperative radiotherapy (5, 29).

Classification after Kovacz and Horvath (40).

pI	TI	Densely granulated
pII	TI	Scarcely granulated with intensive secretion
PIII	TI	Mixed tumor (producing HGH and PRL)
pIV	TI	Acidophylic monomorph bihormonal tumor
pV	TI	Mammosomatotropic tumor
pVI	TI	Prolactin cell carcinoma
pVI	TI	Adenoma of various cells producing several hormones

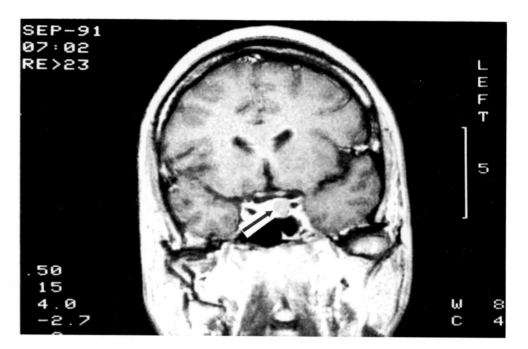

Figure 191. Coronal image (SE 500/15) after gadolinium-DTPA administration. Spheric, clearly demarcated, Macroprolactinoma with low signal intensity, shown intrasellary in the left parasagittal plane - arrow.

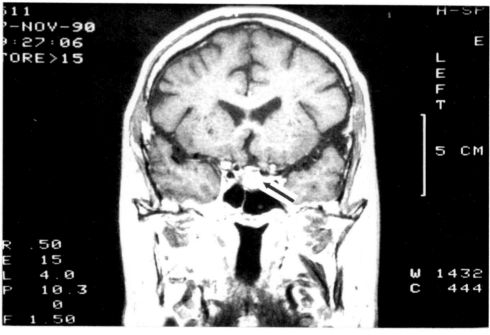

Figure 192. Coronal image (SE 500/15) after gadolinium-DTPA administration. Centrally and paracentrally left inside sellar fossa an ACTH-Producing Adenoma with non-homogenous higher signal intensities is shown - arrow. ACTH-Producing Adenoma slightly distends sellar diaphragm.

d) TSH-Producing adenomas

Extremely rare TSH-producing adenomas can cause relasing hyperthyreosis and thyroid gland enlargement. Subsequent tachycardia, nervousness, fatigue, perspiration and loss of weight are seen. Superimposed symptoms of hyperproduction of HR, ACTH and prolactin could be found as well. Local invasive growth is rarely seen (16, 25).

CT scan is insufficient for the diagnosis of TSH-producing adenomas (18, 20).

Signal intensities are not strictly defined in MR image. Compression and dislocation of hypophysis induced by tumor should be observed, and combined with endocrinology investigation could help to confirm definitive diagnosis (27).

Less than 150 of such tumors have been reported so far, which means that they are quite rare. Macroadenomas with suprasellar propagation are found in 90% of cases.

Medical therapy can decrease TSH level in 75% and diminish tumor in almost 50% (octreotid) or 30% (dopamin agonists) of patients.

Surgery for TSH-producing adenomas combined with drugs and radiotherapy provides for best results (28, 41).

e) FSH and LH-Producing adenomas

Clinical manifestation of FSH-producing adenoma is hypogonadism, i.e. atrophy of testicles, decreased libido, impotence and sterility (40, 42). In elder patients FSH-producing adenomas are usually discovered in macroadenoma phase, because the sexual disorders have been neglected. It is usually seen in males over 50, with hypogonadism. The tumor usually produces alpha-subunit, as well as FSH and LH (12, 48).

There is insufficient experience in CT diagnosis of FSH and LH-producing adenomas. Those tumors have mixed densities in CT scans.

FSH and LH-producing adenomas are shown in mixed, non-specific signal intensities in MR image. Adenoma size and compression to a normal glandular parenchyma by a tumor can contribute to the diagnosis. Therapeutic approach is the same as for non-functional tumors, consisting of surgical resection through transsphenoidal or transcranial access followed by radiotherapy.

f) Hormonally inactive adenomas

Hormonally inactive adenomas of hypophysis or other tumors of sellar region, could be found by neuroradiologic examination in microadenoma stage only accidentally (31).

Patients with hormonally inactive macroadenomas with parasellar and suprasellar propagation have headache, optic chiasm disorders and parasellar cranial nerve impairment.

Bone pathology of sellar fossa could be seen in plane X-ray (1, 3). CT examination is usually sufficient for assessment of hormonally inactive adenomas. Density of those tumors in CT scan depends on pathohistology, regardless of i.v. administration of iodine contrast (28).

MR imaging can display non-secretory tumors with high certainty (50, 51). Signal intensity depends on tumor type, but MR is valuable for volume assessment of the tumor (Figg. 193-195).

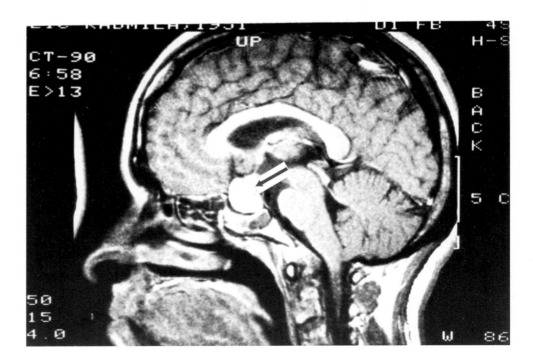

Figure 193. Sagittal image (SE 500/15) after gadolinium-DTPA administration. Hormonally Inactive Adenoma distends sellar fossa and fulfils it completely. Hormonally Inactive Adenoma extends suprasellary, disrupts sellar diaphragm and dislocates optic chiasm cranially. Tumor is isointensive with occasional islets of hyperintensive signal - arrow.

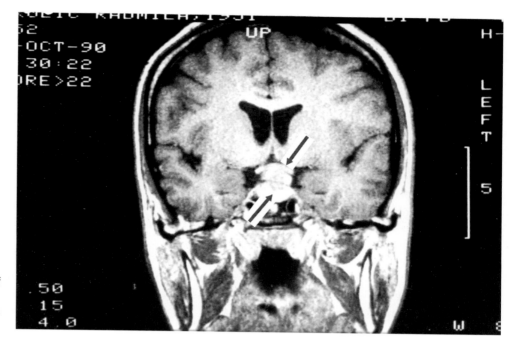

Figure 194. Coronal image (SE 500/15) after gadolinium-DTPA administration. Same patient, N.R., with deviation of optic chiasm due to Hormonally Inactive Adenoma - arrows.

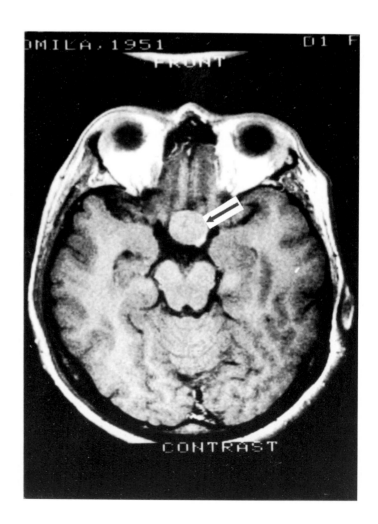

Figure 195. Axial image (SE 500/15) after gadolinium-DTPA administration. Same patient, N.R. with Hormonally Inactive Adenoma clearly demarcated from normal anatomy structures - arrow.

Surgery, through either transsphenoidal or transcranial approach, is applied for hormonally inactive adenomas, as well as for other suprasellar expansive lesions (21). Adequate preoperative medication as well as postoperative monitoring and hormonal substitution is of utmost importance (2).

Generally speaking, transsphenoidal approach is convenient for hypophyseal microadenomas. Transsphenoidal approach has been the method of choice for treatment of all pituitary tumors, even those with considerable suprasellar extension, for the last two decades. Transcranial approach is used occasionally for the eccentric subtemporal or subfrontal growths. Transcranial temporal approach have been abandoned, while pteryonal and subfrontal access are still used.

g) Pathologic lesions of the hypophyseal stalk

Pathology of hypophyseal stalk, such as infarction, tumor, cyst, hypoplasia or rupture is rarely seen, and could be shown by CT or MR examination.

Hormone insufficiency of one or more hormones could be found depending on the pathology of the stalk. Expansive lesions of the stalk could jeopardize optic chiasm and cause visual field deficits. Rupture of the hypophyseal stalk is followed by hypophyseal hormone deficiency, i.e. panhypopituitarism. Posttraumatic rupture of the stalk is followed not only by endocrine disorders, but by a neurologic deficit, caused by craniocerebral trauma, as well.

CT scan in direct coronal plane enables perfect visualization of the hypophyseal stalk. Pathology of the stalk is not clearly seen in the reconstructed axial plane of CT examination. If a pathologic lesion of the hypophyseal stalk is suspected upon CT scan, MR imaging is required to confirm the diagnosis.

MR imaging is a method of choice for the diagnosis of the hypophyseal stalk pathology. MR technique is identical to the one used for the diagnosis of hypophyseal lesions. Substantial advantage of MR imaging is perfect display of hypophysis, its stalk and surrounding structures (49, 53).

MR is ideal for the diagnosis of the tumors of hypophyseal stalk (Fig. 196).

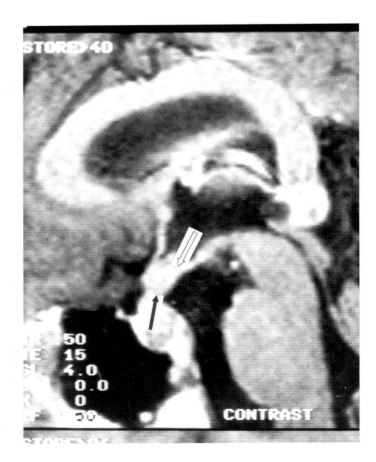

Figure 196. Sagittal image (SE 500/15) after gadolinium-DTPA administration. Tumor with higher signal intensities is shown in the projection of the hypophyseal stalk- white arrow. Tumor with mixed signal intensities is seen inside sellar fossa.

Congenital or posttraumatic rupture of the hypophyseal stalk could be shown optimally by MR tomography (Fig. 197).

h) Empty Sella Syndrome

Empty Sella Syndrome is a separate entity, belonging to pseudotumors of sellar fossa, with extended suprasellar subarachnoidal space with intrasellar liquor drip along the stalk. The term is used when sella is virtually empty, although there is a small plaque of the glandular tissue of hypophysis. Empty Sella could be either primary or secondary. Primary empty sella is congenital malformation combined with agenesis or hypoplasia of sellar diaphragm (17).

Secondary empty sella could be caused by apoplexy of hypophysis, hypophyseal reduction following treatment (conservative, irradiation or surgical), rupture of the intrasellar cyst or hypophyseal reduction seen in multiparas (45).

Increased liquor pressure could cause erosion, distension or even rupture of the sellar fundus, followed by rhinorrhoea.

Usual symptoms of Empty Sella Syndrome are frontal or frontotemporal headache and endocrine disorders, i.e. hypopituitarism. Disorders of optic chiasm, such as bitemporal hemianopsia and central scotoma could be seen in case of the chiasmal prolaps to the sella. Atrophy of the optic nerve papilla could be found exceptionally.

Plane X -ray reveal distended sella and sellar wall erosion.

CT examination with intrathecal injection of air (mini gas cisternography) and intravenous injection of iodine contrast (double contrast CT examination) can confirm the diagnosis of Empty Sella. Disadvantages of this techique are the invasiveness, i.e. being painful for the patient, X ray risk and potential complications such as allergy and infection.

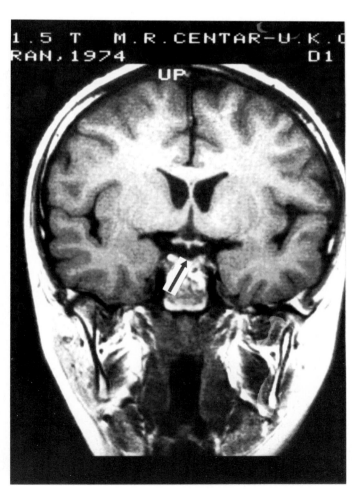

Figure 197. Coronal image (SE 500/15) after gadolinium-DTPA administration. Arrow pointing at hypophyseal stalk rupture.

MR imaging in T-1W sequence, in coronal and sagittal planes, can make the diagnosis of Empty sella without invasion, pain or discomfort as compared to CT examination (Figg. 198, 199).

MR examination is indicated in case of unsuccessful lumbar puncture or inability to get the air into the basal cistern and sellar region, during CT examination, due to technical failure, arachnoidal adhesions and incorrect head position (46).

Double echo sequence could be used for MR diagnosis of *"empty sella syndrome"* as well. Paramagnetic contrast is used in specific cases.

i) MR controls

MR controls are important for monitoring of the evolution of the hypophyseal tumors (22). During conservative medical therapy tumor stagnation or regression is assessed. Further growth, i.e. tumor resistance to the therapy, is an indication for surgery. It is important to define relationship of tumor and surrounding suprasellar and parasellar structures.

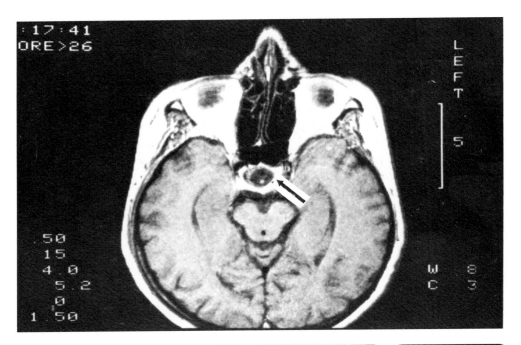

Figure 198. Axial image (SE 500/15). Empty sella syndrome: arrow pointing at low signal intensities of liquor in the sellar fossa.

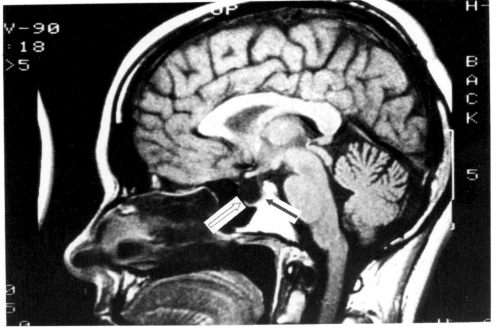

Figure 199. Sagittal image (SE 500/15). Arrows pointing at low signal intensities of liquor filling sellar fossa. Stalk is shown nearby sellar dorsum.

Postirradiation and postoperative MR controls should confirm successful reduction or complete removal of the tumor (Fig. 200).

Conservative treatment is extremely successful, particularly for prolactinomas (Figg. 201, 202).

Further MR controls depend on clinical course, including both endocrine and neurologic manifestations.

Comparative analysis of CT and MR findings in 61 patients with hypophyseal tumors has been done in collaboration of MR center and Institute of endocrinology of Clinical Center of Serbia in Belgrade. Comparative results for eleven different entities were analysed (25).

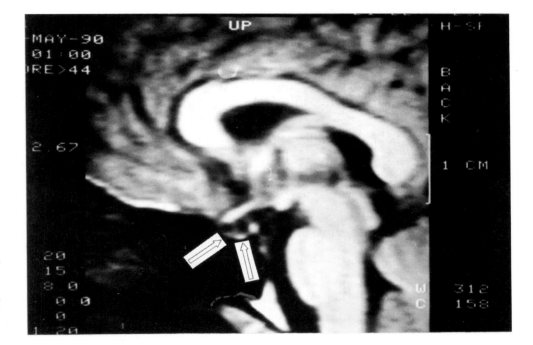

Figure 200. Sagittal image (SE 200/15) Postoperative MR image shows no expansion in the sellar fossa. Hypophyseal stalk is in a correct position. No signs of inflammation in sphenoid region.

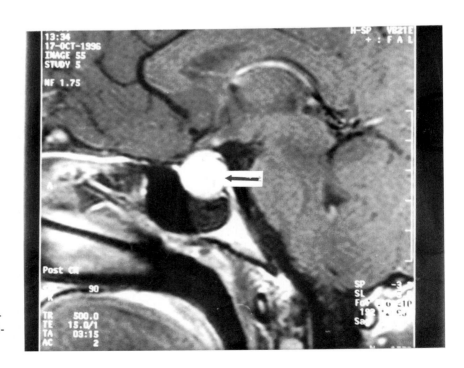

Figure 201. Sagittal image (SE 500/15) after gadolinium-DTPA administration. Patient D.S. Arrow pointing at prolactinoma with suprasellar propagation and sellar diaphragm distension.

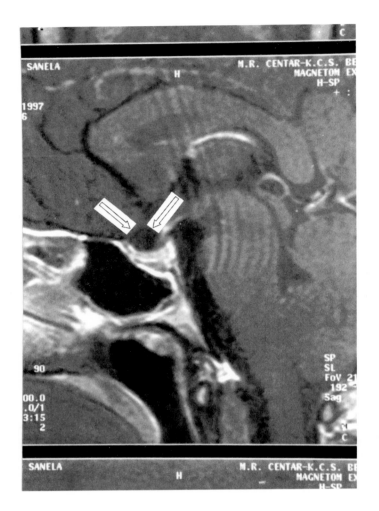

Figure 202. Sagittal image (SE 500/15) after gadolinium-DTPA administration. Same patient, D.S., after six months of conservative treatment. Tumor regression is clearly seen - arrows.

The Table 1 shows comparative analysis of CT and MR findings (CT+ and MR+; CT- and MR-). Findings were usually identical in patients operated on because of hypophyseal tumors, for a total of 27 patients.

CT scan was false positive in 7 patients with suspected tumor, subsequently ruled out by MR imaging and further endocrinologic investigation.

CT scan was negative in 7 cases of microadenoma. CT scan has been dubious in 19 patients with pathologic lesions confirmed by MR examination.

Discrepancy between CT and MR findings was found in 34 patients, but in 15 of patients there was a substantial difference.

Table 1. Has pointed out advantage of MR diagnostic over CT.

GROUP	T+ MR+	T- MR-	T+ MR-	T- MR+	succ.CT S MR+
I. Secreting microadenomas	2	-	-	6	2
II. Secreting macroadenomas	4	-	-	-	1
III. Non-secreting tumors	-	-	-	-	-
IV. Extrasellar tumors	3	-	-	1	3
V. Suspected tumors	-	2	6	-	2
VI. Empty sella syndrome	4	-	1	-	7
VII. Stalk pathology	-	-	-	-	2
VIII. Operated tumors	9	1	-	-	1
IX. Irradiated tumors	1	-	-	-	-
X. Operated and irradiated tumors	1	-	-	-	-
XI. Other entities	-	-	-	-	1
TOTAL	**24**	**3**	**7**	**7**	**19**

REFERENCES

1. Banna M., Schatz SW., Molit MJ., Growes J.: Primary intrasellar germinoma. Br. J. Radiol., 49: 971-973, 1983.

2. Baskin DS., Boggan JE., Wilson CB.: Transsphenoidal microsurgical removal of growth-hormone-secreting pituitary adenomas. A review of 137 cases. J. Neurosurg., 56: 634-641, 1978.

3. Bergland RM., Ray BS., Rorack RM.: Anatomical variations in the pituitary gland and adecent structures in 225 human autopsy cases. J. Neurosurg., 29: 93-99, 1968.

4. Bevan JS., et al.: Factors in the outcome of transsphenoidal surgery for prolactinoma, and non-functioning pituitary tumor, including postoperative bromocriptine therapy. Clin. Endocrinol., 26: 541-556, 1987.

5. Bigos ST., et al.: Chusing's disease; management by transsphenoidal pituitary microsurgery. J. Clin. Endocrinol. Metab., 50: 499-504, 1988.

6. Bilaniuk LT., Zimmerman RA., Weherli WF., Snyder RPJ., Goldberg HI., Grossman RI., Boromley PA., Edelstein WA., Glowe GH., Mac Fall JR., Redington RW.: Magnetic resonance imaging of pituitary lesions using 1,0 to 1,5 T field strenght. Radiology, 153: 415-418, 1984.

7. Bonafe A., Sobel D., Manelfe C.: Relative value of CT and hypocycloidal tomography in the diagnosis of pituitary microadenoma. A radio-surgical correlative study. Neuroradiology, 22: 133-137, 1978.

8. Bonneville JF., Cattin F., Moussa-Bacha K., Portha C.: Dynamic computed tomography of the pituitary gland: the "tuft sign". Radiology, 149: 145-148, 1983.

9. Bonneville JF., Cattin F., Poulignot D., Guiyon JC., Dietemann JL.: Radiographic and Tomographic Evaluation of Prolactinomas. In Tolis G., Mountokalakis T., Stefanis C. and Labrie F. (eds): Prolactin and Prolactinomas. New York, Raven Press, 395-402, 1983.

10. Bonneville JF., Dietemann JL.: Radiology of the sella turcica. Springer-Verlag. Berlin, Heidelberg, New York, 1981.

11. Bonneville JF., Poulignot D., Cattin F., Couturier M., Mollet E., Dietemann JL.: Computed tomographyc demonstration of the effects of bromocriptine on pituitary microadenoma size. Radiology, 143: 451-455, 1982.

12. Borges JL., et al.: Follicule stimulating hormone secreting pituitary tumor with concomita evaluation of serum alfa subunit levels. J. Clin. Endocrinol. Metab., 58: 938-941, 1984.

13. Bruneton JN., Drouillard JR., Sabatier JC., Elie GP., Tavernier JF.: Normal variants of the sella turcica. Radiology, 131: 88-104, 1979.

14. Challa V., Marshal R., Hopkins M.: Pathologic Study of Pituitary Tumors. Report of 62 cases with a review the recent literature. Hum. Pathol., 16: 873-884, 1985.

15. Chamber EF., Turski PA., La Masters D., Newton TH.: Regions of low density in the contrast enhanced pituitary gland: normal and pathological processes. Radiology, 144: 109-13, 1982.

16. Comi RJ., et al: Response of thyreotropin secreting pituitary adenomas to a long-acting somatostatin analogue. N. Engl. J. Med., 317: 12-17, 1987.

17. Daniels D., Pojunas KW., Kilgore DP., Pehl P., Meyer GA., Williams AL., Haughton VM.: MR of the diaphragma sellae. AJRN, 7: 765-769, 1986.

18. Daniels D., et al.: Differential diagnosis of intrasellar tumors by computed tomography. Radiology, 1941: 697-701, 1981.

19. Daughaday W.: The adenohypophysis. In Williams H.R. (ed.): Textbook of Endocrinology. W.B. Saunders Co. Philadelphia, London, Toronto, 85-104, 1984.

20. Davis PS., Hofman JC., Tindal GT., Braun IF.: CT surgical correlation in pituitary adenomas: evaluation in 113 patients. AJRN, 6: 711-6, 1985.

21. Dolinskas CA., Simeone FA.: Transsphenoidal hypophysectomy: Postsurgical CT findings. AJRN, 6: 45-50, 1985.

22. Gillespie JE., Adams JE., Isherwood I.: Tree dimensional computed tomographyc of sellar and paraseller lesions. J. Neuroradiology, 29: 30-35, 1987.

23. Halberg EE., Sheline GE.: Radiotherapy of pituitary tumors. Endocrin, Metab. Clin., North Am., 16: 667-684, 1987.

24. Hartman ML., et al.: Somatotropin pulse fequency and basal concentrations are increased in acromegaly and are reduced bu successful therapy. J. Clin. Endocrinol. Metab., 70: 1375-1384, 1990.

25. Hill SA., Falko JM., Wilson WE., Hunt WE.: Thyrotropin-producing pituitary adenomas. J. Neurosurg., 57: 515-519, 1982.

26. Hosoya T., Kera M., Suzuki T., Yamagushu K.: Fat in the normal cavernous sinus. Neuroradiology, 28: 264-266, 1986.

27. Huk WJ., Fahlsbuch R.: Nuclear Magnetic Resonance Imaging of the Region of the Sella Turcica. Neurosurg. Rev., 8: 141-150, 1985.

28. Ishii K., Waterai J., Hosoua T.: Pituitary adenoma with area of low density on CT surgical pathological correlation. Neuroradiology, 23: 58-67, 1982.

29. Jennings AS., Liddle GW., Orth DN.: Results of treating childhood Chushing's disease with pituitary irradiation. N. Engl. J. Med., 297: 957-962, 1977.

30. Karnaze MG., Sartor K., Winthrop JD., Gado MH., Hodges FJ.: Suprasellar lesions: evaluation with MR imaging. Radiology, 161: 77-82, 1986.

31. Kilbanski A.: Non secretory pituitary tumors. Endocrinol. Metab. Clin. Borth. Am., 16: 793-804, 1987.

32. Kleinberg DL., Noel GL., Frantz AG.: Galactorrhea: a study of 235 cases including 48 with pituitary tumors. N. Engl. J. Med., 296: 589-583, 1977.

33. Kovacs K., Horvath E.: Tumors of pituitary gland. In Hartman W.H. (ed.): Atlas of Tumor Pathology Fascicle 21, 2 and series. Washington D.C.; Arned Forses Institute of Pathology, 1-24, 1986.

34. Kramer S., Fode NC., Erdmond MJ.: Transsphenoidal surgery following unsuccessful prior therapy. An assessment of benefits and risks in 158 patients. J. Neurosurg., 63: 823-829, 1985.

35. Kucharczyk W., Davis DO., Kelly WM., Sze G., Norman D., Newton TH.: Pituitary adenomas: high resolution MR imaging at 1,5 T. Radiology, 1961: 761-765, 1986.

36. Kuuliala I.: CT of pituitary adenomas. Clinical Radiology, 32: 259-264, 1981.

37. Lamberts S., et al.: Bromocriptine and the medical treatment of Cushing's disease. In Miller E.: Neuroactive drugs in Endocrinology. Elsevier-North Holland Biomedical Press, 198: 371-383, 1982.

38. Liessner J., Seider M.: Klinische Kernspintomographie. Enke. Stuttgart, 1987.

39. Lytras N., et al.: Corticotropin releasing factor: responses in normal subjects and patients with disorders of the hypothalamus and pituitary. Clin. Endocrinol., 20: 71-84, 1984.

40. Miura M., Matsukado Y., Kodama T., Mihara Y.: Clinical and histopathological characteristics of gonadothropin-producing pituitary adenomas. J. Neurosurg., 62: 376-382, 1986.

41. Moller DE., et al.: Osteotide suppresses both growth hormone (GH) and GH releasing hormone (GHRH) in acromegaly due to ectopic GHRH secretion. J. Clin. Endocrinolog. Metab., 68: 499-504, 1989.

42. Nicolis G., et al.: Gonadotropin-producing pituitary adenoma in a men with long-standing primary hypogonadism. J. Clin. Endocrinol. Metab., 66: 237-241, 1988.

43. Pelegrini I., et al.: Resistance to bromocriptine in prolactinomas. J. Clin. Endocrinol. Metab., 69: 500-509, 1989.

44. Pomeranz JS.: Craniospinal Magnetic Resonance Imaging. WB Saunders Company. Philadelphia, London, Toronto, Sydney, Tokyo, 1989.

45. Reid RL., Quigley ME., Yen SSC.: Pituitary apoplexy. Arch. Neurol., 42: 712-719, 1985.

46. Reiser M., et al.: Magnet-rezonanz-Tomographie. Springer-Verlag. Berlin, Heidelberg, New York, Paris, London, Tokyo, Hong Kong, 1989.

47. Snow RB., Lavyne MH., Lee BCP., Morgello S., Patterson RH.: Craniothomy versus transsphenoidal excision of large pituitary tumors: the usefulness of MRI in guiding the operative approach. Neurosurgery, 19(1): 59-64. 1986.

48. Snyder PJ.: Gonadotroph cell adenomas of pituitary. Endocrin Rev., 6: 522-563, 1985.

49. Stark D., Bradley GWJR.: Magnetic Resonance Imaging. The C.V. Mosby Company. St. Louis, Washington D.C., Toronto, 1988.

50. Steinberg GK., Koenig GH., Golden JB.: Symptomatic Ratke-s cysts. Report of two cases. J. Neurosurg., 56: 290-295, 1973.

51. Takeuchi J., Hanada H., Nagata I.: Suprasellar germinoma. J. Neurosurg., 49: 41-48, 1978.

52. Wilson CB., Dempsey LC.: Transsphenoidal microsurgical removal of 250 pituitary adenomas. J. Neurosurg., 48: 13-22, 1983.

53. Zawadcki MB., Norman D.: Magnetic Resonance Imaging of the Central Nervous System. Raven Press. New York, 1987.

XI. TEMPORAL LOBE EPILEPSY

Zvonimir Lević, Gradimir Dragutinović, Lukas Rasulić

Epilepsy could be caused by various factors, depending on the age of the patient.

In infants and children under the age of 10, epilepsy could be caused by congenital malformation, metabolic diseases of brain, anoxia, trauma, infection and idiopathic causes.

In the age group ranging from 10 to 30 years temporal lobe epilepsy could be caused by malformations, tumors, trauma, drugs, alcohol, etc. In older patients epileptic seizures could be caused by vascular disorders, trauma, tumors, degenerative diseases of the brain, alcohol and drugs.

Diagnosis of epilepsy could be reached by numerous methods. History obtained from patient or heteroanamnesis, should be followed by physical, neurologic, psychological and psychiatric assessment. Laboratory analyses are necessary as well.

Neurophysiologic and neuroradiologic investigations are essential to discover organic substrate of epilepsy.

Brain scintigraphy, PET (positron emission tomography), SPECT (single photon emission computer tomography) and computerized ultrasound are special methods of investigation of etiology of epilepsy in children. Functional MR imaging have been used recently (3, 8).

One or more epileptogenic foci is found, uni- or bilaterally in the temporal lobes, in case of temporal epilepsy. Temporal lobe has complex functions, and therefore epileptic fits are complex. Lateral and mesial cortex of the temporal lobe contains speech, auditory interpretative functions, whereas mesial and limbic portion control autonomous and behavioral functions. Auditive and visual hallucinations, speech disorders, abdominal sensations, drowsiness, confusion, "dreaming state", vertigo, olfactory sensations, visceral sensations, anger, fear, depression, pleasure, depersonalization, derealization and mnestic disorders could be seen during epileptic discharge.

Typical temporal seizure is manifested by a lack of contact, complex or simple automatisms, like scratching, buttoning, unbuttoning, taking off the clothes, chewing and swallowing. Brief seizures are followed by complete amnesia.

Following neuroradiologic methods of examination are used: Plane X- ray, angiography, computer tomography and magnetic resonance imaging.

Classic radiographs could show bone pathology and endocranial calcifications.

Angiography is indicated for vascular pathology, such as A-V malformation, angioma, etc.

Doctrine suggest that MRI should follow CT examination if the cause was not discovered or remains unclear. MRI should be applied if precise or multiplanar display is needed for planning the surgery or conservative treatment adjustment.

MR imaging is five times as successful as CT in detecting expansive lesions that have caused epilepsy (5).

MR imaging could reveal following organic lesions, that have caused temporal lobe epilepsy: scars, tumors, calcifications, cysts, ischemic lesions, demyelination changes, metastases, parasitoses, a-v malformations, thickened meninges, etc. Considering the fact that temporal lobe epilepsy could be induced by various factors, a number of sequences should be used for the diagnosis (4).

a) Arachnoidal cyst

Small arachnoidal cyst of the left temporal lobe was discovered by MR examination of a patient suffering from epileptic fits since childhood. CT scan could not show temporobasal structures precisely, because of the artifacts induced by massive bones of the cranial base (Fig. 203).

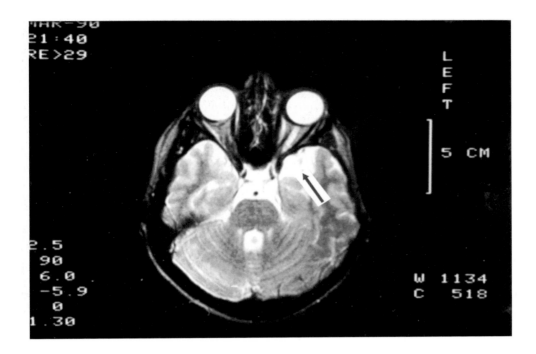

Figure 203. Axial image (SE 2500/90). Small arachnoidal cyst with high signal intensities in the left temporo-basal region - arrow.

b) Spontaneous intracerebral hemorrhage

Acute spontaneous intracerebral hemorrhage in a 39 year old patient was manifested by neurologic deficit and epileptic fits (2). MR examination have shown a smaller collection of blood (Fig. 204).

c) Aneurysm of the internal carotid artery

Calcified and partly thrombosed aneurysm of the left internal carotid artery was discovered by MRI in a patient with long-standing Grand mal epilepsy (Fig. 205).

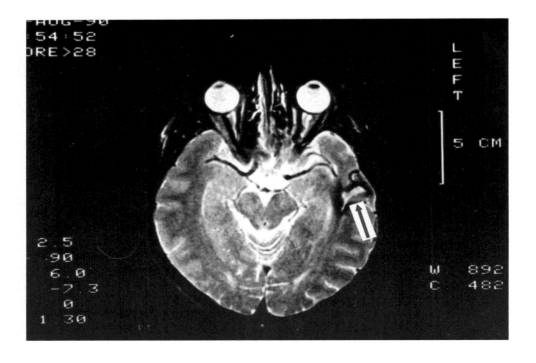

Figure 204. Axial image (SE 2500/90). Intracerebral hematoma with high signal intensities, surrounded by hemosiderin edge with low signal intensity, without marked perifocal edema, is shown in the left temporal region - arrow.

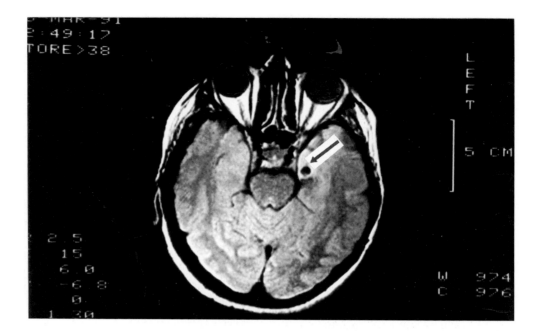

Figure 205. Axial image (SE 2500/15). Left parasellar circular zone of low signal intensity corresponding to the aneurysm of the internal carotid artery. Increased signal intensity perifocally suggests the suffering of the brain tissue in the vicinity of the aneurysm - arrow.

d) Cavernoma

Patient has been referred to neuroradiology after two year history of epileptic seizures. CT scan have revealed partly calcified cavernoma, as a small hypodense zone. MR examination was indicated to confirm the diagnosis and rule out other pathology.

MR image in T-2W sequence have shown cavernoma with the typical features (Fig. 206). Necessary sequences, such as T-1W, T-2W and FLASH, were used (5).

e) Trauma

A thirty eight year old male has suffered from epileptic fits caused by a craniocerebral trauma six moths ago. In spite of antiepileptic therapy the seizures frequency was increased, including an episode

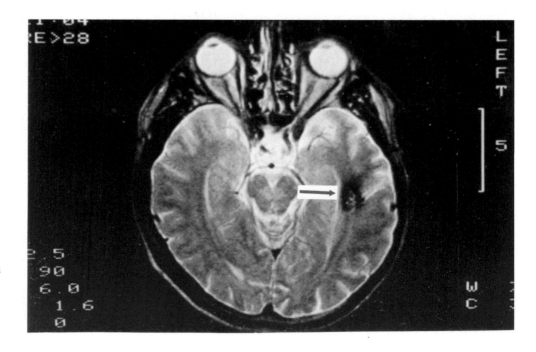

Figure 206. Axial image (SE 2500/90). Small zone of mixed higher signal intensities, surrounded by a hemosiderin edge with low signal intensities is shown in the left temporal region - arrow.

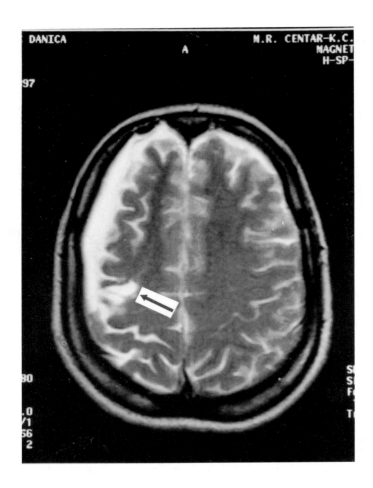

Figure 207. Axial image (SE 4000/99). Markedly dilated `subarachnoidal space with high signal intensities and ribbon of the high signal intensities, corresponding to post- traumatic encephalomalatic cyst is shown in the right parietal area - arrow.

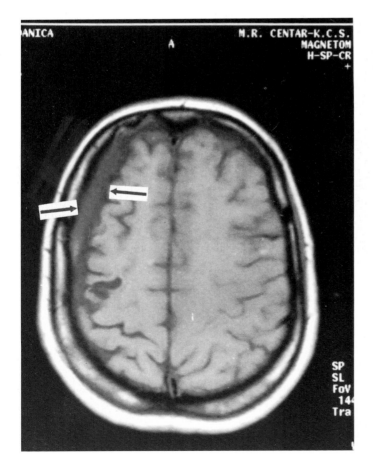

Figure 208. Axial image (SE 500/15). Hygroma in the right parietal region, clearly separated from liquor - arrows. Posttraumatic lesion has low signal intensities.

of *status epilepticus.* CT examination done immediately after the injury was negative (7).

MR image have shown hygroma in the right parietal area, as well as posttraumatic lesion high in the right parietal region. MR tomographs (Figg. 207, 208) show advantages of certain sequences and justifies their use in standard procedures.

f) Tumor

CT examination was performed in a 38-year old patient with sudden onset of epilepsy. MR was indicated because of the negative CT scan. MR image in T-2W sequence have discovered tumor in the right temporo-basal region (Fig. 209). Tumor have caused *Grand mal* epileptic fits.

g) Postoperative defect

Arachnoidal cyst was discovered by CT in a patient who has had epilepsy since early childhood. Epileptic fits have continued after surgical removal of the arachnoidal cyst and cortical resection (1, 6).

MR·control have displayed postoperative defect multiplanary in T-2W sequence (Fig. 210).

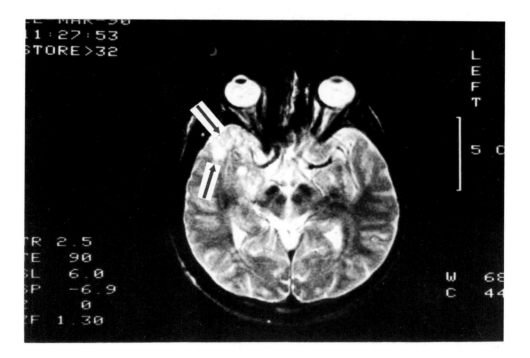

Figure 209. Axial image (SE 2500/90). Tumor of the right temporo-basal area is shown as non-homogenous, poorly defined zone of the high signal intensity - arrows. Astrocytoma, grade II, was pathohistologically confirmed after the surgery.

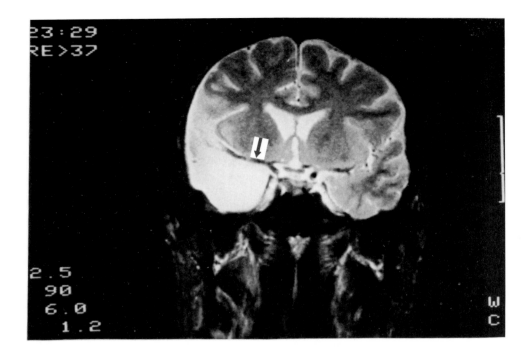

Figure 210. Coronal image (SE 2500/90). Huge post-operative defect, filled with hyperintensive liquor, is shown in the right temporal zone. Distal part of the right internal carotid artery, as well as arteria cerebri media and part of arteria cerebri anterior are well defined in MR tomograph - arrow.

REFERENCES

1. Horsley V.: Brain Surgery. Brit Med. J., 2: 670-675, 1986.
2. Kertesz A., McLachlan RS., Black SE., Nicholson LR., Carr T., Blume TW.: Magnetic Resonance Imaging and the Epileptic Focus. Edited by HG Wiser and CE Elger. Springer-Verlag. Berlin, Heidelberg, 1987.
3. Latack JT., About-Khalil BW., Siegl GJ., Sackellares JC., Gabrileson TO., Aisen AM.: Patients with partial seizures: evaluation by MR, and PET imaging. Radiology, 1986: 159-163, 1986.
4. McLachlan RS., Nicholson RL., Black S., Carr T., Blume WT.: Nuclear Magnetic Resonance Imaging, a New Approach to the Investigation of Refractory Temporal Lobe Epilepsy. Epilepsia, 15: 55-80, 1974.
5. Ormson MJ., Kispert DB., Sharbrough FW., Huoser OW., Earnest F., Scheithauer BW., Laws ER.: Cryptic Structural Lesions in Refractory Partial Epilepsy: MR imaging et CT Studies. Radiology, 160: 215-219, 1986.
6. Radtke RA., Mc Namara JO., Lewis DV., Heinz ER.: Usefulnes of MRI in pre-surgical evaluation of intractable partial seizures. Epilepsia, 27: 612-618, 1986.
7. Schorner W., Meenecke HJ., Felix R.: Temporal-Lobe Epilepsy: Comparison of CT and MR imaging. AJR, 149: 231-239, 1987.
8. Stefan H., Pawlik G., Bocher-Schwarz H., Biersack HJ., Burr W., Penin H., Heiss WD.: Functional and morphological abnormalities in temporal lobe epilepsy: a comparison of interctal and ictal EEG, CT, MRI, SPECT, and PET. J. Neurol., 234: 377-384, 1987.

XII. MR ANGIOGRAPHY OF THE ENDOCRANIUM AND NECK

Gradimir Dragutinović, Vaso Antunović, Miodrag Rakić

MR angiography (MRA) was enabled by development of a new software and powerful MR machines, thus evading disadvantages of classic angiography. MRA is non-invasive, potentially hazardous iodine contrast is not needed, various complications induced by examiner error are avoided, there is no ionizing irradiation, it could be applied in outpatients, etc.

Flow measurement techniques applied in MR angiography have enabled display of the fluid movement. Adjusted techniques in angiography include phase-sensitive methods and Time-of-flight, with specific features depending on the MR equipment manufacturer (4, 6, 11).

Patient should be perfectly still during examination.

Rapid sequences have been used nowadays to display blood vessels in a target plane, thus obtaining basic tomograph for the development of further procedures (10).

Generally speaking, it is important for the examiner that various angiography phases (arterial, parenchymatous and venous) could be obtained in certain sequences in two or three planes, by the use of appropriate software. Both angiographs are in a subtraction form, obtained by avoiding bone and soft tissue, i.e. only blood vessels are displayed (like in digital subtraction angiography). Three-dimensional display of blood vessels by MIP technique enables rotation of the blood vessels and choosing the best angle for differentiation of lesions (2, 8). The fact is very important for the diagnosis of subocclusion, visualization of the "neck" or infundibulum of the aneurysm, etc. All those MR procedures and software manipulation take no more than ten minutes, so that the patient presence inside MR machine is not required for further software operations (Figg. 211-213) (9).

MR angiography is used on a wider scale in clinical practice. Indication for visualization of endocranial blood vessels, both major arteries and major veins, is decided upon neurologic findings, CT scan and MR image. Subocclusion and occlusion of the major blood vessels are usually found (Figg. 214-217).

Display of the aneurysms of endocranial blood vessels is a special discipline. Giant aneurysms are easily seen, but visualization of smaller aneurysms depends on their location (12).

Following routine has been currently used in the Institute of neurosurgery in Belgrade: once the smaller aneurysm is shown by MRI, DSA (digital subtraction angiography) should be applied to confirm the diagnosis prior to the surgery (Fig. 220). Reverse procedure is applied for giant aneurysm found by conventional angiography, when a goal of MR angiography is to provide for multiplanar display of the relationship between the aneurysm and surrounding structure (for example, in the cavernous sinus region) (Figg. 218-221).

MR angiograms are important for the display of A-V malformations. MR angiography is usually sufficient for the diagnosis of inoperable A-V malformation (Figg. 222, 223).

MR angiography is used to determine afferent and efferent blood vessels in occult A-V malformations (3, 5, 7).

It is important to display pathologic vascularization nearby expansive lesion, as well as to define the relationship between tumor and major blood vessels (Fig. 224).

MR angiography of the extracranial segment of the major blood vessels includes visualization of a. carotis communis, its bifurcation and complete carotid arteries up to the terminal branches bilaterally (1, 13) (Fig. 225).

Subocclusion or occlusion of those blood vessels could be shown and measured (diameter or flow percentage in the stenosis) (Figg. 226, 227).

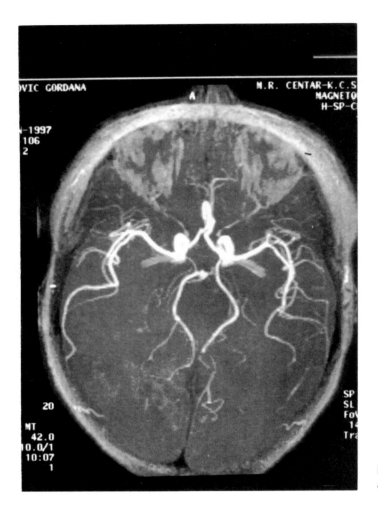

Figure 211. Normal MR angiogram produced with MIP algorithm (Axial section).

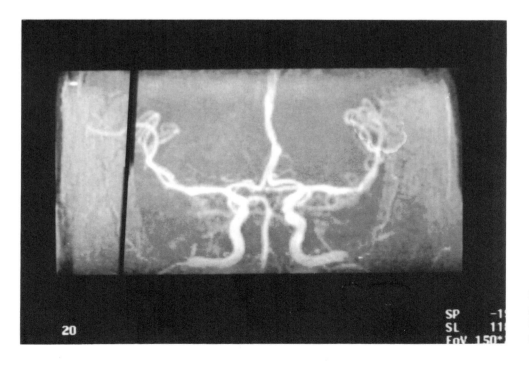

Figure 212. Normal MR angiogram produced with MIP algorithm (Coronal section).

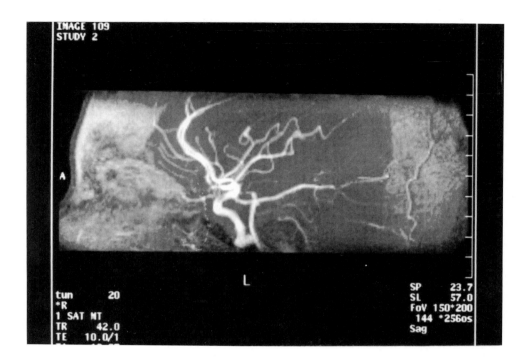

Figure 213. Normal MR angiogram produced with MIP algorithm (Sagittal section).

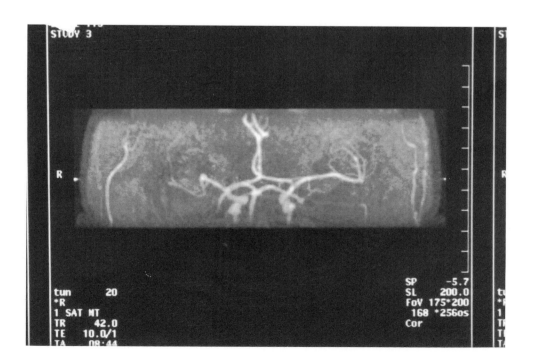

Figure 214. MR angiogram produced with MIP algorithm (Coronal section) Occlusion of the right a. cerebri media.

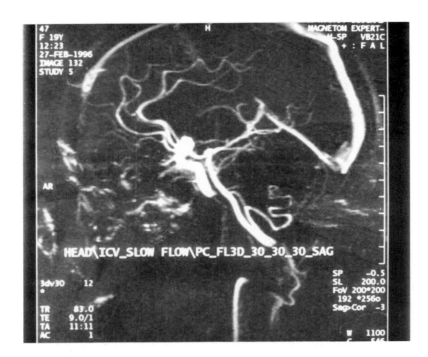

Figure 215. MR angiogram produced with MIP algorithm (Sagittal section).
Occlusion of the right a. cerebri media.

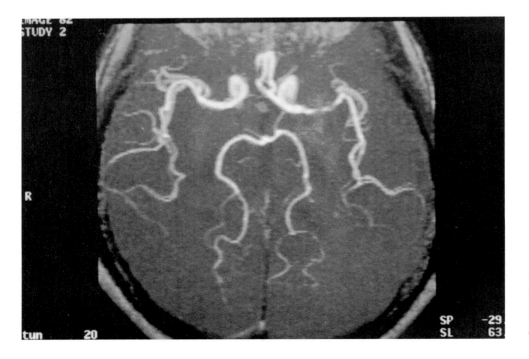

Figure 216. MR angiogram produced with MIP algorithm (Axial section).
Subocclusion of the left a. cerebri media.

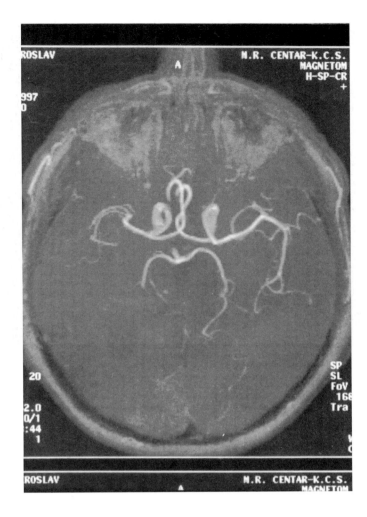

Figure 217. MR angiogram produced with MIP algorithm (Axial section). Occlusion of the right a. cerebri media and right a. cerebri posterior.

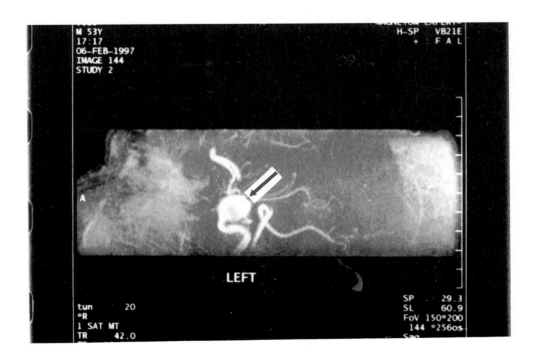

Figure 218. MR angiogram produced with MIP algorithm (Sagittal section). Giant aneurysm of the internal carotid artery in a 53 year old man - arrow.

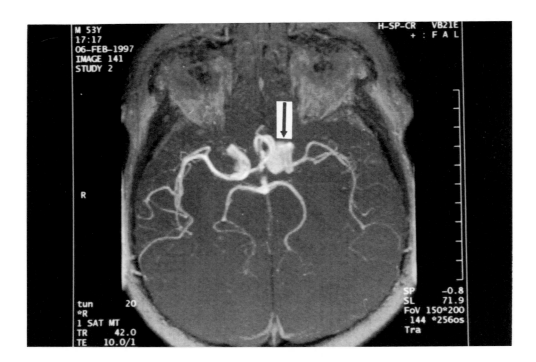

Figure 219. MR angiogram produced with MIP algorithm (Axial section). Giant aneurysm of the internal carotid artery in a 53 year old man - arrow.

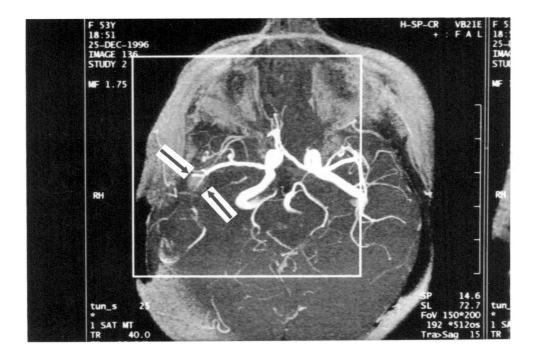

Figure 220. MR angiogram produced with MIP algorithm (Axial section). Saccular aneurysm of the right arteria cerebri media - arrows.

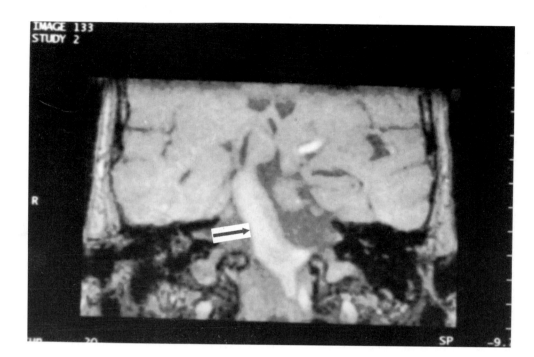

Figure 221. MR angiogram produced with MIP algorithm (Coronal section). Fusiform aneurysm of the basilar artery in a 65 year old man- arrow.

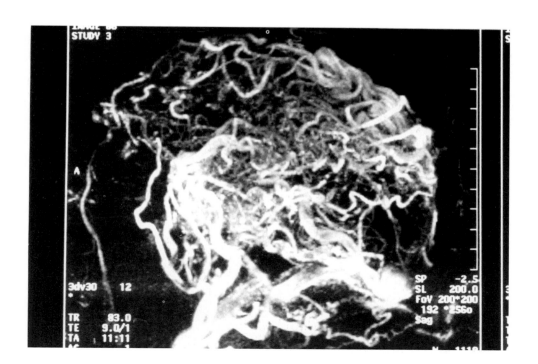

Figure 222. MR angiogram produced with MIP algorithm (Sagittal section). Giant AVM.

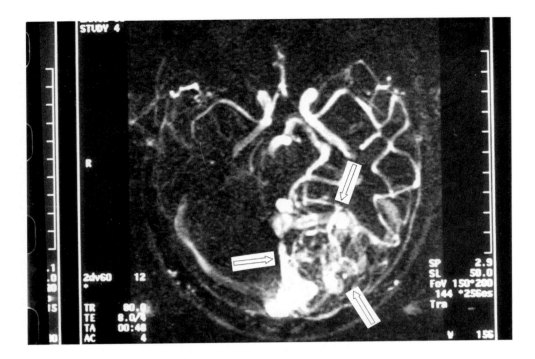

Figure 223. MR angiogram produced with MIP algorithm (Axial section). AVM of the left parieto-occipital region -arrows.

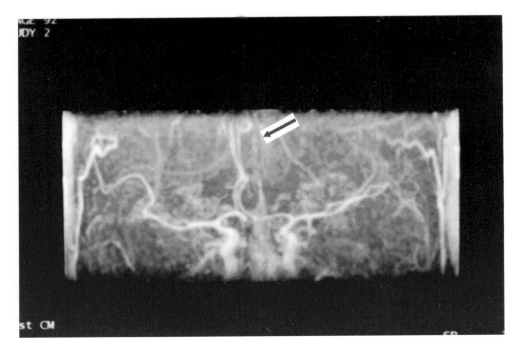

Figure 224. MR angiogram produced with MIP algorithm (Coronal section). Tumor of the left temporal region - scarce pathologic vascularization with elevated a. cerebri media - arrows and dislocation of both anterior cerebral arteries to the right - black arrow.

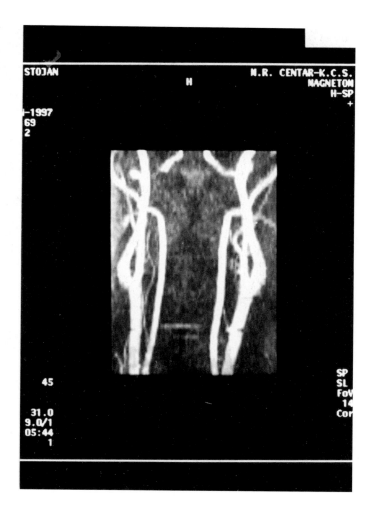

Figure 225. Normal MR angiogram produced with MIP algorithm (Coronal section).
Bifurcation of common carotid artery.

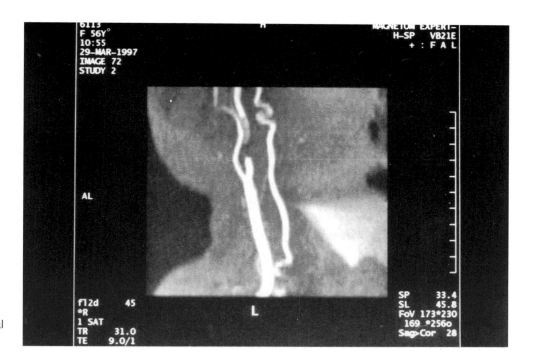

Figure 226. MR angiogram produced with MIP algorithm (Coronal section).
Occlusion of the right internal carotid artery.

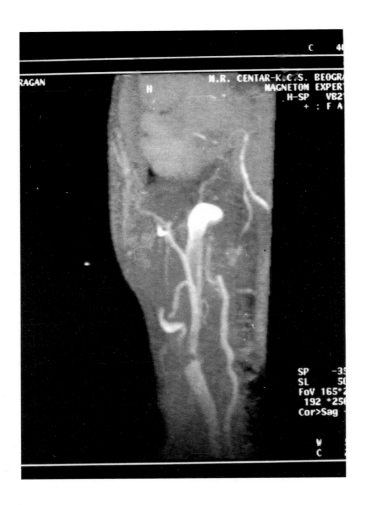

Figure 227. MR angiogram produced with MIP algorithm (Coronal section).
Subocclusion of the right internal carotid artery.

REFERENCES

1. Alfidi RJ., et al.: MR angiography of peripheral, carotid and coronary arteries. AJR, 149: 1097-1112, 1987.
2. Anderson SC., Shah CP., Murtagh FR.: Congested deep cortical veins as a sign of dural venous thrombosis: MR and CT correlations. J. Comput. Assist. Tomogr., 11: 1059-1066, 1987.
3. Cammarata C., Han JS., Haaga JR., Alfidi RJ., Kaufman B.: Cerebral venous angiomas imaged by MR. Radiology, 155: 639-643. 1985.
4. Dumoulin CL., et al.: Three-dimensional phase contrast angiography. Magn. Reson. Med., 9: 139-143, 1989.
5. Edelman RR., et al.: Intracerebral arteriovenous malformations: evaluation with selective MR angiography and venography. Radiology, 173: 831-840, 1989.
6. Keller PJ., et al.: MR angiography with twodimensional acquisition and three-dimensional display. Radiology, 173: 527-538, 1989.
7. Kucharczyk W., Lemme-Plaghos L., Uske A., Brant-Zawadzki M., Dooms G., Norman D.: Intracranial vascular malformations: MR and CT imaging. Radiology, 156: 383-389. 1985.
8. Macchi PJ., et al.: High field MR imaging of cerebral venous thrombosis. J. Comput. Assist. Tomogr., 10: 10-17, 1986.
9. Marchal G., et al.: Intracranial vascular lesions: optimization and clinical evaluation of the 3D time of flight MR angiography. Radiology, 175: 443-451, 1990.
10. Masaryk TJ., et al.: Intracranial circulation: prelimanary clinical results with three-dimensional (volume) MR angiography. Radiology, 171: 793-801, 1989.
11. Rippe DJ., et al.: Demonstration of dural sinus occlusion by the use of MR angiography. Am. J. Neuroradiol., 11: 199-201, 1990.
12. Ross JS., et al.: Intracranial aneurysms: evaluation by MR angiography. Am. J. Neuroradiol., 11: 449-462, 1990.
13. Ruskowski JT., et al: MRI angiography of the carotid artery. Magn. Reson. Imaging, 4: 497-511, 1986.

XIII. MR CONTROLS FOLLOWING THERAPY

Gradimir Dragutinović, Ljiljana Djordjić, Lukas Rasulić

MR controls are indicated upon clinical manifestations in patient or brain pathology:
In patients without definitive diagnosis and progressive disease.

During and after conservative therapy for neurologic, infectious, neuroendocrine, ENT diseases, etc.

MR controls are used postoperatively in case of postoperative complications or when residual or recurrent tumor is suspected. High resolution of MR enables early diagnosis of residual and recurrent tumors. It is of utmost importance to determine radiological features of the tumor upon the first MR examination and pathohistology, so that early detection of the residual or recurrent tumor is alleviated (1).

In patients treated by radiotherapy, MR can show the effects of irradiation on both expansive process and normal anatomy structures. Irradiation can cause degenerative lesions, necrosis and brain hemorrhage (2).

If endocranial secondary deposits are suspected, with primary tumor already known and discrete neurologic finding, MR of CNS can help the early detection and treatment of metastases.

MR controls should be done under same conditions as the initial one, using identical planes, slice thickness, slice distance and sequence. Administration of paramagnetic contrast is decided upon the previous MR findings.

High cost of the examination is a limiting factor for MR controls (7).

Examples:

1-a) Progressive M.S.
Patient with clinical and laboratory confirmation of M.S. in a relapse was examined on MR. SE 500/15 with and without gadolinium-DTPA administration and SE 2500/90/15 were used.

MR tomographs in SE 500/15 after gadolinium-DTPA administration have shown big multiple sclerosis focus in a left temporo-parietal region. Lesion with low signal intensities has the margin with high signal intensities (disturbed hematoencephalic barrier) and perifocal edema with low signal intensity. The rest of small, older M.S. lesions are shown as low signal intensity foci (8).

MR image confirms clinical exacerbation of M.S., showing precise location and size of the recent lesion (Fig. 228).

1-b) Remission of the M.S.
After eight months of conservative therapy patients condition was improved both objectively and subjectively, so that MR control was performed (6). Regression of the pathologic lesions is obvious: the volume of the M.S. lesion is reduced, hyperintensive edge is gone and signal intensity of the cystic lesion is moderately decreased (Fig. 229).

2-a) Tumor denial
Cystic tumor of the left cerebellar hemisphere was found in CT scan of a 6 year old child with acute cerebellar symptomatology.

MR was indicated to confirm the diagnosis (3). MR tomographs in T-2W sequence have revealed big edema of the left cerebellar hemisphere. Diagnosis of cystic tumor was denied (Fig. 230).

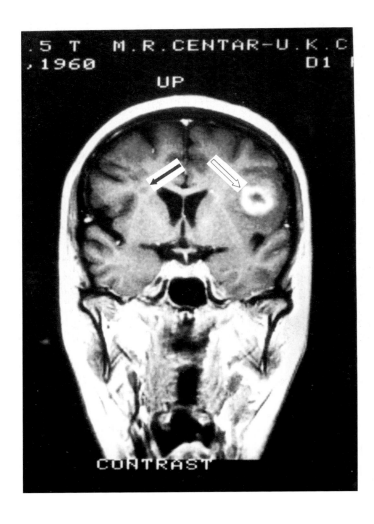

Figure 228. Coronal image (SE 500/15) after gadolinium-DTPA administration.
Big, acute cystic M.S. plaque - white arrow. Older M.S. plaques have low signal intensities - black arrow.

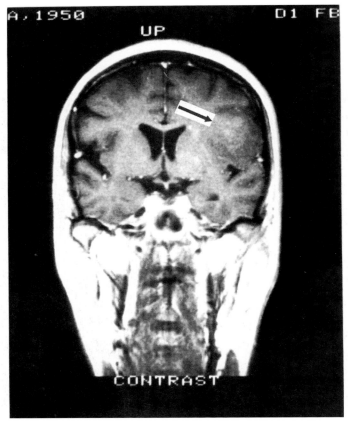

Figure 229. MR control - Identical coronal image (SE 500/15) after gadolinium-DTPA administration. Black arrow pointing at the area of previous acute M.S. focus. Regression of the lesion is obvious.

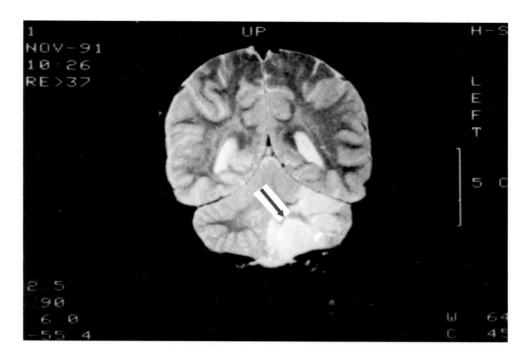

Figure 230. Coronal image (SE 2500/90). Arrow pointing edematous left cerebellar hemisphere.

Non-homogenous signal enhancement of the gyrus edge, and partly in the deeper cerebellar structures was observed in SE 500/15 after gadolinium-DTPA administration. MR image was not convincing about the expansive lesion (Fig. 231).

Surgery was postponed on the basis of MR findings, although the patients condition remained unchanged. It took several weeks of conservative treatment to get the patient better and, finally, completely cured.

MR control, three months later, has discovered incarceration of the left cerebellar hemisphere (Fig. 232). Etiology have remained unknown.

3-a) Tumor controls

In a 25 year old patient parasagittal falx meningioma was confirmed by MR examination. Diagnosis was established upon the CT finding. MR has been done because multiplanar assessment of the relationship between tumor and superior sagittal sinus was needed (Fig. 233).

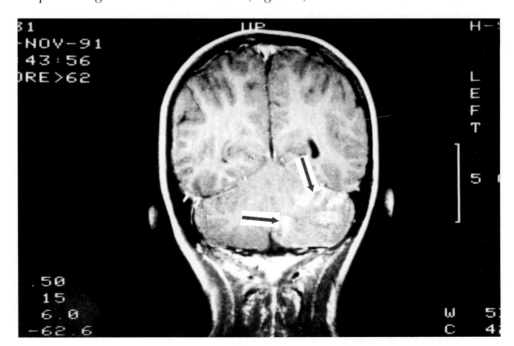

Figure 231. Coronal image (SE 500/15) after gadolinium-DTPA administration. Arrows pointing at signal intensity enhancement in the left cerebellar hemisphere.

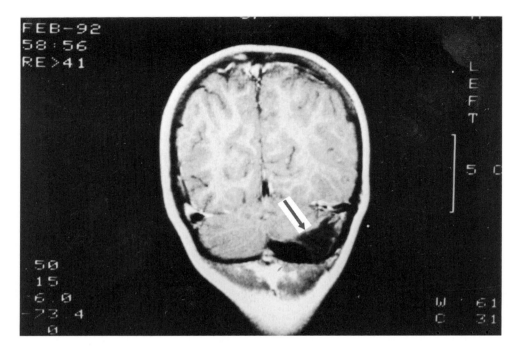

Figure 232. MR control - Coronal image (SE 500/15) after gadolinium-DTPA administration. Arrow pointing at the reduction of the cerebellar parenchyma in the left side (low signal intensity).

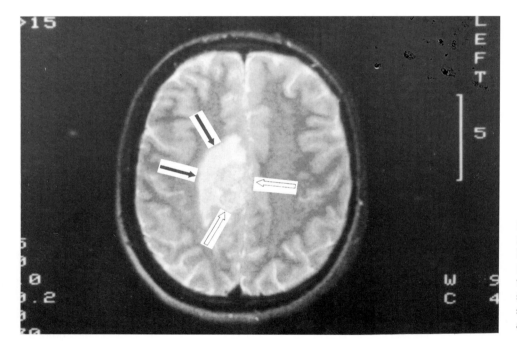

Figure 233. Axial image (SE 2500/90). Tumor has signal intensities similar to the normal anatomy structures - white arrows, whereas intensive perifocal edema has high signal intensities - black arrows.

MR control, six months after extremely successful surgery, did not reveal residual or recurrent meningioma. There is no marked postoperative defect (Fig. 234).

3-b) Diagnostic controls of residual and recurrent tumors

Patient with bilateral hemianopsia and descendent atrophy of both optic nerves, with no deficit of pituitary hormones, CT diagnosis of non-functional adenoma was made. Multiplanar display of tumor and parasellar brain structures was needed, so that MR examination was indicated (4, 5).

Huge hormone-inactive adenoma extending intrasellary, parasellary and suprasellary was found (Fig. 235).

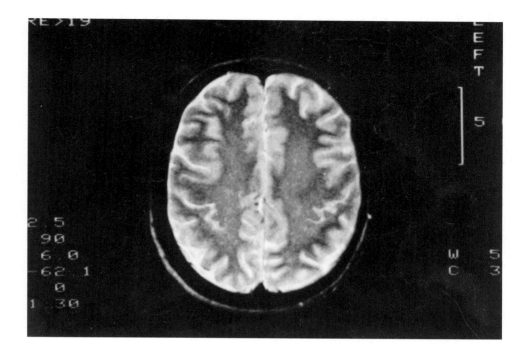

Figure 234. Axial image (SE 2500/90). Postoperative assessment of the brain structures was done in the identical section plane, using the same slice thickness and distance, as well as the identical sequence. Brain recovery is tremendous. Edema regression is complete.

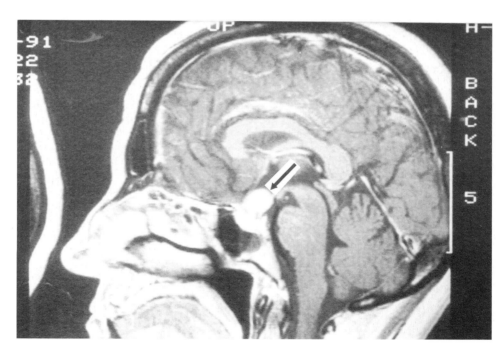

Figure 235. Sagittal image (SE 500/15) after gadolinium-DTPA administration. Huge intrasellar adenoma with high signal intensities and considerable suprasellar propagation - arrow.

Neurologic status was not improved three months after the surgery. MR control have revealed big residual tumor with critical tumor mass located in suprasellar region (Fig. 236). Possibility of reoperation or eventual radiotherapy have arised.

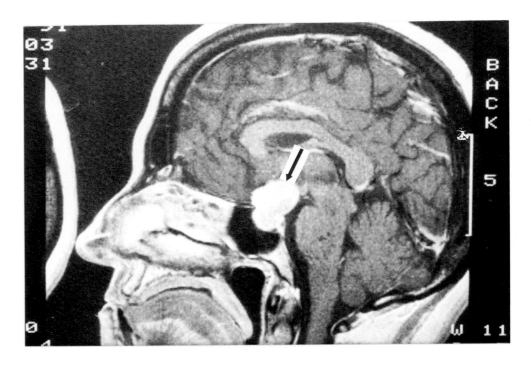

Figure 236. MR control - Sagittal image (SE 500/15) after gadoli- nium-DTPA administration. Arrow pointing at a big residual/recurrent tumor, whereas intrasellar tumor mass was reduced.

REFERENCES

1. Halbsgut A., Lechner B.: Magnetresonanz-Tomographie (NMR). Frankfurt, 1986.
2. Huk WJ., Gademann G., Friedman G.: Magnetic Resonance Imaging of Central Nervous System Diseases. Springer Verlag, Berlin, New York, Heidelberg, Tokyo, Paris, London, 1989.
3. Liessner J., Seider M.: Klinische Kernspintomographie. Enke. Stuttgart, 1987.
4. Pomeranz JS.: Craniospinal Magnetic Resonance Imaging. W.B. Saunders Company. Philadelphia, London, Toronto, Sydney, Tokyo, 1989.
5. Reiser M., et al.: Magnet-rezonanz-Tomographie. Springer-Verlag. Berlin, Heidelberg, New York, Paris, London, Tokyo, Hong Kong, 1989.
6. Stark D., Bradley GWJR.: Magnetic Resonance Imaging. The C.V. Mosby Company. St. Louis, Washington D.C., Toronto, 1988.
7. Zawadcki MB., Norman D.: Magnetic Resonance Imaging of the Central Nervous System. Raven Press. New York, 1987.
8. Zeitler E.: Kernspintomographie. Deutsche Artze Verlag. Koeln, 1984.

XIV. MR IN CHILDREN

Gradimir Dragutinović, Zvonimir Lević, Vaso Antunović

MR examination in children is very important. Special open MR systems have been designed in order to make the examination and eventual anesthesia easier, to enable the presence of parents and to improve the communication with little patients (4-6, 8).

Magnetom Open 0.2 T was among the first open systems (Fig. 237).

Practical advantages of MR examination are:
-no ionizing radiation
-early detection and perfect visualization of the pathology
-all advantages of MRI mentioned in adults

Disadvantages of MR examination are:
-long duration
-anesthesia needed to keep the children still
-high cost of the examination.

Indications in children are similar to those in adults. Computer tomography is still in the front-line of diagnosis, and MR examination, being a complementary method, is used for the diagnosis of congenital malformations, white matter diseases, intra- and postpartum trauma and. (See the following images) (1, 9).

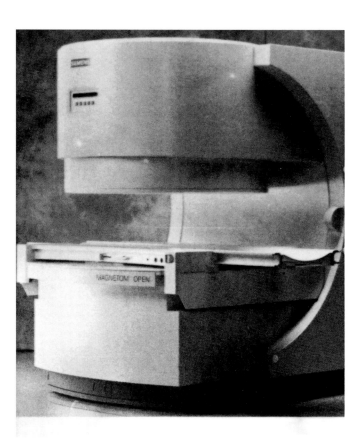

Figure 237. MAGNETOM OPEN 0.2 T.

a) Retrocerebellar arachnoidal pouch

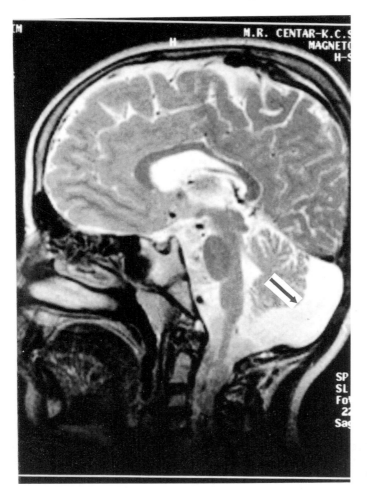

Figure 238. Sagittal image (SE 4000/99). Retrocerebellar arachnoidal pouch without hydrocephalus in a 9-year old boy-arrow.

b) Arachnoidal Cyst

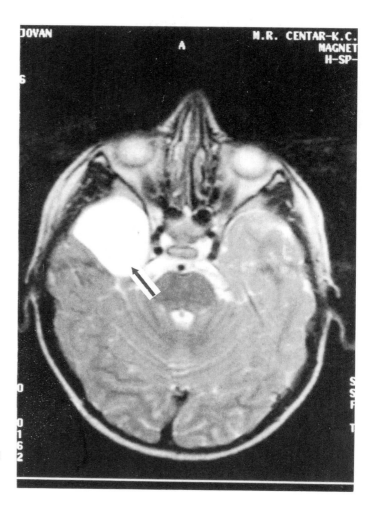

Figure 239. Axial image (SE 4000/99). Large arachnoidal cyst of the right temporal region in a 4-year old boy with epilepsy-arrow.

c) Cryptic AVM

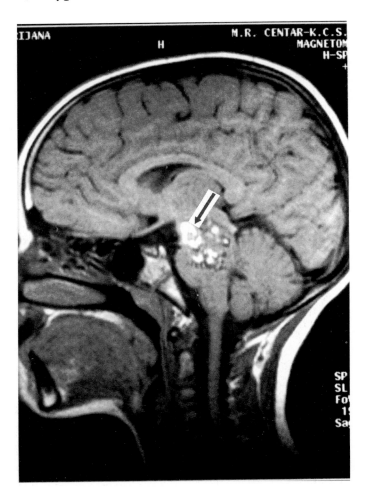

Figure 240. Sagittal image (SE 570/15). Cryptic AVM with tetraparesis chronica in 6-year old boy-arrow.

d) Borreliosis

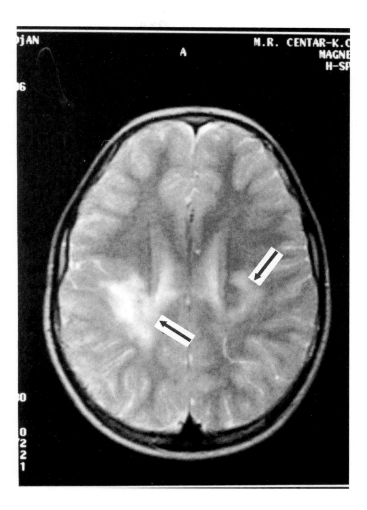

Figure 241. Axial image (SE 4000/90). Bilateral periventricular large hyperintensive lesion in 8-year old boy-arrows.

e) Leukodystrophy

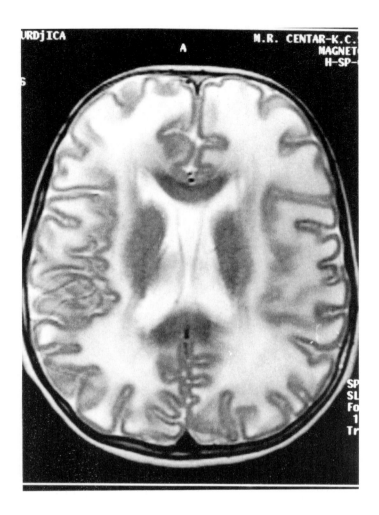

Figure 242. Axial image (SE 4000/99). Leukodystrophy in a 7-year old girl with metal deterioration, apathy and hypotonia.

f) Meningiomas

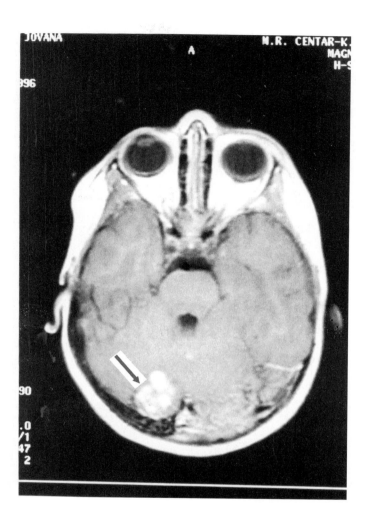

Figure 243. Axial image (SE 570/15) after gadolinium-DTPA administration. Infratentorial, solid, well delineated tumor in a 5-year old girl - arrow.

g) Pilocytic Astrocytomas

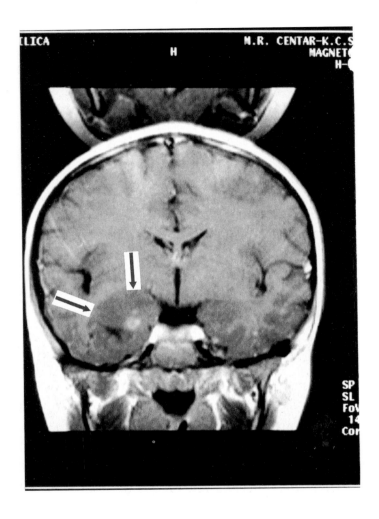

Figure 244. Coronal image (SE 570/15) after gadolinium-DTPA administration. Tumor of the right temporal region in a 6-year old girl.

h) Craniopharyngiomas

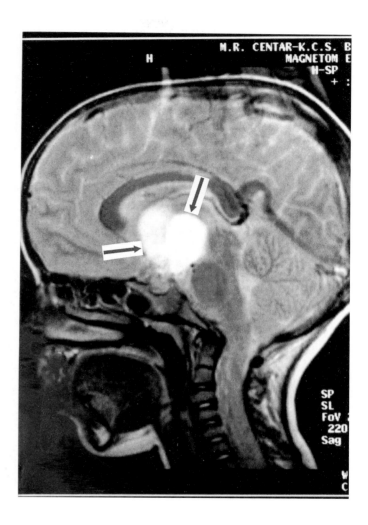

Figure 245. Sagittal image (TSE 2200/88).
Craniopharyngioma in a 7-year old boy with deterioration of vision.

i) Astrocytoma of the cervical cord

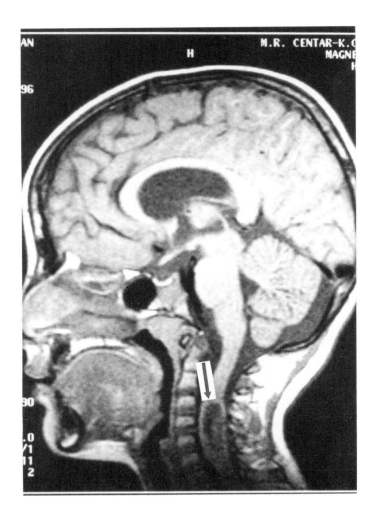

Figure 246. Sagittal image (SE 560/15). Tumor of the cervical cord in a 7-year old boy-arrow.

REFERENCES

1. Banna M.: Arachnoid cysts on computed tomography, AJR, 127: 979-988, 1976.
2. Barkovich AJ., et al.: Revised classification of posterior fossa cysts and cystic malformations based on the results of multiplanar MR imaging. Am. J. Neuroradiol., 10: 977-987, 1989.
3. Coates TL., et al.: Pediatric choroid plexus neoplasms: MR, CT and pathologic correlation, Radiology, 173: 81-87, 1989.
4. Curnes JT., Oakes WJ., Boyko OB.: MR imaging of hindbrain deformity in Chiari II patients with and without symptoms of brainstem compression. Am. J. Neuroradiol., 10: 293-301, 1989.
5. Jinkins JR., Whittemore AR., Bradley WG.: MR imaging of callosal and corticocallosal dysgenesis. Am. J. Neuroradiol., 10: 339-342, 1989.
6. Kemp SS., et al.: Magnetic resonance imaging of the cerebral aqueduct. Neuroradiology, 29: 430-431, 1987.
7. Packer RJ., et al.: Magnetic resonance imaging of lesions of the posterior fossa and upper cervical cord in childhood. Pediatrics, 76: 84-92, 1985.
8. Pojunas K., et al.: Syringomyelia and hydromyelia: magnetic resonance evaluation. Radiology, 153: 679-688, 1984.
9. Zimmerman RA., Bilaniuk LT.: Applications of magnetic resonance imaging in diseases of the pediatric central nervous system. MRI Pediatr., 4: 11-17, 1986.

B. MAGNETIC RESONANCE IN THE DIAGNOSIS OF THE PATHOLOGY OF THE SOFT TISSUES INSIDE SPINAL CANAL

Gradimir Dragutinović, Vaso Antunović, Zvonimir Lević

GENERAL PRINCIPLES

1. Introduction

MR examination is superior to any other complementary neuroradiologic method for the diagnosis of the bone and soft tissue pathology of spine in numerous indications, that are still being updated. MR imaging of the spine is different from the brain examination as we are going to explain in the following chapters.

2. Neuroradiologic examination of the spine

It is necessary to examine the patient clinically in details and perform routine paraclinical examinations (EMG, laboratory analyses, etc.) prior to setting the indication for MR imaging.

Radiological examination used for assessment of soft tissues and bone pathology of the spine are: X-ray plane, myelography, angiography, CT scan and MR.

X-ray plane of spine are necessary for the incipient diagnosis even nowadays. Anterior-posterior (AP or frontal), latero-lateral (LL or profile), semioblique and polytomographic radiographs can contribute enormously to the definitive diagnosis of the spinal condition.

Myelography is a special radiological technique of examination of the pathology inside the spinal canal. The first myelography with negative contrast (air), was performed by Dandy in 1919. Advances in the pharmaceutical industry have introduced in clinical practice liposoluble iodine contrast, that have enabled better radiological diagnosis without intrathecal application of the air.

Liposoluble iodine contrast have been abandoned, because of the numerous disadvantages, such as adhesions, toxic effect on dura, spinal epilepsy, etc., and less toxic iodine contrast were introduced, but in spite of a lot of complications caused by liposoluble contrast diagnostic improvement was enormous. Liposoluble contrast has not been used during the last two decades, but replaced with hydrosoluble iodine contrast that practically has no complications. Hydrosoluble iodine contrast has low toxicity and potential complications, although rarely seen, are spinal epilepsy, anaphylactic shock, etc.

Myelographic examination requires intrathecal injection of 5 ml of hydrosoluble iodine contrast in the lumbar region (lumbar myelography) or suboccipitally (suboccipital myelography). Cervical radiculography through lateral puncture of the neck is a special technique of examination.

Lumbar myelography is used for the diagnosis of spatio-compressive processes on the nerve roots (therefor it is called lumbar radiculography) or tracing the contrast up to the thoracic spine in Trendelenburg position, to detect the stop of contrast in thoraco-lumbar region. Contrast could be led to the cervical segment of spine by the use of special positioning of the patient, thus enabling the exploration of the whole spinal canal. Positioning of the patient enables cranio-caudal and vice versa movement of the contrast through subarachnoidal space using gravitation support, so that various segments of the spine could be explored.

If there is a stop of contrast, for example in case of intraspinal expansion compromising the liquor circulation as well, inferior pole of the tumor is determined. Suboccipital myelography is needed to determine a superior pole. A special, complicated and risky technique is needed for suboccipital intrathecal injection of 5 ml of iodine contrast. Contrast is drawn caudally, because of gravitation, and when it reaches the stop, the superior pole of the tumor is defined.

Suboccipital puncture is performed if the lumbar puncture is not possible because of the arachnitic adhesions, bigger tumor mass in the site of attempted puncture in the lumbo-sacral (LS) region, etc, obstructing the passage of the iodine contrast to the superior spinal segments.

Lateral puncture of the cervical spine with intrathecal injection of hydrosoluble iodine contrast is complicated and inconvenient for the patient, because he lays face downwards. After the premedication, lateral puncture is done under radioscopy control and the contrast injected to achieve good distribution around the nerve roots. Therefore the examination is also called cervical radiculography.

Cervical and lumbar radiculography are used for indirect confirmation of spatio-compressive processes, such as discus hernia, tumor, periradicular cyst, etc.

Although the myelography is an indirect method of visualization, it is still widely used even nowadays all over the world, as well as in our country.

Disadvantages of myelography are that it is invasive and painful, requirements for highly skilled radiologist and technician, indirect visualization of lesions, irradiation, etc.

Angiography is rarely performed. Superselective angiography of spinal blood vessels enables imaging of the tiny vessels inside the spinal canal and it is important for the diagnosis of arterio-venous malformation, hemangioma, aneurysm, occlusion, etc. Those examinations are rarely performed, unless the embolization in the second act is planned. Intervention radiology and therapy are associated with a high risk for the patient.

CT was a real breakthrough in the direct visualization that have enabled definitive diagnosis of the numerous pathologic conditions of bone and soft tissues of the spine.

After the **Scout scan** in LL view of the target segment of the spine, the axial sections are made. Slice thickness 1-2, 3-5 mm and there is additional possibility of the reconstruction of perpendicular planes, i.e. coronal and sagittal. **Extended** scale is very suitable for the display of normal anatomy structures, as well as for the pathology of the spinal bones.

CT examination could be done with intravenous administration of the iodine contrast, when it is required. Iodine contrast enhances the density of the pathologic lesions of the medulla spinalis, like it does in brain pathology. Expansive processes, such as meningioma, ependymoma, etc. are a usual indication for i.v. application of contrast.

Combination of myelography and CT, so called **Myelo-scan**, is a special technique of CT examination following intrathecal injection of hydrosoluble contrast. This is highly precise, although a complicated neuroimaging technique, that enables demarcation of medulla spinalis from subarachnoidal space. Indications for **Myelo-scan** should be determined by neuroradiologist, in order to improve differential diagnosis.

If the above mentioned neuroradiologic examination are insufficient for the definitive diagnosis, MR imaging is indicated. Dependent on clinical appearance and neurologic status, MR could follow the other neuroradiologic examinations, but in certain pathologic conditions of medullae spinalis, MR imaging could be done immediately, avoiding all other radiological examinations (2, 3, 16).

3. Magnetic Resonance of normal anatomy structures

The following sequences are used for the exploration of the spine: **T-1W**, double echo and special rapid **FLASH** and **FISP** sequences. Additional software enables spinal MR angiography (4, 5).

T-1W sequence is used for the differentiation of anatomic details of bone and soft tissues, the same way it is used for MR imaging of the brain (Figg. **247-249**).

Advantage of double echo sequence is the same for the pathology of medulla spinalis, as it is for the brain pathology (Fig. 250).

Same sequences are used for the display of normal anatomy details of thoracic (Th) and lumbo-sacral spinal segment (Figg. 251-256).

Beside **T-1W** and double echo sequence, used for the display of normal anatomy of soft tissue and bone, varieties such as **FLASH** and **FISP** sequence are used to confirm discus hernia, bony fragments, blood collections, fat, etc. can be applied (Fig. 257).

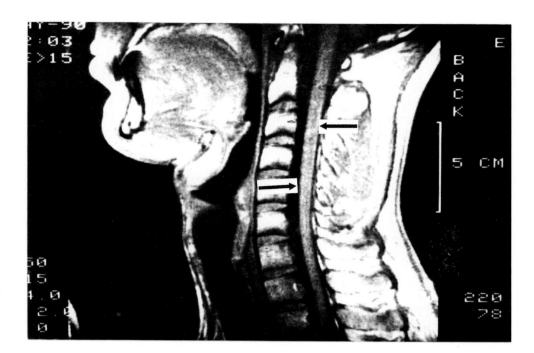

Figure 247. Normal cervical canal. Sagittal image (SE 500/15). Normal cervical spinal cord - arrows.

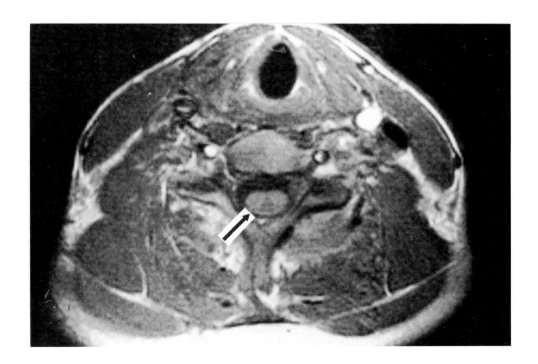

Figure 248. Normal cervical canal. Axial image (SE 500/15). Normal cervical spinal cord - arrow.

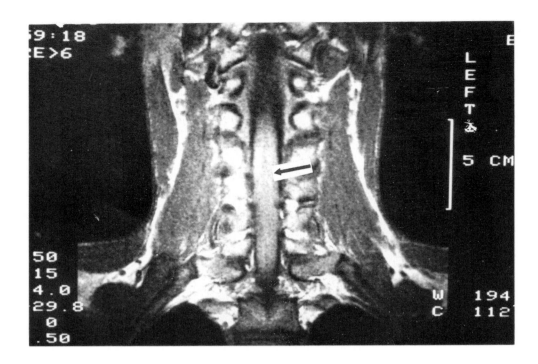

Figure 249. Normal cervical canal. Coronal image (SE 500/15). Normal cervical spinal cord - arrow.

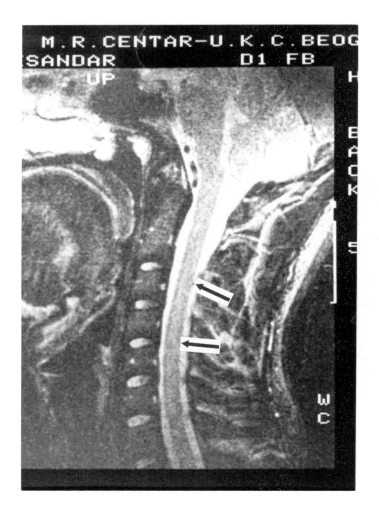

Figure 250. Normal cervical canal. Sagittal image (SE 2500/90). Normal cervical spinal cord - white arrows. High intensity signal of CSF produces a myelograph effects - black arrows.

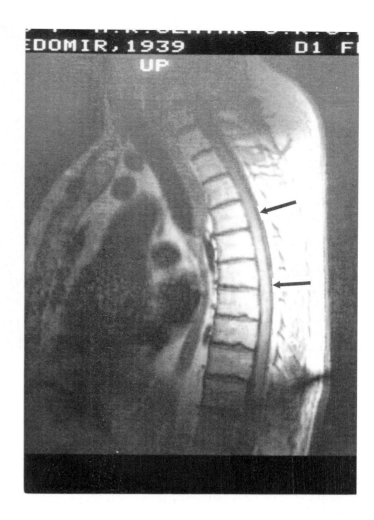

Figure 251. Normal thoracic spinal cord and canal.
Sagittal image (SE 500/15). Normal spinal cord -

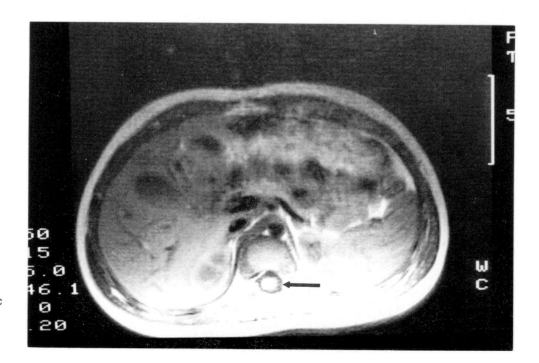

Figure 252. Normal thoracic
spinal cord and canal. Axial
image (SE 500/15). Normal
spinal cord - arrows.

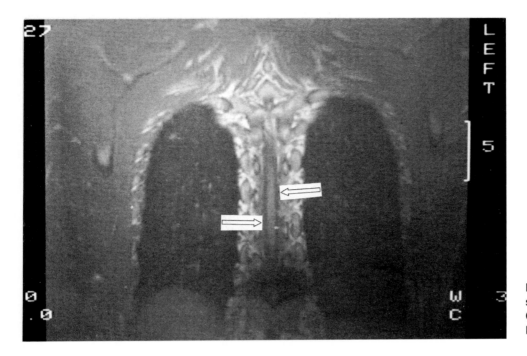

Figure 253. Normal thoracic spinal cord and canal. Coronal image (SE 500/15). Normal spinal cord - arrows.

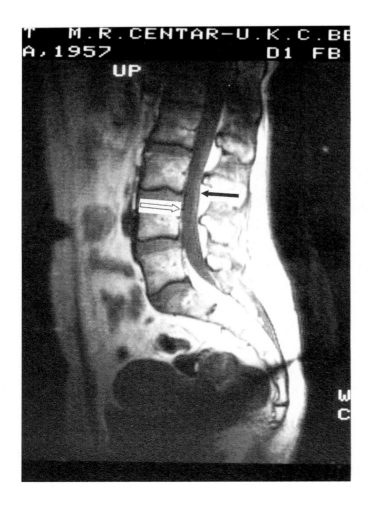

Figure 254. Normal lumbar spine. Sagittal image (SE 500/15). Normal spinal canal - arrows.

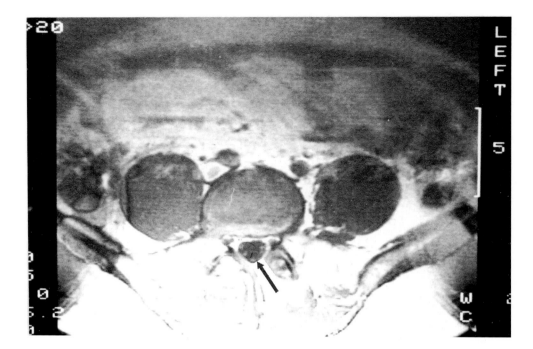

Figure 255. Normal lumbar spine. Axial image (SE 500/15). Normal spinal canal - arrow.

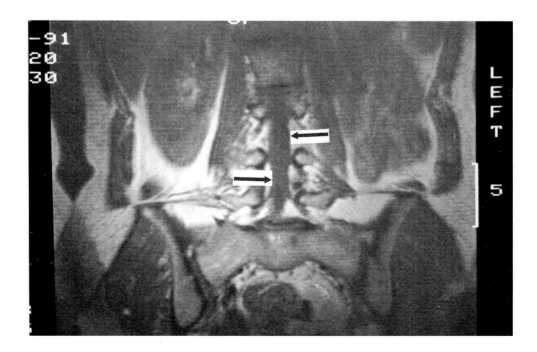

Figure 256. Normal lumbar spine. Coronal image (SE 500/15). Normal spinal canal - arrows.

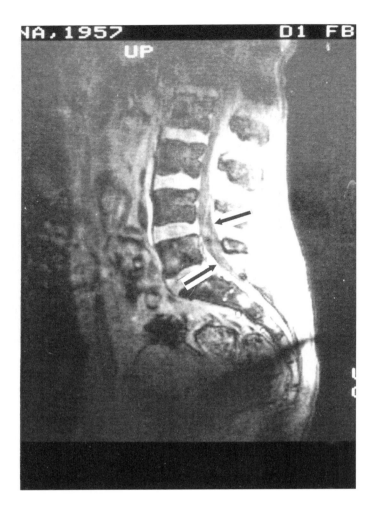

Figure 257. Normal lumbar spine. Sagittal image (FA 50, TR 0.19, TE 7). Mediosagittal view of normal dural sac - arrows.

This sequence is used exclusively for confirmation of the disc pathology.

New software for MR myelography are developed and performed in fi3d TR 71.0, TE 21.0/1 sequence. MR myelography shows nerve roots as well in MIP technique, but this technique is rarely used because it needs further improvement (Figg. 258, 259).

4. Artifacts

Identical artifacts are found in MR examination of the spine and head. Patient movement during the imaging is the crucial problem. Respiratory movement, heart beating, major blood vessels pulsation and intestinal peristaltic could interfere with computer tomography. **"Cardiac triggering"** and **"Respiratory gating"** techniques are used to avoid harmful effect of those movements. Sometimes, patient should be immobilized by straps, if sedation proves insufficient (1).

5. Technique of MR examination

After the patient has been prepared, the same way as for the brain examination, respective segment of the spine is explored on **MR** machine. Patient should lay on his back on the **MR** table in the **MR** room. Cranio-caudal diameter of the field is 15 cm. Antero-posterior and latero-lateral diameter of the field encompasses the dimensions of the neck, thorax, abdomen or pelvis. Blow up of certain details can "expel" tissues and organs surrounding the spine form MR tomograph. Special spinal coils are used for MR imaging of the spine. Newest coils (Array coil) are capable of imaging the whole spine at once.

Spinal coil could be round or ellipsoid plate that should be put beneath the respective segment of the spine (Fig. 260).

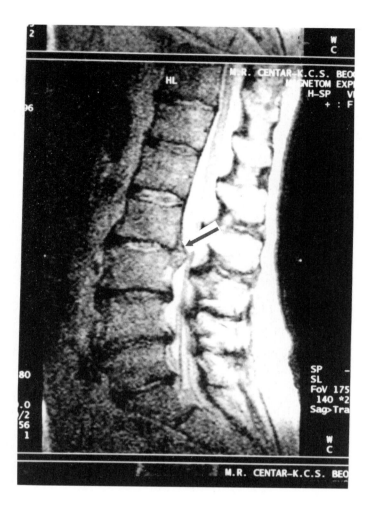

Figure 258. Lumbar spine. Sagittal image (TSE 4000/90). Discus hernia L2 - L3 in patient T.M., aged 63 - arrow.

Best resolution in MR imaging of cervical spine is achieved by the use of **"Helmolz"** coil made of two receiving and emitting antennae (6) (Fig. 261).

"Body" coil, as a part of MR machine, is used if the imaging of the whole spine with lower resolution is needed, for example in case of multiple bone metastases, abnormal spinal curves, various deformities and anomalies, in children, etc. **"Body"** coil is in standard use for MR imaging of abdomen, thorax, etc. (8).

Total time of examination is 5-15 minutes. Absolute and relative contraindications for MR examination, preparation, premedication, anesthesia, etc. are the same as for MR examination of the brain.

6. Choice of sequences for MR imaging

Slice thickness is 2,3 up to 4 mm for direct imaging in sagittal, coronal and axial views. Paraxial views are used also for MR examination of the spine, depending on pathologic and physiologic spinal curves, to display target structures precisely and avoid geometric distortion, such as square into the rectangle, or circle into the ellipse, etc. This fact is very important for subsequent interpretation of the shape of lesion in the tomographs (15).

Slice distance is 0.1-0.2 Reduction of the slice thickness provides for the display of smaller lesions and tiniest details of normal anatomy structures within spinal canal.

Scout scan is always done in T-1W sequence in sagittal view. Five to seven sections of certain thickness are recorded simultaneously. Those section planes are valuable for the diagnosis and therefore they could not be regarded as **Scout scan** only.

According to the pathology revealed by sagittal sections and assumed diagnosis, additional axial and/or coronal planes and respective sequences are used.

Protocol of MR imaging of the spine includes following sequences: **T-1W, T-2W, proton density,** and special rapid sequences **FLASH** and **FISP**, when needed to confirm discus hernia, bony fragments, hemorrhage, etc. (7, 10).

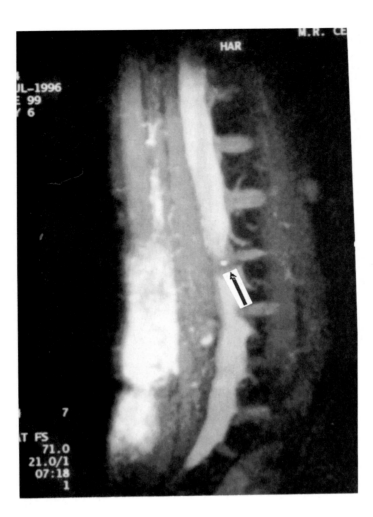

Figure 259. Lumbar spine. Sagittal image (fi3d 71.0, 21.0/1). MR myelograph - Discus hernia L2-L3 in patient T.M, aged 63 - arrow.

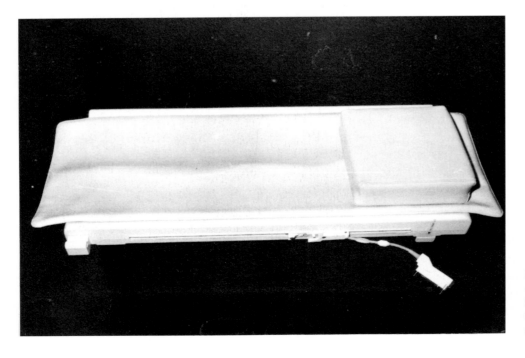

Figure 260. Round and ellipsoid coils for MR imaging of thoracic and lumbo-sacral segments of the spine.

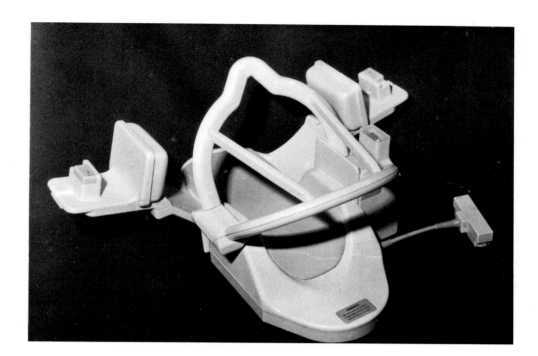

Figure 261. "Helmholz" coil for the imaging of cervical spinal segment.

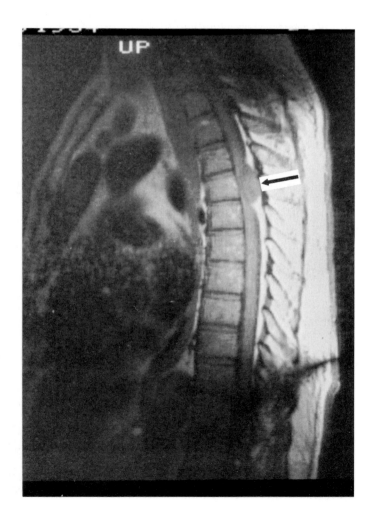

Figure 262. Thoracic spinal cord and canal in a 63 year old man. Sagittal image (SE 500/15). Neurinoma of the thoracic spine. Extramedullar, intradural, medium intensity nodular mass at T5-T6 with anterior displacement of the spinal cord - arrow.

Inversion recovery is a special sequence of signal intensity inversion that takes 10-14 minutes and has no special advantage, so that it is seldom used all over the world and in our country as well.

MR myelography has become possible by the use of 3D reconstruction and MIP technique for the desired view in MR myelograph. Technologic advantage of MR myelography has not been fully evaluated yet (12).

MR angiography is a possibility to perform non-invasive angiography without the contrast or any peril for the patient, and reach the precise diagnosis using MIP technique of blood vessels positioning. MR angiography still enables approximative assessment and could not replace invasive spinal angiography.

Time is not critical, so that full arsenal of sequences should be used until the final diagnosis is reached. Paramagnetic contrast administration is indicated for special cases.

7. Paramagnetic contrast in the MR imaging of the spine

Paramagnetic contrast Magnevist is used for exploration of the soft tissue structures inside spinal canal and extravertebrally. Effect and signal enhancement in pathologic lesions is based on the same principles as in brain pathology (14).

Administration of paramagnetic contrast, dose and timing of MR imaging are identical as well. Imaging is always done in T-1W sequence. Contraindications for contrast application are the same as for the diagnosis of brain pathology (5, 9, 11).

Indications for Magnevist application depend on the diseases of medulla spinalis and it is usually used for optimal triplanar display and full demarcation of tumor from normal structures (Figg. 262, 263).

Same patient has been examined in other sequence (SE 500/15) after gadolinium-DTPA administration (12, 13).

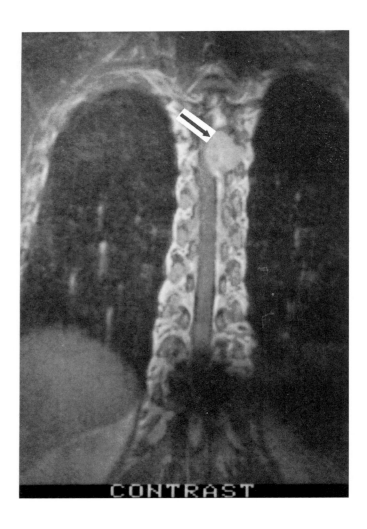

Figure 263. Thoracic spinal cord and canal in a 63 year old man. Coronal image (SE 500/15) after gadolinium-DTPA administration. Rapid and marked enhancement of the neurinoma - arrow.

REFERENCES

1. Bellon EM., Haake EM., Coleman PE., Sacco DC., Steiger DA., Gangarosa RE .: MR artifacts: a review. AJR, 147: 1271-1281, 1986.
2. Berger PE., et al.: High-resolution surface coil magnetic resonance imaging of the spine: normal and pathologic anatomy. Radiographics, 6: 573-577, 1986.
3. Brant-Zawadzki M., Norman D., Newton TH., Kelly WM., Kjos B., Mills CM., Dillon W., Sobel D., Crooks LE.: Magnetic resonance of the brain: the optimal screening technique. Radiology, 152: 71-77, 1984.
4. Han JS., et al.: NMR imaging of the spine. AJNR, 4: 1151-1179,1983.
5. Hueftle MG., et al.: Lumbar spine: postoperative MR imaging with Gd-DTPA. Radiology, 167: 817-827, 1988.
6. Kalkarni MV., Patton JA., Price RR.: Technical considerations for the use of surface coils in MRI. AJR, 147: 373-378, 1986.
7. Mayer JS., Kulkarni MV.: MR imaging of incisional spinal cord injury. AJNR, 8: 925-940, 1987.
8. McArdle CB., et al.: Surface coil MR of spinal trauma: preliminary experience. AJNR, 7: 885-893, 1986.
9. Michel D.: Grundlagen und Methoden der kernmagnetischen Resonanz. Akademie Verlag. Berlin, 1981.
10. Modic MT., et al.: Nuclear magnetic resonance imaging of the spine. Radiology, 148: 757-769, 1983.
11. Sze G., et al.: Gadolinium DTPA in the evaluation of intradural extramedullary disease. Am. J. Neuroradiol., 9: 153-160, 1988.
12. Sze G., Krol G., Zimmerman RD., Deck MDF.: Gadolinium-DTPA: malignant extradural spinal tumors. Radiology, 167: 217-226, 1988.
13. Sze G.: Gadolinium-DTPA in spinal disease. Radiol. Blin. North Am., 26: 1009-1019, 1988.
14. Valk J.: Gadolinium-DTPA in MR of spinal lesions. AJNR, 9: 345-361, 1988.
15. Van Dyk C., et al.: Gradient echo MR imaging of the cervical spine: evaluation of extradural degenerative disease. AJNR, 10: 627-641, 1989.
16. Walker HS., et al.: Magnetic resonance imaging of the pediatric spine. Radiographics, 7: 1129-1144, 1987.

I. MALFORMATIONS

Ljiljana Djordjić, Gradimir Dragutinović, Lukas Rasulić

Congenital malformations of the spine in general could be divided into two groups: malformations of the bone and malformations of soft tissues inside spinal canal. Bone structures are perfectly visualized directly by radiological techniques. Classic radiography and CT examination are the methods of choice for the diagnosis of bone malformations of the spine. This is particularly true for the new generation of CT machines (helical CT). MR examination can add to the precise multiplanar visualization of the pathologic lesions of the bones (3).

MR is superior to CT for the multiplanar display of malformations of the spinal canal and medulla spinalis. Precise diagnosis of abnormality is enabled by optimal demarcation of normal anatomy of medulla spinalis, white and gray matter, liquor space, spinal nerve roots and paravertebral soft tissues by MR imaging. MR examination could provide the information on the bone malformation as well (1, 8).

Rare spinal cord malformations, that could be associated with bone malformations, are: amyelia, myelodysplasia, diplomyelia, diastematomyelia, *Arnold-Chiari* malformation, syringomyelia, A-V malformation, etc. Certain malformation of spinal bones, such as *Klippel-Feil* syndrome, platybasia, etc, could be associated with neurologic findings, although no abnormality of medulla spinalis has been observed.

A) Midline closure defects of the spine (I) and of the spinal cord (II)

I Of the spine
—a- Spina bifida occulta
—b- Spina bifida cystica
—c- Meningocele
—d- Myelomeningocele
—e- Ventral spinal defects

II Of the spinal cord
—a- Syringomyelia and hydromyelia
—b- Duplication of the spinal cord
　　dimyelia
　　diplomyelia
　　diastematomyelia
—c- Tethered cord
—d- Lipoma
—e- Dermoid, epidermoid, dermal sinus
—f- Teratomas

I —a- Spina bifida occulta

Spina bifida occulta is formed because of the abortive laminar fusion in a part of spinal canal, usually lumbo-sacral segment. It is found accidentally in 20% of adults. It is important to diagnose the anomaly prior to the surgical exposure of the spinal canal.

Myelodysplasia is a malformation that could be associated with spina bifida as well.

I —c- Meningocele

Meningocele are quite rare malformations with cystic lesion containing meninges and cerebrospinal liquor and no nerve tissue whatsoever.

CT examination enables precise diagnosis of myelopdysplasiae. **Myelo-scan** is required sometimes.

MR tomography optimally shows various forms of myelodysplasia multiplanary.

Features of myelocele with subcutaneous spread, could be precisely assessed in MR tomographs (13).

MR confirms meningocele mutiplanary in classic sequences, displaying vertebral bone abnormalities at the same time (Fig. 264).

I—d- Meningomyelocele

Meningomyelocele are the most frequent and most important type of spinal dysraphism found in approximately 2/1000 newborn children. It is caused by a defective formation of the neural tube, which is embryonic precursor of the vertebral column and spinal cord. It is manifested by a protrusion of the neural elements of the spinal cord through a vertebral defect to the meningeal sac. Spinal cord fusion have not occurred, but the spinal cord exists in a flat embryonic shape, with nerve roots arising from the ventral surface and open spinal cord dorsally.

Irreversible neurologic deficit is caused by a spinal cord anomaly in meningomyelocele. Spinal cord, conus or cauda equina could be affected dependent on the level of the defect.

Prenatal diagnosis could be made by ultrasound examination and alpha 1 fetoprotein measurement in amniotic fluid between 14. and 16. weeks of pregnancy.

Meningomyelocele are usually associated with other congenital malformations, such as Arnold-Chiari type II, aqueduct stenosis or hydromyelia (syringomyelia) (15).

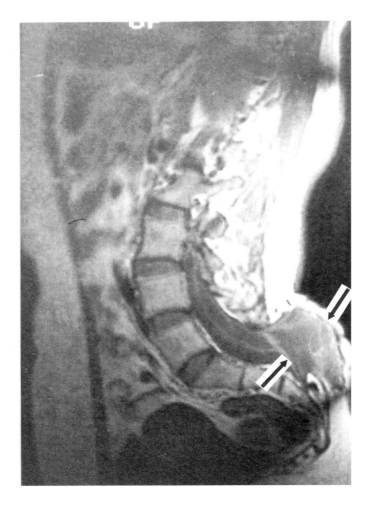

Figure 264. Lumbar spine. Sagittal image (SE 500/15). Sacral meningocela with subcutaneous spread is optimally shown - arrows.

Clinical manifestation and neurologic deficit in meningomyelocele are determined by various forms of the extraspinal meningeal prolapse, involvement of the portions of medulla spinalis in the prolapsed segment and cystic cavity inside prolapsed medulla.

Computer tomography can show meningomyelocele quite well.

Magnetic resonance is a method of choice for the diagnosis of this anomaly in children (18).

Surgical treatment should provide for:

a. Neural tissue preservation and its reposition to the spinal canal.

b. Watertight closure of dural sac.

c. Covering of the defect by muscle, fascia and skin.

Criteria for the surgical therapy are:

a. Paralysis beyond L2, L3 or higher level

b. Marked hydrocephalus

c. Kyphosis

d. Other significant malformations or perinatal trauma.

II—a- Syringomyelia and hydromyelia

Syringomyelia is a cavity inside a spinal cord with gradual accumulation of fluid. Syringomyelic cavity can involve the whole AP or LL diameter of the spinal cord with cranio-caudal extension through one or more spinal cord segments (2).

Term syringomyelia is related to a closed cavity, separated from the spinal canal, without any communication. Lack of communication could be caused by previous trauma, neoplasm or associated with arachnitis spinalis. Pathologic process that have caused syringomyelia is sometimes unknown (5).

Dilation of the central canal communicating with other CSF liquor cavities is called hydromyelia. Hydromyelia (Communicant syringomyelia) can be caused by Arnold-Chiari I or II malformation and basilar arachnitis sometimes (7).

Syringomyelia can be classified as a) primary and b) secondary

a) Primary syringomyelia is caused by a developmental disorder, trauma or dilation of the preexisting cyst due to the transudation of liquid from surrounding tissue.

b) Secondary syringomyelia is caused by a direct trauma, following resorption of the blood in hematomyelia or arachnoiditis, i.e. in certain forms of expansive process with or without cystic component.

Idiopathic syringomyelia in adults is associated with lost sensation of pain and weakness of the arms, because of the distribution of the spinothalamic and corticothalamic fibers. Progressive syndrome of dislocated loss of sensibility with shoulder distribution is seen in such cases (f.e. lack of pain sensation and preserved tactile sensation). Lack of sensibility is accompanied by a muscular mass reduction and muscular weakness, beginning in the arms. Cranial extension of the syrinx can cause other impairments such as dysphagia and nystagmus.

Natural history of the disease is gradual deterioration.

CT scan can detect bigger syringomyelic cavities, usually situated in the cervical segment. Subarachnoidal injection of hydrosoluble contrast during CT examination has been abandoned. Myelography is not indicated for the diagnosis of syringomyelia.

MR is a method of choice for the diagnosis of syringomyelia. Intramedullar cavity in any spinal segment is displayed by MR. Complete medulla spinalis is shown by MR imaging, without artifacts, which is of special importance for the craniocervical junction and cervico-thoracic region, inaccessible to the CT exploration (10, 17).

MR imaging is done in sagittal and eventually axial views (Fig. 265).

Syringomyelic cavity with low signal intensity is shown in the cervical and partly thoracic segments of the spinal cord, extending from C1 to Th3 level - arrows.

MR controls are of utmost importance for already diagnosed syringomyelic cavities. Fluid pressure inside the cavity is equal or higher than the liquor pressure inside the spinal canal. Syringomyelic cavity dilation could be caused by elevated pressure of its fluid contents. If progressive syringomyelia is discovered by a MR control after several months, neurosurgical drainage of the fluid from the cystic cavity should be performed (11).

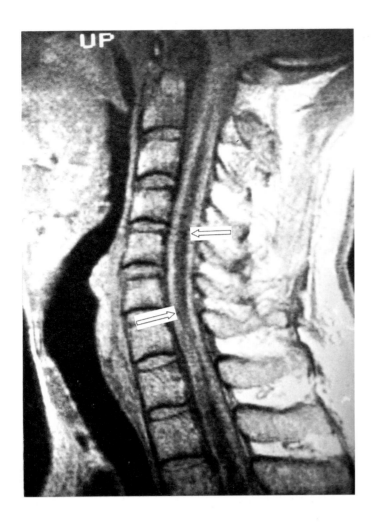

Figure 265. Cervical canal. Sagittal image (SE 2000/15)-syringomyelic cavity-arrows.

Two principle types of surgical treatment are:
1. Decompression of the posterior cranial fossa
2. Shunting of the intramedullar cavity
Choice of the best surgical procedure and role of the surgery are still controversial (4, 19).

If there is associated Arnold-Chiari malformation with incarceration of the tonsil in foramen magnum, decompression and dural plastic should be done (16). If there is no such malformation, syrinx could be drained to subarachnoidal space, peritoneal or pleural cavity. In case of hydrocephalus ventricular drainage could be performed.

Some Authors advocate opening of the dilated central canal to subarachnoidal space at the level of filum terminale.

II—b- Diastematomyelia

In diastematomyelia, spinal cord is split in two semimedullae separated by a bony ridge or dural septum. Progressive neurologic deficit develops because of the spinal cord traction due to fixation and inability to grow.

Spinal cord traction is sometimes caused by a short, thick filum terminale (hypertrophied filum terminale) associated with spina bifida and hairy zone above lower spine as the only abnormalities.

Radiological examination include X-ray radiography, CT scan with iodine contrast application and MRI.

Various vertebral abnormalities are seen in X-ray plane, such as spina bifida, hemivertebrae, abnormal spinal curves, diastematomyelic ridges and increased interpedicular distances (6).

Magnetic resonance is indicated as a complementary method for the diagnosis of diastematomyelia (9).

Surgical treatment for this malformation includes removal of the pathologic substrate with neural elements preservation mobilization of the spinal cord.

Intraneural fibromatosis is less frequent than cutaneous form, usually affecting major nerves with possible malignant alteration. It is usually found in the cervical, brachial or lumbo-sacral plexus and manifested by a radicular syndrome of the involved nerve and progressive development of the spinal syndrome with respective symptomatology of the spinal level affected by neurofibroma. Tumor arises from the intraneurally proliferated Schwanns cells with diffuse transformation of long neural segments. They compress the nerve but don't invade the neural substance, with axon penetration of neurofibroma body unlike eccentric position of the tumor body axon in schwannoma.

Microsurgical resection of the tumor is still controversial. Although approximately 10% of neurofibroma undergo malignant alteration it should be kept in mind that radical surgical excision can cause serious neurologic deficit. Initial partial resection of the tumor is advocated, with subsequent radical excision in case of malignant alteration.

II —d- Lipoma

Lumbo-sacral lipoma is manifested at birth as a soft subcutaneous mass in the midline. Lipomeningomyelocele are far more serious, with lipoma involving neural tissue and protruding through spina bifida. Less severe forms are associated with low position of the conus and spinal cord traction over enlarged filum terminale and fat tissue (Fig. 266).

II —e- Dermoid, epidermoid, dermal sinus
II —f- Teratomas

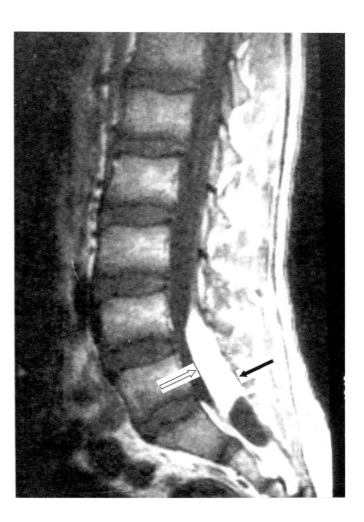

Figure 266. Lumbar spine. Sagittal image (SE 500/15). Lipoma shown in high intensity - arrows.

Dermoid, epidermoid, dermal sinus, teratoma, lipoma, etc., according to some Authors, represent the tumors which accompany occult spinal dysraphism. Those malformations lead to numerous spinal disorders, usually in lumbar region with eventual neurologic impairment because of the spinal cord traction. They are usually associated with cutaneous manifestations above, such as skin spots, sinus tract, lipoma, hemangioma or abnormal hirsutism.

Malformations are usually manifest in childhood or youth with slowly progressive neurologic dysfunction, such as:

disturbed sphincter function
progressive leg weakness and feet deformities
back pain
impaired sensibility in lower extremities
progressive scoliosis

CT and MRI are the methods of choice for the diagnosis (14).
MRI is superior for triplanar visualization of malformation (Figg. 267, 268).
Those malformations can be surgically treated.

B) Neuroectodermal dysplasias

—a- Neurofibromatosis

Neurofibromatosis - Morbus Recklinghausen is representant of neuroectodermal dysplasia. Skin pigmentation, multiple cutaneous neurofibromata (*"mollusca fibrosa"*), hyperplasia of the skin and subcutaneous tissue, abnormal hirsutism, hyperostosis or bone rarefaction with cyst formation (*osteitis fibrosa cystica*) as

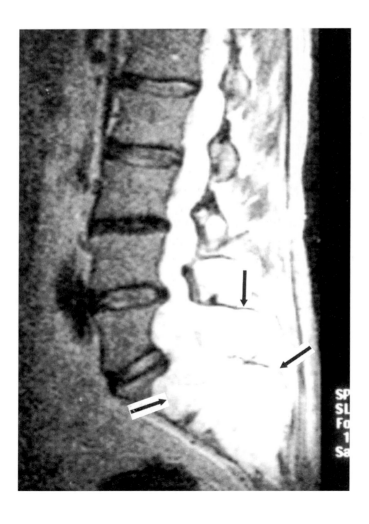

Figure 267. Lumbar spine. Sagittal image (SE 4000/90). Teratomas in a 45 year old man - arrows.

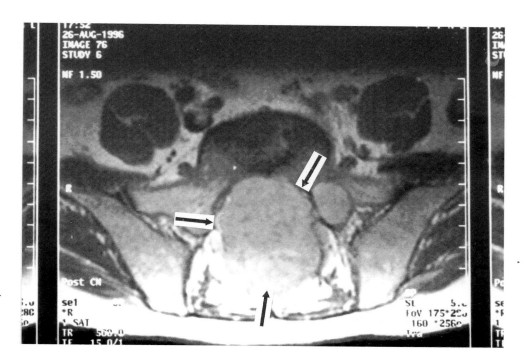

Figure 268. Lumbar spine. Axial image (SE 500/15) after gadolinium-DTPA administration. Teratomas in a 45 year old man - arrows.

well as multiple neurofibromata of spinal and cranial nerves are found. Acoustic and trigeminal nerves are usually involved among cranial nerves. Spinal neurofibromata affect nerve roots paravertebrally. Neurofibroma is slow growing of variable size up to 10 mm and their number could surpass several thousand. They are made of Schwanns cells, fibroblasts, myelinated and non-myelinated nerve fibers and collagen and hyaline degenerated connective tissue. Malignant alteration is exceptional, with rapid lethal outcome.

The disease is progressive and asymptomatic for quite a long time. The diagnosis is usually made upon cutaneous spots and tumors. In type II neurofibromatosis or "central neurofibromatosis" bilateral acoustic neurinoma and other endocranial tumors are found, without peripheral manifestation of the disease. Symptoms depend on the size and location of neurofibromata.

Neuroradiologic aspect relates to the total volume and location of neurofibromas, both in intracranial and intraspinal localization.

CT with i.v. injection of iodine contrast is usually sufficient for the display of neurofibromas in various locations. MR imaging is important for the diagnosis of smaller neurofibromas and multiplanar display of multiple tumors (12, 20).

In our patient, tumor has caused compression of the cervical segment of medulla spinalis. Neurofibroma is clearly demarcated, located paravertebrally and invading spinal canal. Coronal MR tomographs after i.v. injection of paramagnetic contrast optimally displays neurofibroma with high signal intensities. Multiplanar view of the expansive formation enables correct choice of the operative approach (Fig. 269).

Treatment of tumor is by neurosurgical removal.

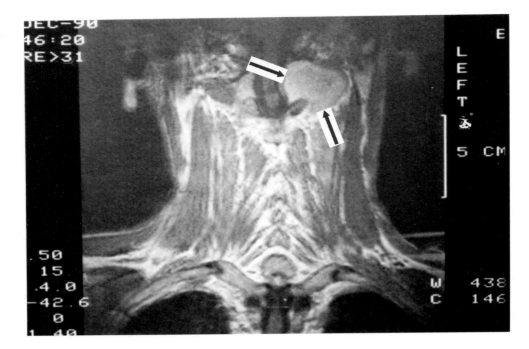

Figure 269. Cervical spine. Coronal image (SE 500/15) after gadolinium-DTPA administration. Extradural, paravertebral, well defined neurofibroma with high signal intensities is shown at the level of C2 vertebral body. Tumor makes impression on the cervical spinal cord - arrows.

REFERENCES

1. Baleriaux O., Oeroover N., Hermanus N., Segebarth C.: MRI of the spine. Diagn. Imag. Clin. Med., 55: 66-71, 1986.
2. Ball MJ., Dayan AD.: Pathogenesis of syringomyelia. Lancet II, 799-801, 1972.
3. Bewewrmeyer H., et al.: MR imaging of familiar basilar impression. J. Comput. Tomogr., 8: 953-971, 1984.
4. Davis PC., et al.: Spinal abnormalities in pediatric patients: MR imaging findings compared with clinical, myelographic, and surgical findings. Radiology, 166: 679-691, 1988.
5. Donaner E., Rascher K.: Syringomyelia: A brief review of ontogenic, experimental and clinical aspects. Neurosurg. Rev., 16: 7-13, 1993.
6. Dunsber SB., Brown O., Thompson N.: Craniovertebral anomalies. Clin. Neurosurg., 27: 430-439, 1980.
7. Eggers C., Hamer I.: Hydrosyringomyelia in childhood. Clinical aspects pathogenesis and therapy. Neuropediatric, 10: 87-99, 1979.
8. Friedburg H., Schumacher M., Hennig J.: Pathologie des kraniozervikalen Uberganges in der magnetischen Resonanztomographie. ROFO, 145: 315-320, 1986.
9. Han JS., et al.: Demonstration of diastematomyelia and associated abnormalities with MR imaging. AJNR, 6: 215-229, 1985.
10. Kohler D., Treisch J., Hertel G., Schorner W., Fiegler W.: Die magnetische Resonanztomagraphie der Syringomyelie. ROFO, 143(6): 617-622, 1985.
11. Lee BCP., Zimmerman RD., Manning JJ., Deck MDF.: MR imaging of syringomyelia and hydromyelia. AJR, 144: 1149 1985.
12. Lewis TT., Kingsley DP.: Magnetic resonance imaging of multiple spinal neurofibromata-neurofibromatosis. Neuroradiology, 29: 562-571, 1987.
13. Modic MT., et al.: Nuclear magnetic resonance imaging of the spine. Radiology, 148: 757-786, 1983.
14. Monajati A., Spitzer RM., LaRue WJ., Heggeness L.: MR imaging of a spinal teratoma. J. Comput. Assist. Tomogr., 10: 307-310, 1986.
15. Paul KS., et al.: Arnold-Chiari malformations. Review of cases. J. Neurosurg., 58: 183-187, 1983.
16. Samuelsson L., et al.: MR imaging of syringohydromyelia and Chiari malformations in myelomeningocele patient with scoliosis. AJNR, 8: 539-546, 1987.
17. Sherman JL., Brkovich AJ., Citrin CM.: The MR appearance of syringomyelia: new observations. AJNR, 7: 985-999, 1986.
18. Sklar EM., Quencer RM., Gren BA.: Posttraumtic spinal meningocele: MR and clinical features. AJNR, 11: 1184-1211, 1990.
19. Williams B.: Syringomyelia. Neurosurg. Clin. North Am., 1: 653-685, 1990.
20. Zanella FE., Steinbrich W., Friedmann G., Koulouskis A.: Magnetische Resonanztomographie (MR) bei spinalen Raumforderungen. ROFO, 145: 326-330, 1986.

II. VASCULAR DISEASES OF MEDULLA SPINALIS

Zvonimir Lević, Gradimir Dragutinović, Vaso Antunović

Clinical and neuroradiologic diagnosis of vascular diseases of medulla spinalis and spinal canal is quite difficult. The same vascular diseases are found in the brain and medulla spinalis.

CT and angiography are not selective enough for the visualization of smaller lesions. Therefore MR is the dominant method of acquiring informations on these lesions.

a) Infarction of the medulla spinalis

Infarction of the medulla spinalis or myelomalacia is usually caused by ischemia in the vascularization bed of anterior spinal artery. Ischemia involves two thirds of the spinal cord.

Infarction of the medulla spinalis is clinically manifested by paralysis, loss of sensibility of syringomyelic type, inferior to the affected spinal cord level, and impaired sphincter function. Onset of symptomatology is usually accompanied by intensive pain in the back and legs. Flaccid palsy is initially found, with development of the spasticity within several weeks.

Axial CT scan of the infarction of the medulla spinalis is usually overlapped by artifacts and blurred by movement, so that it is hard to establish the diagnosis.

MRI could make the diagnosis of the infarction the medulla spinalis in a form of progressive or complete infarction. Milder ischemia is impossible to recognize or differentiate in MR tomographs. Neurologist makes a final diagnosis of the infarction of the medulla spinalis according to clinical, laboratory and MR findings (4).

MR features of the lesions caused by impaired arterial or venous circulation, in classic sequences and section planes, are identical to those found in the brain (10).

Neurologic examination should determine the site of lesion precisely, to enable the detection of smaller lesions in MR tomographs.

Infarction zone has lower signal intensities in T-1W and higher signal intensities in T-2W sequence. MR finding is non-specific so that myelomalacia, cyst, infiltrative tumor, etc, should be ruled out in differential diagnosis (Fig. 270).

b) Hemorrhage

Hemorrhage is rarely found in the spinal canal or spinal cord. It is usually caused by trauma and exceptionally in A-V malformation, aneurysm, tumor, etc.

Hemorrhage in epidural or subdural space is seen in hemorrhagic diathesis, anticoagulant therapy or vascular malformations. Onset of compressive syndrome is acute.

Intramedullar hemorrhage induces sudden lesion of the spinal cord with subsequent palsy, loss of sensibility and impaired sphincter function. Recent bleeding or xanthochromia is found in liquor.

Angiography can detect a cause of bleeding and lesion of the spinal blood vessels in intramedullar and extramedullar hemorrhage.

CT and MR examination are diagnostic methods for display of blood collections due to the damaged blood vessels. Both methods have similar resolution, with CT being the superior method. Numerous reasons for CT supremacy are explained in the Chapter on the brain hemorrhage.

CT is indicated as a first neuroradiologic examination for posttraumatic or spontaneous hemorrhage.

In patient J.S., aged 22, with CT diagnosis of extradural hemorrhage, MR was indicated for the confirmation of CT diagnosis (9).

Falciform, hyperintensive blood collection is shown in sagittal MR tomographs in T-1W sequence (Fig. 271).

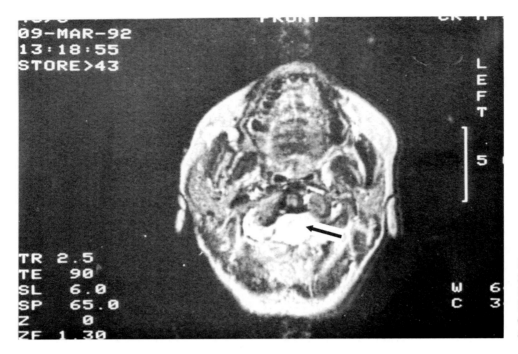

Figure 270. Axial image (SE 2500/90). Infarction lesion of high signal intensity is shown in the initial portion of the cervical spinal cord - black arrow.

c) A-V malformations

Vascular malformations are rarely found in spinal canal.

There are three principle types of arterio-venous malformations:

Dural arterio-venous fistula, with a nidus of A-V fistula located in the dural sheath of the root and adjacent spinal dura. They are almost always found in elderly males.

Intradural vascular malformation with nidus located in the spinal cord or pia mater. Those are juvenile or glomus A-V malformations.

Cavernous angioma

Arterio-venous malformations (AVM) are the most frequent spinal vascular malformations, making 4% of all spinal tumors. They are four times more frequent in males than in females. Other unusual types are telangiectasia (angioma capillare) and venous malformations made exclusively of veins.

Macroscopic appearance of AVM is highly variable. It could be simple with a single blood vessel making fistulous communication or "juvenile" with multiple, nutritive arteries vascularizing extensively dilated vascular mass that invades spinal canal and penetrates spinal cord. This type is usually seen in children. "Glomus" type consists of one or more blood vessels converging to strictly delineated vascular plexus, draining through one or more arteriolyzed veins.

Spinal arterio-venous malformations could be found practically anywhere in the spine, affecting not only the spinal cord surface, but having intramedullar component as well. (Fig. 271).

Spinal AVM can cause real compression of the spinal cord only occasionally, so that manifest lesions are usually due to the primary spinal cord involvement, imitating compressive lesions in such a case.

A-V malformations following spontaneous or posttraumatic bleeding have positive neurologic finding. Alterations of the liquor contents and color depend on the site of bleeding.

Clinical manifestations of spinal AVM are due to numerous mechanisms. Steal phenomenon is caused by rerouting of the blood flow from normal neural tissue through a shunt to the AVM, with subsequent spinal cord ischemia. Thrombosis could cause a disastrous clinical appearance. Compression, i.e. pulsatile compression, is of little importance in the clinical course. Progressive myelomalacia could be explained by a chronic elevation of the venous pressure. Hemorrhage is a mechanism of clinical manifestation as well (7).

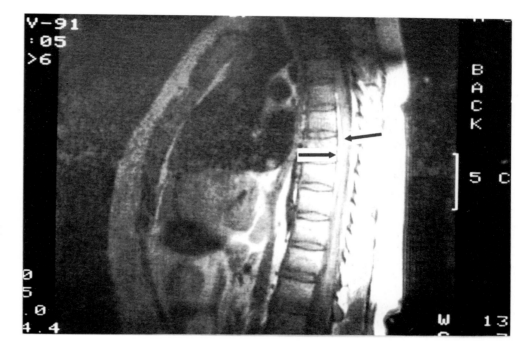

Figure 271. Thoracic spinal cord and canal in a 22 year old man. Sagittal image (SE 500/15).
Falciform, hyperintensive blood collection is shown extradurally in the ventral side of medulla spinalis, extending from Th4 to Th 9 vertebral body - arrows.

Clinical manifestations are:
Back pain and radicular pain
Progressive neurologic deficit with
    a. Paresis
    b. Impaired sensibility
    c. Impaired sphincter function
    d. Impotence
3. Sudden disastrous neurologic stroke due to the hemorrhage or thrombosis in the spinal cord.
4. Subarachnoidal hemorrhage.

Pain frequently accompanys the spinal AVM. Majority of patients have progressive neurologic deficit, intermittent and recurrent in one half of them.

In case of subarachnoidal hemorrhage with sudden, intensive pain in the back, spinal cord AVM should be suspected. Subarachnoidal hemorrhage is seen in 15% of patients. Diagnosis is quite clear if the hemorrhage is followed by paraplegia or quadriplegia, but could be complicated if spinal cord manifestations are absent.

Invasive spinal angiography is needed for neuroradiologic confirmation of A-V malformation inside the spinal canal. Non-invasive CT scan is inconclusive for smaller A-V malformations.

Magnetic resonance (MRI) have substituted myelography as the initial diagnostic procedure in patient with spinal AVM. Serpentinous area of low signal intensity are seen in the subarachnoidal space as a reflection of the blood flow through dilated blood vessels. However, MRI could have normal or non-specific abnormal signal in patients with dural AVM. It is the most frequent type of AVM and, at the same time, the most suitable for the treatment. If MRI is performed as a single diagnostic procedure, without subsequent examination for myelopathy or radiculopathy, such patients could remain undiagnosed (1-3).

Unlike MRI, myelographs are always abnormal in all types of spinal AVM, except for cavernous angioma. Angiography is not indicated in patients with negative myelography. However, if AVM is suspected on the basis of MRI or myelography, spinal angiography should follow in order to get anatomy details of the malformation (5, 6).

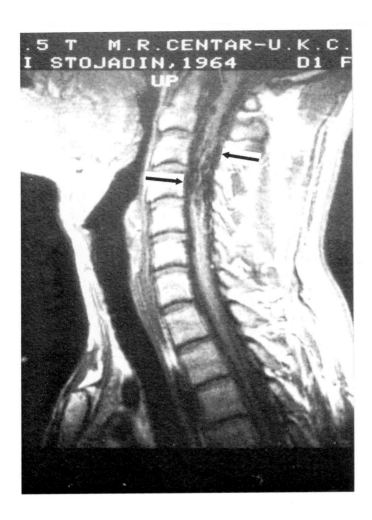

Figure 272. Cervical spine and spinal cord. Sagittal image (SE 500/15). Intramedullar AVM - arrows.

Combination of MR and spinal angiography enable spatial display of A-V malformation, its relationship with adjacent normal anatomy structures, afferent and efferent pathologic blood vessels, i.e. the whole system of abnormal vascularization (9).

Standard and special sequences are used for MR examination (Figg. 272, 273).

Recent software have enabled non-invasive MR angiography without the contrast administration (Fig. 274). This method of AVM visualization is not still incorporated in the diagnostic battery (8).

Treatment of the patients with dural AVM should eliminate venous congestion by hemilaminectomy, followed by exposition of the proximal ganglion of the nerve root, opening of dura and identification of intradural penetration of the drainage vein. Blood vessel is usually located nearby dural penetration of the nerve root. Coagulation of the intradural drainage vessel by bipolar diathermy is usually sufficient to eliminate venous congestion without damage to the spinal cord vascularization or nerve root function.

Surgical treatment of true intradural AVM with considerable intramedullar component is a high risk procedure. Reliable identification of drainage vessels of the malformation with careful microsurgical resection is required to preserve normal spinal cord tissue.

Extended, intramedullar juvenile type of the malformation is usually inoperable, for any attempt of the surgical excision can cause severe neurologic sequels. Therefore, surgery should be combined with spinal angiography embolization in such cases.

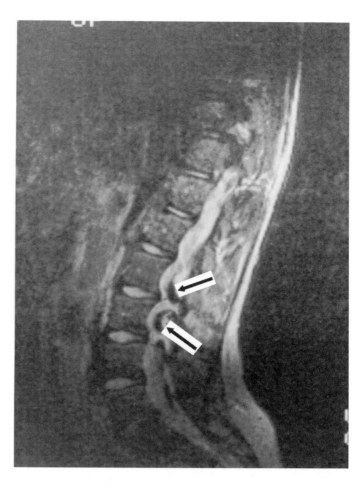

Figure 273. Lumbar spine. Sagittal image (SE 2000/90). AVM - wide, tortuous pathologic blood vessel if low signal intensity is show in the spinal canal - arrows.

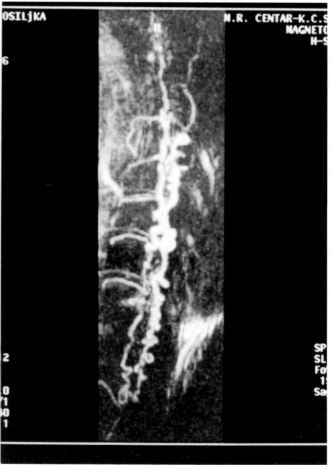

Figure 274. MR angiography - AVM.

REFERENCES

1. Dechiro G., et al.: Tumors and arteriovenous malformations of the spinal cord: assessment using MR. Radiology, 156: 689-701, 1985.
2. Doppman J., et al.: MR imaging of spinal arteriovenous malformations. J. Neuroradiol., 14: 351-372, 1987.
3. Dormont D., et al.: MRI study of spinal arteriovenous malformations. J. Neuroradiol., 14: 351-366, 1987.
4. Fox AJ., et al.: Magnetic resonance imaging of small medullary infarctions. AJNR, 7: 229-242, 1986.
5. Kulkarni MV., et al.: Diagnosis of spinal arteriovenous malformation in a pregnant patient by MR imaging. J. Comput. Assist. Tomogr., 9: 171-188, 1985.
6. Lee BCP., et al.: MR imaging of cerebral vascular malformations. AJNR, 6: 863-877, 1985.
7. Linden D., Berhit P.: Spinal arteriovenous malformations: clinical and neurophysiological findings. J. Neurol., 243: 9-12, 1996.
8. Minami S., et al.: Spinal arteriovenous malformation MR imaging. Radiology, 169: 109-116, 1988.
9. Russel NA., Benoit BG.: Spinal subdural hematoma. A review Surg. Neurol., 20: 133-137, 1983.
10. Satran R.: Spinal cord infarction. Stroke, 19: 529-532, 1988.

III. SPINAL TRAUMA

Lukas Rasulić, Gradimir Dragutinović, Miroslav Samardzić

Incidence of spinal trauma is approximately 2-5/100000 inhabitants, although in the majority of cases spinal trauma involve only bones and ligaments, without injury to the nerve roots or spinal cord. Quadriplegia occurs in 10% of cases.

Adolescents and younger population are usually affected. Severe spinal cord trauma is usually caused by traffic accidents, but sport injuries are also frequently seen.

Spinal injury should be ruled out in all patients with severe head trauma. Spinal injury should be suspected if the patient complains of spinal pain, numbness or weakness of one or more extremities, neck deformity, etc.

Open wounds, caused either by puncture or bullets from the weapons, can damage a medulla by blast, vascular impairment or direct injury by a bullet or bony fragment.

Although severe spinal trauma usually causes serious neurologic deficit, it is not always possible to find a correlation between the degree of the bone injury and spinal cord lesion. Minor injuries to the spine usually does not cause neurologic deficit, but severe neurologic deficit could be seen occasionally.

Type of spinal trauma and neurologic deficit depends on the mechanism of trauma. Spinal cord could be damaged by a direct compression by bony fragments, ligament particles or intervertebral disc, impaired vascularization and/or traction.

Neurologic findings can vary depending on the level and degree of the injury. Careful neurologic examination should detect the level and degree of the injury and implicate further investigation, such as native radiography, CT and MR examination (1).

Basic issue of the neurologic status is to determine whether the injury has caused complete functional section of the spinal cord with subsequent loss of motor and sensor functions distally to the injured level. Motor deficit is verified when a patient is asked to move the extremities against the resistance, and the function is ranked from 0 to 5. Sensibility is investigated by touching arms, legs and perineum by point of a needle. Reflexes are tested in the end. Rectal touché is always done. If the patient is unconscious, muscle tone and spinal reflexes are tested to find eventual asymmetry.

Areflexia is found immediately below the level of the injury. Hyperreflexia could indicate incomplete spinal cord injury or medullar contusion. Dysfunction of the autonomous nerve system distally to the level of the injury will be manifested by a lack of perspiration and vasomotor response, with subsequent impairment of the urinary bladder and rectum tone, and occasional priapism.

There are several syndromes associated with spinal cord injury:
a) complete spinal cord section syndrome
b) anterior section syndrome
c) central medullar injury syndrome
d) various partial sections

a) Features of the complete section syndrome are complete absence of the voluntary movement and any sensibility below the injured level. Systemic hypotension and depressant drugs could exacerbate the syndrome, so that they should be discontinued before the final diagnosis of complete lesion is made. Paraplegia or quadriplegia is seen, depending on the site of lesion, accompanied by autonomous function impairment, such as urinary bladder and rectal function.

Spinal cord injuries induce upper motor neuron paralysis with absence of voluntary movements, hypertonus and hyperreflexia. Lumbar spine injuries involve cauda equina and cause paralysis of the lower motor neuron with reduced muscular tone and absent reflexes. Combined lesion of upper and lower motor neurons is seen in thoraco-lumbar injury.

Afferent fibers transmitting various sensibility modalities, such as touch, pain, temperature, position and tactile discrimination, are severed inferior to the level of the complete lesion. Visceral sensation can occur as well. Occasionally hyposensibility along several spinal segments can precede a total loss of function. Abnormal hypersensibility, hyperesthesia or hyperalgia are seen sometimes at the level or just below the lesion.

Insufficient termoregulation is seen in patients with complete spinal lesion, because of the damaged autonomous mechanisms of vasoconstriction and vasodilatation.

Cervical or high thoracic lesions beyond the sympathicus outlet at Th5 level can cause hypotension. Interruption of the sympathetic splanchnic vasomotor control can cause severe postural hypotension induced by impaired venous reflux, in the beginning.

b) Anterior section syndrome cause bilaterally loss of the movements with preservation of the posterior columns function. Vascular lesion following direct anterior trauma, occlusion of the anterior spinal artery or acute herniation of a disc, can cause this syndrome.

Emergency diagnosis is needed in patients with this syndrome, to rule out disc rupture with subsequent compression. Injury to the corticospinal and spinothalamic pathways causes motor paralysis below the lesion with loss of the pain, temperature and touch sensation and relative preservation of the sensations of the light touch, proprioceptive and position, because of their pathways in the posterior medullar columns.

c) Syndrome of central medullar injury is seen in elderly patients after the fall; it is usually caused by hyperextension of the cervical spine with compression of medulla between degenerated disc in front and thickened ligamenta flava posteriorly. Spinal cord lesion is centrally situated, with centrally located cervical tract damage and subsequent predominant motor and sensory deficit in upper extremities. Gait troubles and urinary incontinence are present as well.

d) Various forms of partial section are seen as a incomplete partial section syndrome. Numerous asymmetric motor and sensory deficits are seen. Brown-Sequard syndrome due to hemisection of medulla is usually caused by penetrant wound, but occasionally seen in closed injuries as well. Limb paralysis below the lesion level with contralateral loss of sensibility for pain, touch and temperature is seen.

Direct and indirect spinal and medullar injuries should be examined by classic radiography in emergency diagnosis.

X-ray plane reveal bone destruction in case of direct trauma caused by various weapons. Traumatic lesions of medulla spinalis, hemorrhage, foreign bodies and bony fragments are visualized by CT scan.

Indirect wounds of the spine are best assessed by X-ray plane and CT examination, with precise determination of the type and severity of the injury to the bone and soft tissues of spine (10).

MR is used for delayed, precise diagnosis of the spinal cord trauma. MR is indicated if the previous neuroradiologic examination was insufficient, i.e. the finding is not conclusive or there is discrepancy between neurologic finding, general condition of the patient and neuroradiological findings (2, 3, 6).

As compared to the CT, MR has higher selectivity for detection of smaller lesions, such as small foci of myelomalacia, cysts, syringomyelic cavities, intramedullar hemorrhage, etc. (4, 5, 9).

MR examination is contra-indicated for the diagnosis of spinal trauma with metal foreign bodies because of feromagnetic effect and heating of non-ferromagnetic metals (7, 8, 11, 13).

There are several examples of posttraumatic sequels in medulla spinalis where the MR examination was indicated:

1. Patient have suffered direct sclerotherapy wound of Th3 vertebra. Inferior paraplegia was manifest immediately after the trauma. Classic radiographs and CT scan have determined damage to Th3, without any detail on medullar lesion. There were no bony fragments inside the spinal canal, that could have had spatio-compressive effect thus indicating surgical removal. MR imaging was aimed to determine the type and site of lesion in the medulla spinalis. Traumatic lesion of the medulla spinalis correlates with neurologic finding and general condition of a patient (Fig. 275).

2. Female patient have had direct penetrant wound by sharp wooden object in the region of the tho-

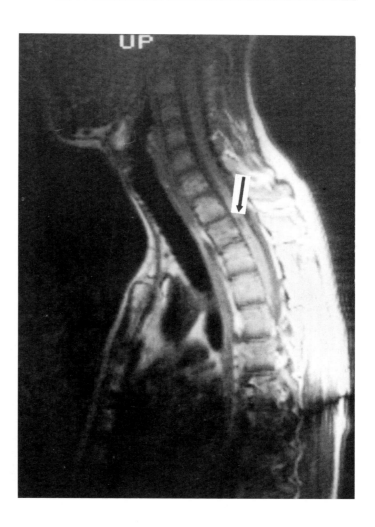

Figure 275. Thoracic spinal cord and canal in a 27 year old man. Sagittal image (SE 500/15). Traumatic myelomalatic cyst with low signal intensities is seen at Th3 level - arrow.

racic spine. Sudden weakness and numbness of the left leg was found. Neurologic examination have revealed monoparesis of the left leg. Liquor was yellowish, with elevated number of leukocytes, corresponding to the later phase of subarachnoidal hemorrhage.

Classic radiographs were negative. CT scan was not conclusive about the site, type and quality of the lesion. MR was indicated. This example has proven capability of MR imaging for precise diagnosis of intramedullar traumatic lesions and early detection of asymptomatic bone pathology (Fig. 276).

3. Patient with explosive fracture of C5 have developed complete quadriplegia. There was no improvement after several months of conservative treatment.

Apart from vertebral lesions seen in classic radiographs and CT scan, MR tomograph in T-1W sequence have revealed intramedullar cystic cavity at C5 – C6 level. AP diameter of the cyst involves the complete width of the cervical segment of medulla spinalis. Pathoanatomic substrata correlates with clinical course and neurologic finding of quadriplegia (Fig. 277).

4. Patient suffered L3 fracture when he fell from a motorcycle 4 years ago. After two operations aimed to achieve L3 fixation and removal of intraspinal bony splinters, deterioration with severe flaccid paraparesis and neurogenic urinary bladder have occurred.

MR imaging in T-1W sequence have revealed syringomyelic cavity, secondary to the indirect trauma of corresponding spinal segment (12). This example confirms the superiority of MR over CT for the diagnosis of lesions in the critical zone of the craniocervical junction (Fig. 278).

5. Female patient, aged 47, suffered intensive pain with development of acute inferior paraparesis, following a fall on her back. X-ray plane and CT scan were negative.

MR image in (SE 4000/90) have shown myelomalacia in Th6 - T 7 segment. Examination was repeated in SE 500/15 after i.v. injection of paramagnetic contrast (Fig. 279).

6. A patient has a history of thoraco-lumbar pain for one year following stumbling and falling to the floor. Another fall has enhanced the pain. Pathologic fracture of L1 vertebra was discovered by classic

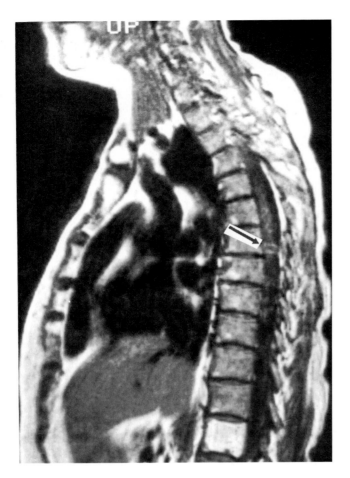

Figure 276. Thoracic spinal cord and canal in a 69 year old man. Sagittal image (SE 500/15)-intramedullar traumatic lesion-arrow.

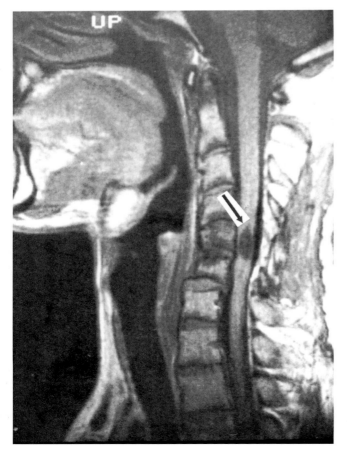

Figure 277. Cervical spine. Sagittal image (SE 500/15) Arrow pointing at intramedullar cyst of the cervical spinal cord.

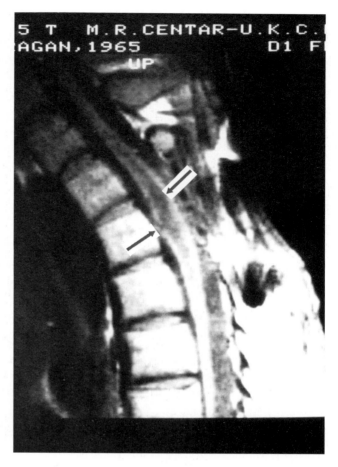

Figure 278. Thoraco-lumbar spine. Sagittal image (SE 500/15). Arrows pointing at spindle like syringomyelic cavity in the medulla spinalis extending from C 6 to Th 2 vertebra.

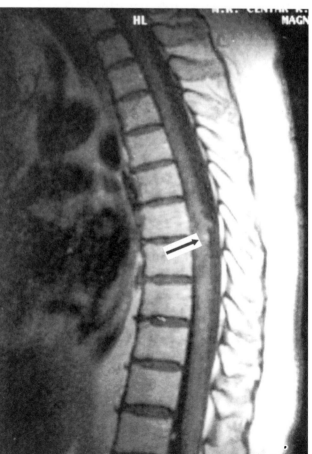

Figure 279. Thoracic spine. Sagittal image (SE 500/15) after gadolinium-DTPA administration.
Arrow pointing at hyperintensive zone within medulla spinalis due to the impaired hematoencephalic barrier (myelomalacia).

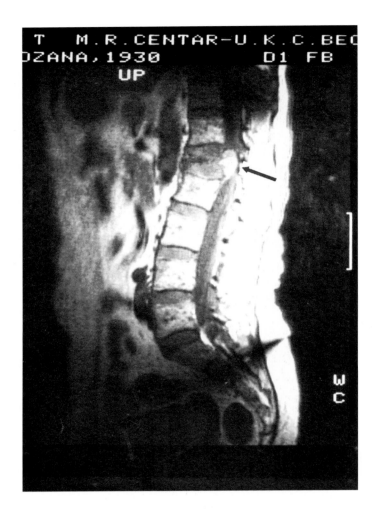

Figure 280. Lumbar spine. Sagittal image (SE 500/15). Black arrow pointing at the site of spatio-compressive lesion.

radiography and CT scan. Secondary deposit in that vertebra was suspected. Apart form pain on palpation in thoraco-lumbar segment, painful and limited movement, no other abnormality was found by neurologic examination.

MR was indicated for planning of corporectomy, biopsy and stabilization. MR tomograph have shown reduced height of L1 vertebra, with changed uneven signal intensity and extension of the posterior vertebral corpus and tumor into the spinal canal, thus causing the compression to the terminal segment of medulla spinalis and its dislocation backwards and to the left. Other vertebrae, particularly L2, L3 and L4 have altered signal intensities, i.e. reduced in T-1W, corresponding to the secondary deposits as well (Fig. 280).

REFERENCES

1. Baker LL., Goodman SB., Perksash I.: Benign versus pathologic compression fractures of vertebral bodies: assessment with conventional spin-echo, chemical shift and STIR MR imaging. Radiology, 174: 495-505, 1990.
2. Baleriaux D., et al.: MRI of the spine. Diagn. Imag. Clin. Med., 55: 66-74, 1986.
3. Chakeres DW., et al.: MR imaging of acute spinal cord trauma. AJNR, 8: 5-12, 1987.
4. Hackney DB., et al.: Hemorrhage and edema in acute spinal cord compression: demonstration by MRI imaging. Radiology, 161: 387-401, 1986.
5. Masaryk TJ., et al.: Cervical myelopathy: a comparison of magnetic resonance and myelography. J. Comput. Assist. Tomogr., 10: 184-199, 1986.
6. McArdie CB., et al.: Surface coil MR of spinal trauma: preliminary experience. AJNR, 7: 885-899, 1986.
7. Mirvis SE., et al.: Acute cervical spine trauma: evaluation with 1,5T MR imaging. Radiology, 166: 807-820, 1988.
8. Modic MT., et al.: Nuclear magnetic resonance imaging of the spine. Radiology, 148: 757-767, 1983.
9. Naseem M., Zachariah SB., Stone J., Russell E.: Cervicomedullary hematoma: diagnosis with MR. AJNR, 7: 1096-1107, 1986.
10. Post MJD.: Computed tomography of spinal trauma. In Post MJD. (ed.): Computed Tomography of the Spine. Williams and Wilkins. Baltimore, 782-821, 1984.
11. Sklar EM., Quencer RM., Gren BA.: Posttraumatic spinal meningocele: MR and clinical features. AJNR, 11: 1184-1199, 1990.
12. Takahashi M., Yamashita Y., Sakamoto Y., Kojima R.: Chronic cervical cord compression: clinical significance of increased signal intensity on MR images. Radiology, 173: 219-233, 1989.
13. Tarr RW., et al.: MR imaging of recent spinal trauma. J. Comput. Assist. Tomogr., 11: 412-423, 1987.

IV. INFLAMMATORY DISEASES

Gradimir Dragutinović, Zvonimir Lević, Vaso Antunović

Inflammatory diseases of medulla spinalis and soft tissues within spinal canal are rarely seen. It is a challenge for a radiologist, along with clinical neurologist, to detect inflammatory lesions within spinal canal.

Classic neuroradiologic examination is usually negative in inflammation of the spinal canal contents. Myelography can reveal spatio-compressive effect of the extradural abscess. CT examination is a method of choice for the diagnosis of inflammatory lesions of the bony structures and extramedullar foci with compression effect. Intramedullar lesions are hard to detect by CT scan.

MR in various sequences is capable of precise detection of inflammatory lesions and clear demarcation of epidural from subdural space. Detailed differentiation of the soft tissue contents within spinal canal is required for the detection of the pathologic lesions of medulla spinalis (intradural and extradural) (3).

a) Myelitis

Myelitis is bacterial, viral or specific (*lues, tbc*) inflammation of the white and gray matter of the spinal cord. *Myelitis* could be secondary to the systemic or generalized disease of CNS, such as *sclerosis multiplex*. Etiology of *myelitis* is frequently unknown.

Pathologic process can involve the whole segment of medulla spinalis (*myelitis transversalis*), part of the segmental section (*myelitis partialis*) or several segments (*myelitis diffusa*).

Acute transversal myelitis usually commences with pain in the back and high fever. Spinal symptomatology, such as paresthesia, weakness of the legs and trunk, and sphincter control impairment arises 2-3 days later. If the complete section of the spinal cord is involved in inflammation, syndrome of complete medullar lesion with flaccid paraplegia, anesthesia below the level of the lesion and incontinentia alvi et urinae will develop. Discrete proteinorachy and pleocytosis are found in CSF, but the absence of the inflammation syndrome in clinical appearance or liquor does not exclude myelitis (5).

Pathologic process is rarely ascendant (Landrys ascendant paralysis), affecting all proximal muscles, thus causing respiratory paralysis and death, which is inevitable in such cases.

CT scan is usually negative in myelitis.

MR can detect subtle lesions, seen in transversal myelitis, if the lesion level is determined correctly. Lesions of higher signal intensities are seen in sagittal, coronal and, eventually axial plane in T-2W sequence. Signal intensity can be enhanced by a contrast administration in T-1W sequence. MR image is non-specific and does not implicate the etiology of myelitis (1).

In patient, aged 44, with tbc meningomyelitis, MR tomography of thoracic spinal cord is done. MR image is non-specific for tbc meningomyelitis. MR tomographs in (SE 500/15) have shown signal enhancement of granulomatous arachnoiditis in spinal canal after i.v. administration of paramagnetic contrast (4).

Bigger, irregular area of high signal intensity (granulomatous arachnoiditis) is seen in thoracic segment of medulla spinalis - arrows. Signal intensity is homogenous, involving partial or complete spinal cord section in various segments (Fig. 281).

Spinal cord abscess is extremely rare. Diagnosis of the abscess is complicated. Those lesions could be displayed by direct methods of examination: CT and particularly MR. Their features are identical to the brain abscess (5).

Tuberculous abscess in the spinal canal combined with destruction of Th 11 vertebral body is shown in patient C.D., aged 23 (Fig. 282).

MR examination is indicated in patients with clinical appearance of transversal myelitis and negative CT scan.

Non-specific lesion of high signal intensity at Th 8 - Th 9 level, is seen in MR tomographs in sagittal view in T-2W sequence. According to its features, the lesion corresponds to transversal myelitis of unknown etiology (Fig. 283).

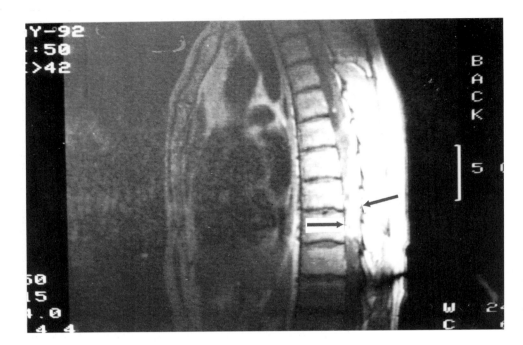

Figure 281. Thoracic spinal cord and canal. Sagittal image (SE 500/15) after gadolinium-DTPA administration (arrows).

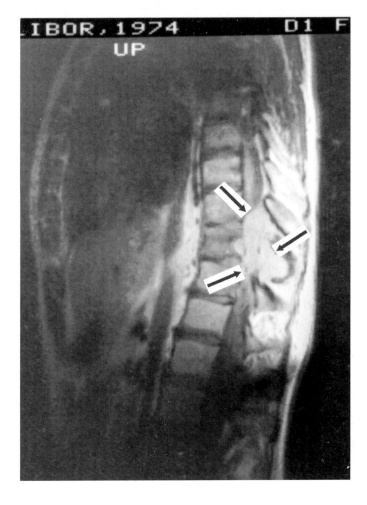

Figure 282. Thoracic spinal cord and spine. Sagittal image (SE 500/15). Tuberculous abscess with confirmed tuberculosis - arrows.

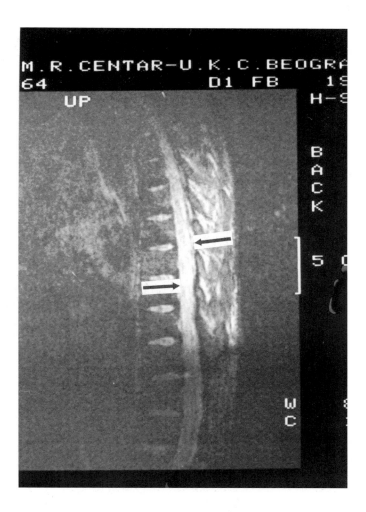

Figure 283. Thoracic spinal cord and canal. Sagittal image (SE 2000/90). Arrows pointing at hyperintensive lesion of transversal myelitis.

b) Parasitoses

Parasitoses of the spinal vertebrae or spinal canal are rarely seen. Parasites usually affect other organs (liver, brain, lungs, heart, etc). Parasitosis of the spine or spinal canal should be suspected on the basis of positive neurologic and laboratory findings. Symptoms depend on location, size and type of parasites.

Methods of direct visualization, CT and MR are indicated for the diagnosis of parasitoses.

Echinococcus has implanted in the vertebral bodies of Th 9 and Th 10 in patient D.R., aged 58. Classic radiography and CT scan are the methods of choice for the diagnosis of echinoccocus cysts in the spinal bones. In this case MR was indicated because of the inferior paraparesis in order to determine relationship between lesions in the spine caused by a parasite and parenchyma of medulla spinalis in the critical region (Fig. 284).

High signal intensities of echinococcus implanted in the vertebral body are seen in MR tomographs in sagittal view, in T-1W sequence. Disrupted corticalis and pathologic fracture are shown. Some of the vertebral bodies underwent degeneration, and cystic and necrotic zones are seen as well.

Compression effect by affected vertebrae, formed in a gibbus, have caused a lesion of the thoracic segment of the spinal cord. Low signal intensities of myelopathy/myelomalacia (cysts) are seen inside the medulla spinalis.

Accidental MR finding is reduced height of Th 6, Th 7 and Th 8 vertebrae. Alteration of signal intensities corresponds to lysis, partly cystic and partly diffuse. Secondary deposits should be considered in differential diagnosis (2).

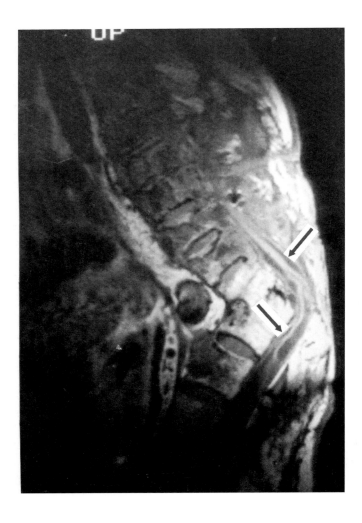

Figure 284. Thoracic spinal cord and canal. Sagittal image (SE 500/15). Arrows pointing at cystic alteration of medulla spinalis at the level of gibus.

REFERENCES

1. Barakos JA., Mark AS., Dillon WP., Norman D.: MR imaging of acute tranverse myelitis and AIDS myelopathy. J. Comput. Assist. Tomogr., 14 (1): 45-58, 1990.
2. Berger PE., et al.: High-resolution surface coil magnetic resonance imaging of the spine: normal and pathologic anatomy. Radiographics, 6: 573-590, 1986.
3. Modic MT., et al.: Nuclear magnetic resonance imaging of the spine. Radiology, 148: 757-781, 1983.
4. Sze G.: MR of the spine: contrast agents. Radiol. Clin. North Am., 26: 1009-1022, 1988.
5. Valk J.: Gadolinium-DTPA in MR of spinal lesions. AJNR, 9: 345-358, 1988.

V. DEMYELINATION DISEASES

Zvonimir Lević, Gradimir Dragutinović

a) Sclerosis multiplex

Multiple sclerosis is a disease which can be seen by MR imaging as demyelination plaques in the medulla spinalis. M.S. plaques in the brain are associated with solitary or multiple plaques in the medulla spinalis. Sometimes, M.S. plaques are seen only in the spinal cord.

If M.S. plaques affect only the spinal cord, symptomatology is limited to the medulla spinalis. Progressive spastic paraparesis in middle aged patients is usually seen. According to Mc Alpine criteria it is classified as "possible M.S." Sensitive disorders and sphincter function impairment is found along with spastic paraparesis. Spinal symptomatology is usually found in other forms of M.S. due to demyelination changes in medulla spinalis.

Lower cervical region and craniocervical junction are predilection sites for M.S. plaques. It has been assumed that repeated microtrauma and flexibility of this segment of spinal cord can induce this. Lhermittes phenomenon ("electricity" felt in the extremities during head tilt) is explained by this location of demyelination lesion (Fig. 285).

M.S. plaques could not be usually seen in CT scan. MR tomography of the certain segment of medulla spinalis in sagittal and coronal views, using double echo sequence (**T-2W and proton density**) with slice thickness of 3 mm have discovered demyelination focus with high signal intensity (Figg. 285, 286).

Non-specific appearance of M.S. plaques makes it hard to differentiate from myelopathy/myelomalacia, some of intramedullar expansive processes, etc. Like M.S. plaques in the brain, the recent ones become enhanced by paramagnetic contrast injection, while the older ones remain unchanged (4, 5, 8, 9).

b) Myelopathy and myelomalacia

Myelopathy encompasses wide range of etiologically or pathohistologically undefined lesions or diseases of medulla spinalis. Myelopathic lesions in the spinal cord could be caused by various pathology, such as stenosed spinal canal, vascular diseases, trauma, degenerative diseases, etc.

Myelomalacia is colliquation of the spinal cord caused by the vascular impairment (emboly, thrombosis); direct trauma to the medulla spinalis; compression caused by fractures and luxation of vertebrae and disci; inflammation of vertebrae (tbc spondylitis); incipient tumors, etc. Myelomalatic segment of medulla spinalis is edematous, colliquated and its structure is blurred. Pathohistologically it is similar to encephalomalacia. Postmyelomalatic pseudocyst of medulla spinalis is a sequel of myelomalacia.

Cervical myelopathy due to compression of the spinal cord in the stenosed spinal canal is of utmost clinical significance.

Stenosis of the spinal canal can be caused by various factors:
– congenital stenosis,
– cervical spondylosis with hypotrophic facet joints and osteofits,
– hypertrophy of ligamenta flava,
– prolapse of intervertebral cervical disc,
– excessive mobility, usually accompanied by cervical spondylosis.
In all those cases myelopathy is caused by:
– direct pressure on the spinal cord,
– spinal cord ischemia due to compression and obstruction of small blood vessels inside the spinal cord or compression of the nutritive radicular arteries in intervertebral foramina.
Neural changes in the spinal cord consist of:
– degeneration and loss of neurons, cavitation and glial proliferation in the gray matter,
– demyelination of the posterior columns.
Waller's degeneration of ascendant tracts beyond, and descendent pathways below the site of com-

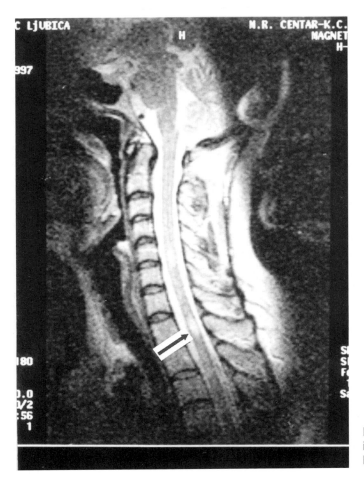

Figure 285. Cervical canal and spinal cord. Sagittal image (TSE 4000/90). Hyperintensive M.S. plaque at a level of Th 1 vertebral body - arrow.

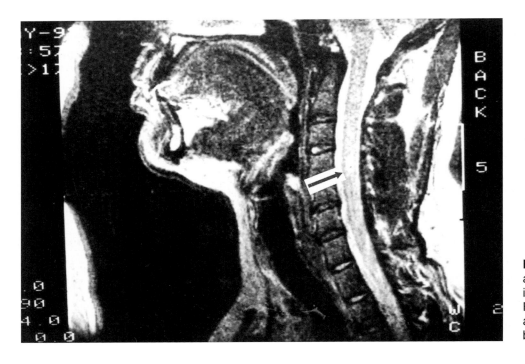

Figure 286. Cervical canal and spinal cord. Sagittal image (SE 2000/90). Hyperintensive M.S. plaque at a level of C 4 vertebral body - arrow.

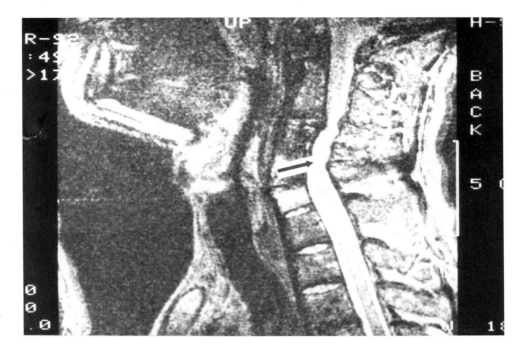

Figure 287. Cervical spine and spinal cord. Sagittal image (SE 2000/90). Posttraumatic compressive hyperintensive myelopathy/myelomalacia of the cervical spinal cord at C 3 - C 4 level - arrow.

pression, proliferation of small blood vessels with thickened walls, exceptional involvement of anterior columns.

Clinical course is slowly progressive, but sudden deterioration could be seen, especially after the trauma. Pain and neurologic deficit are clinical manifestations. Pain in the neck is not caused by myelopathy itself, but rather by degenerative changes of the spine. Stenosis of intravertebral foramina with subsequent pressure to the neural roots will cause radicular pain in case of cervical myelopathy and brachial neuralgia.

Initial neurologic deficit is muscular weakness, usually in lower extremities. Depending on the level and extent of lesion the deficit in upper extremities could be peripheral or central, accompanied by spastic paraparesis of lower extremities. Weakness or hypotrophy of suboccipital spinal muscles, shoulder muscles, biceps and triceps, with occasional fasciculation could be seen as well. Tendon reflexes in upper extremities are reduced with distal hyperreflexion, dependent on lower or upper motor neuron involvement.

Lesion of upper motor neuron is seen in lower extremities because of the corticospinal tract involvement with hyperreflexion and Babinski sign.

Sensibility impairment in form of numbness and hands and fingers can also occur. Severe sensibility deficit or complete loss of sensibility is rarely seen in cervical myelopathy. Deficit could have dermatome characteristic due to compression of a certain nerve root. Loss of sensation of position and vibration will arise in case of compression of posterior medullar columns.

Classic radiography and myelography are negative in myelopathy and myelomalacia. CT scan is insufficient for visualization of myelopathy or myelomalacia of the spinal cord in comparison with MR, especially for the lesions of the craniocervical junction where they are hidden by artifacts of bone origin (7).

MR is a method of choice for the diagnosis of myelopathy/myelomalacia. Myelopathy can not be differentiated from myelomalacia in MR tomographs. The outcome of myelopathy is possible recovery including *restitutio ad integrum*, whereas myelomalacia will end as pseudocyst (1).

Myelomalacia/myelopathy is seen in MR tomographs following various spinal cord diseases, such as trauma, vascular impairment, disease of white and gray matter of medulla spinalis, infectious diseases, degenerative diseases of spine, etc. (2, 3, 6).

Myelomacia or myelopathia are best displayed in double echo sequences. Sagittal, axial and, eventually, axial views are used. Myelopathic or myelomalatic lesion is shown in high signal intensities (Fig. 287).

Postmyelomalatic pseudocyst as the worst outcome of myelomalacia of medulla spinalis is easily diagnosed by MR examination.

REFERENCES

1. Barakos JA., Mark AS., Dillon WP., Norman D.: MR imaging of acute tranverse myelitis and AIDS myelopathy. J. Comput. Assist. Tomogr., 14(1): 45-59, 1990.
2. Gebarski SS., et al.: Post traumatic progressive myelopathy. Radiology, 157: 379-394, 1985.
3. Han JS., et al.: NMR imaging of the spine. AJNR, 4: 1151-1177, 1983.
4. Larsson EM., Holtas S., Nilsson O.: Gd-DTPA enhancement of suspected spinal multiple sclerosis, AJNR, 10: 1071-1092, 1989.
5. Maravilla KR., et al.: Magnetic resonance demonstration of multiple sclerosis plaques in the cervical cord. AJNR, 5: 685-699, 1984.
6. Ramsey RG., Zachrias CE.: MR imaging of the spine after radiation therapy: easily recognizable effects. AJNR, 6: 247-266, 1985.
7. Ross JS.: Myelopathy. Neuroimaging Clin. N. Am., 5: 367-384, 1995.
8. Sze G.: Gadolinium-DTPA in spinal disease. Radiol. Blin. North Am., 26: 1009-1022, 1988.
9. Valk J.: Gadolinium-DTPA in MR of spinal lesions. AJNR, 9: 345-357, 1988.

VI. TUMORS

Vaso Antunović, Gradimir Dragutinović, Miodrag Rakić

S. J. Pomeranz have classified primary spinal tumors as intramedullar, extramedullar, intradural, extradural and others. Expansive lesions of bony structures of spine, as well as paravertebral tumors with invasion of vertebrae or medulla spinalis, belong to a separate group. Secondary deposits are found in medulla spinalis or extramedullary in vertebral bones (21).

a) Intramedullar tumors

Intramedullar tumors are rarely found in spinal tumors.

Ependymoma and astrocytoma are usually seen, whereas hemangioblastoma and other histological types are found exceptionally.

Ependymoma, making up 60% of intramedullar tumors, usually originates from filum terminale causing compression of cauda equina. Mixopapillary type is found in the majority of cases. Ependymoma arises from ependymal cell remnants in the central spinal canal. Incidence in children is higher than in adults. Cervical canal or conus medullare are frequently affected.

Astrocytoma originates from the glial elements in the spinal cord. Gradual onset of motor and sensory deficit distal to a site of lesion is typical. They could be found at any level, with cervical location being the most frequent. Low grade of malignancy is seen in the beginning.

Epidermoid, dermoid and hemangioblastoma could be found occasionally in the spinal cord. Epidermoid could develop from cellular implants during lumbar puncture. Complete excision is hard to achieve. Dermoids could be connected to dermal sinus on the surface of the skin. Hemangioblastoma could be found in Hippel-Landau disease, so that other features of the disease, such as renal cell carcinoma, should be searched for.

Clinical manifestations of intramedullar tumors depend on the involved spinal cord level. Progressive limb weakness, loss of sensibility inferior to the tumor level and sphincter dysfunction. Syringomyelic dissociation of sensibility is seen in dermatomes corresponding to the spinal cord portion involved by tumor. Compression to the anterior cornua of the spinal cord gray matter causes the weakness and atrophy of muscles in corresponding myotomes. Tumor level is defined by a level of impaired sensibility. However, it could be overlooked or absent, especially in high cervical lesions.

For example, ependymoma arising form filu terminale will cause compression of cauda equina. History of a pain in the lower back and along the leg is present, followed by progressive weakness of legs (radicular type), sensibility impairment in gluteal region and eventual sphincter disorders.

Usual symptoms of intramedullar tumors in children, and occasionally in adults, are spinal rigidity and pain, progressive motor deficit and sensibility impairment inferior to the tumor level.

Progression of the clinical course and spinal cord involvement depend on the hystologic type of the tumor.

Enlarged medullar contour is seen in myelography in case of intramedullar tumors. Myelography could be negative if an intramedullar tumor is so small that it does not affect diameters of medulla spinalis.

Diagnosis of intramedullar tumor can be achieved by CT scan and it is usually done prior to MR examination (1, 7).

MRI is a method of choice for the diagnosis of these tumors, because it can show the structure of medulla and not only boundaries.

MR diagnosis of intramedullar tumors consists of classic sequences, additional FLASH and FISP sequence, and paramagnetic contrast injection as well. Medullar glioma signal is changed by a contrast administration like in brain tumors (3).

MR examination can reveal not only solid tumors, but the cysts, hemorrhage, necrosis, syringomyelia, peritumoral edema, etc., as well.

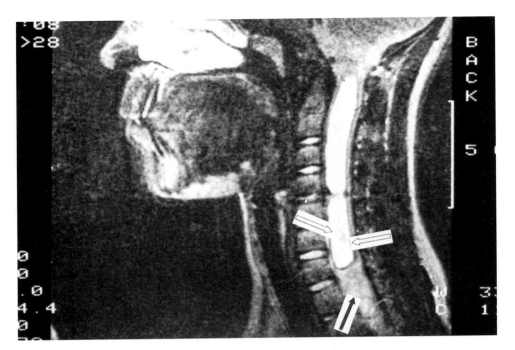

Figure 288. Cervical spine and spinal cord. Sagittal image (SE 2000/90). Ependymoma. Cystic lesions have high signal intensity - white arrows. Solid tumor of a small volume, has slightly lower signal intensities than medulla spinalis - black

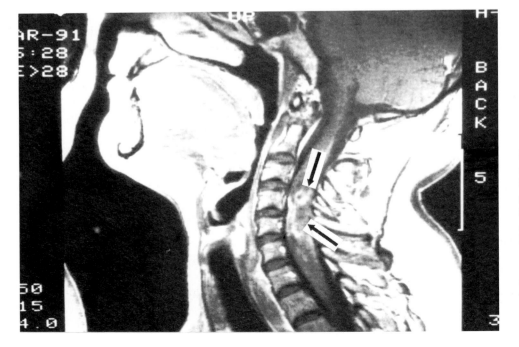

Figure 289. Cervical spine and spinal cord. Sagittal image (SE 500/15) after gadolinium-DTPA administration.
Astrocytoma (grade I and II) has low signal intensities. Paramagnetic contrast administration have enhanced signal intensities in certain portions of the tumor, in a form of irregular islets - arrows.

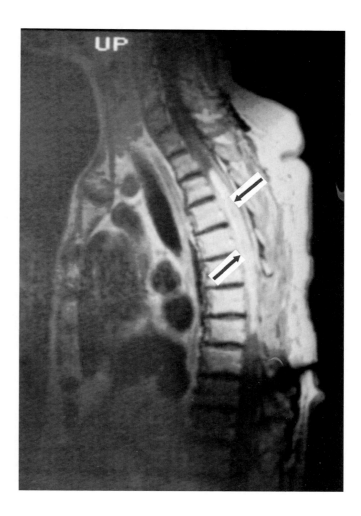

Figure 290. Thoracic spine and spinal cord. Sagittal image (SE 500/15) after gadolinium-DTPA administration. Fusiform pilocytic astrocytoma (WHO grade 2) infiltrates several thoracic segments of medulla spinalis - black arrows. Small syringomyelic cavity is seen above superior pole of ependymoma.

a-1 Ependymoma

In patient M.M., syringomyelic cavity was suspected upon CT, but no differentiation of a solid tumor tissue was possible. MR tomograph has revealed ependymoma of cervical medulla spinalis extending to the upper thoracic medulla spinalis (Fig. 288).

a-2 Astrocytoma

MR tomography of patient M.A. have shown low grade astrocytoma (grade I-II) of the cervical spinal cord. Tumor extends craniocaudally from C-1 to C-7, A-P diameter is enlarged, particularly in the segment between C-3 and C-6 (Fig. 289).

In a patient N.N. CT scan of astrocytoma of thoracic medulla spinalis was insufficient for determination of upper and lower pole of the tumor or syringomyelic cavity. Numerous artifacts caused by bone structures in CT scan, are avoided in MR images in sagittal plane (SE 500/15) with i.v. injection of paramagnetic contrast. Astrocytoma is optimally displayed (Fig. 290).

Additional sequence (SE 2000/90/15) was needed for confirmation of the syringomyelic cavity (Fig. 291).

Low grade astrocytoma is seen in MR tomographs of 11-year old boy M.M. in sequence (SE 2000/90) (Fig. 291).

Therapy for intramedullar tumors is neurosurgery combined with radiotherapy, depending on type, size and malignancy grade of the tumor.

b) Intradural extramedullar tumors

Intradural extramedullar tumors are neoplasm which lie inside dura and compress spinal cord and nerve roots. They are usually benign.

Neurinoma (neurofibroma, schwannoma) is the most frequent, affecting adults 30-50 year old.

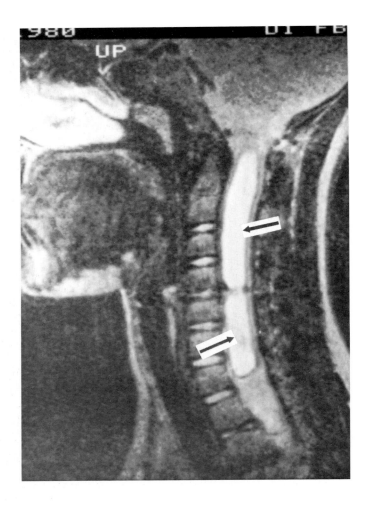

Figure 291. Cervical spine and spinal cord. Sagittal image (2000/90). Pilocytic astrocytoma (WHO grade 1-2) in the cervical and cervico-thoracic region with marked cystic cavity - arrows.

Intraspinal meningiomas are usually seen in elderly females. They are always intradural, usually in the thoracic region, with considerable spinal cord compression. They are slow growing, with a long-standing history of undefined back pain and slow onset of motor deficit and sensory impairment.

Intraspinal lipoma is important for children, usually seen in conus region and associated with dermal sinus.

There are several rarely seen intradural extramedullar expansions, such as liquor metastases of medulloblastoma and ependymoma. Arachnoidal or neuroenteric cyst, probably originating from alimentary tract embryonic elements, could be found as extramedullar intradural expansive mass.

Intradural extramedullar tumors are slowly progressive, with radicular pain present for years and gradual onset of medullar compression.

Although minor symptoms and signs of medullar compression could be present for weeks or even months, rapid neurologic deterioration with paralysis, sensibility impairment and sphincter disorder is usual.

Long standing history of cervical radix involvement could precede obvious signs of spinal cord compression in the cervical region. If tumor is located laterally, Brown-Sequard syndrome is seen.

Native radiographs in intradural extramedullar tumors show dilation of neural intervertebral foramina, of the affected nerve root. Pedicular erosion, due to long-standing compression, could be seen in native radiography in case of spinal meningioma.

Myelography could discover expansive process, make rough estimate of the site of lesion and differentiation between extra- and intramedullar tumors, indirectly. It is insufficient for modern neurosurgery. Differentiation of expansive lesion from the hemorrhage, adhesions, etc. is extremely complicated or even impossible.

Technical difficulties and obstacles in intrathecal application of hydrosoluble iodine contrast in myelography, should be considered as well.

CT scan could reveal bone destruction undiscovered by native radiography. CT examination is usually sufficient for the diagnosis of extramedullar tumors, especially if iodine contrast and Myelo-scan are applied, further details on tumor and its relationship to the surrounding structures could be acquired. Artifacts and low

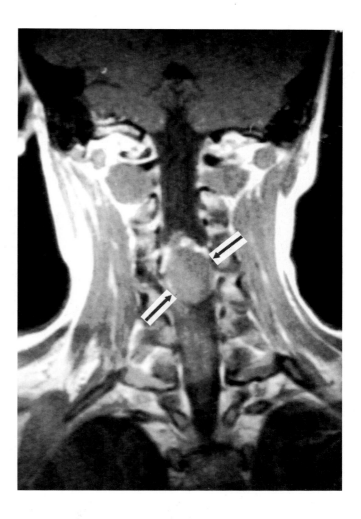

Figure 292. Cervical spine and spinal cord. Coronal image (SE 500/15) after gadolinium-DTPA administration. Neurinoma - arrows.

resolution could interfere with precise CT diagnosis in cranio-cervical junction, cervico-thoracic junction or in thoracic segments.

MR imaging is valuable for the diagnosis of primary and secondary expansive lesions of spine and is indicated for all dubious, insufficient and uncertain cases (9, 16, 17).

MR can optimally show extramedullar tumors, delineating tumors from medulla spinalis and revealing postcompressive lesions of medulla (6, 29).

MR is the ultimate diagnostic procedure for confirmation of the expansive process prior to surgical, radiation or, rarely, medical treatment (12, 18, 23).

MR features of the tumors of medulla spinalis, with or without paramagnetic contrast application, are practically identical to the tumors of the same type located intracranially (5, 20, 25, 26).

Early detection of extramedullar tumors is essential, because it can reduce postoperative sequels to the minimum or avoid them completely.

b-1 Neurinoma

Extramedullar intradural neurinoma, dorsal to the medulla spinalis, at a level C6-C7, is found in a 15-year old boy. Medulla was shifted anteriorly and to the right, thus inducing gradual onset of clinical symptoms (Fig. 292).

Intradural neurinoma, at L3 and L4 level, that have caused incontinence, beside radicular neurologic deficit, was found in patient, M.M., aged 66. Onset of symptoms was very slow. MR tomograph have shown clearly demarcated tumor with higher signal intensities. In case of clearly seen meningioma or neurinoma, paramagnetic contrast, Magnevist, is not required (Fig. 293).

b-2 Meningioma

In patient D.R., with neurologic deficit typical for the cervical medullar lesion, MR tomograph in sagittal plane and sequence (SE 500/15), extramedullar intradural meningioma is shown (Fig. 294).

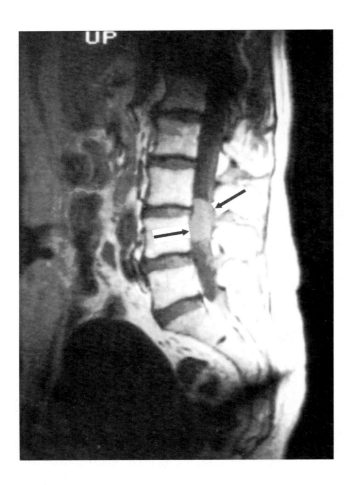

Figure 293. Lumbar spine. Sagittal image (SE 500/15). Arrows pointing at neurinoma, which have filled dural sac completely.

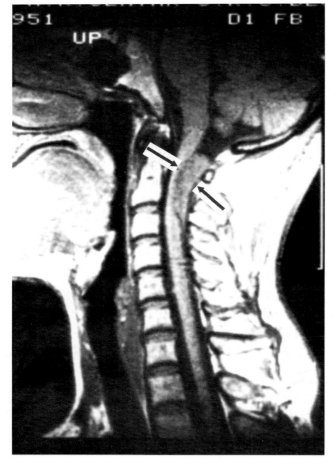

Figure 294. Cervical spine and spinal cord. Sagittal image (SE 500/15). Clearly demarcated meningioma of lower signal intensities, as compared to medulla spinalis. AP diameter of cervical medulla spinalis is considerably reduced dorsally by a tumor. Meningioma extends craniocaudally from craniocervical junction to the level of the caudal plate of C3 vertebra in the axial plane - arrows.

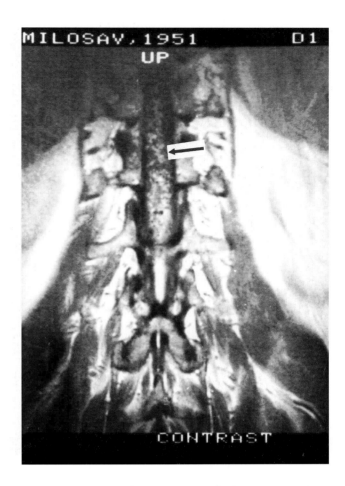

Figure 295. Thoracic and lumbar spine. Sagittal image (SE 500/15) after gadolinium-DTPA administration. Arrow pointing at honeycomb appearance of hemangioblastoma.

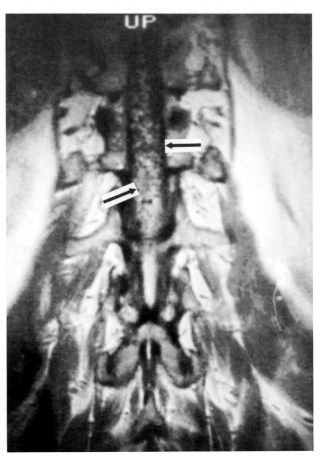

Figure 296. Thoracic and lumbar spine. Coronal image (SE 500/15) after gadolinium-DTPA administration. Arrows pointing at honeycomb appearance of hemangioblastoma.

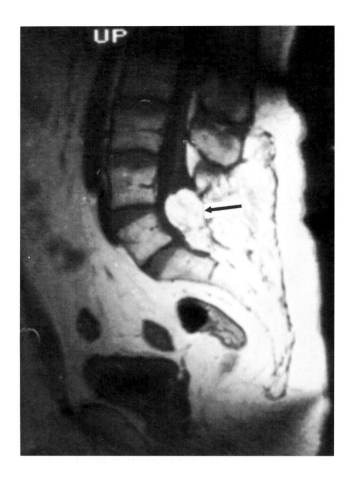

Figure 297. Lumbar spine. Sagittal image (SE 500/15). Arrow pointing at clearly demarcated hyperintensive lipoma inside spinal canal.

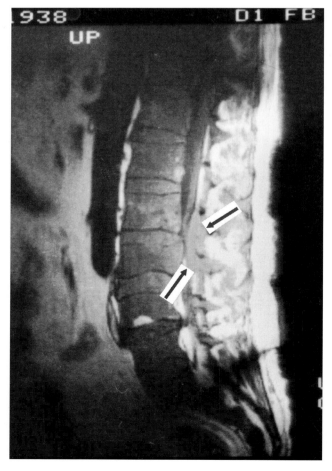

Figure 298. Lumbar spine. Sagittal image (SE 400/15). Plasmacytoma propagates along dorsal side of LS spine, invading spinal canal. Plasmacytoma is homogenous, clearly demarcated in a dural sac, shown in discretely higher signal intensities - arrows.

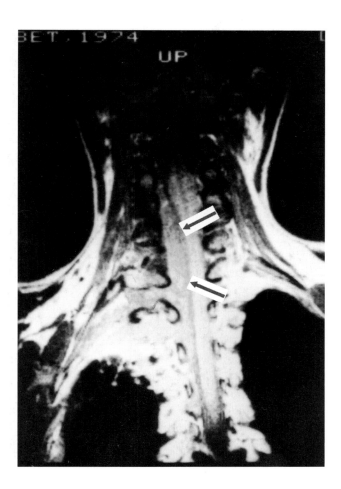

Figure 299. Cervico-thoracic spine. Coronal image (SE 500/22). Solid portion of the tumor tissue in the spinal canal has irregular higher signal intensities and extends cranio-caudally. Cervico-thoracic segment of medulla spinalis is dislocated by the tumor and LL diameter is reduced - arrows.

b-3 Hemangioblastoma

Hemangioblastoma is made up of blood vessel mass and bigger ovoid and polymorph cells resembling honeycomb because of high lipid contents. Blood vessels are thin walled, usually capillaries.

Hemangioblastoma is intramedullar in 50% of cases, but intra- and extramedullar form could be seen, as shown in the following example. Terminal medulla spinalis is usually affected by hemangioblastoma.

MR imaging gives more details on the general features as compared to CT scan.

In patient M.S., aged 20, extramedullar hemangioblastoma, engulfing thoracic spinal cord like a honeycomb, was diagnosed. MR tomographs in sequence (SE 500/15) have shown enhancement of the solid tumor signal after i.v. injection of paramagnetic contrast, Magnevist (29) (Figg. 295, 296).

b-4 Lipoma

Lipoma is a benign tumor usually located in the dural sac and clearly demarcated (intradurally extramedullary).

Lipoma is hypodense in CT scan. MR image show lipoma with typical high signal intensities in all sequences applied (Fig. 297). Both examination are valid for the diagnosis of lipoma without contrast administration (13, 30).

Treatment of extramedular intradural tumors is usually neurosurgery. MR controls are valuable for early detection of residual/recurrent tumors.

c) Extradural tumors

Extradural tumors are positioned out of dura, compromising dura and intradural structures, i.e. medulla spinalis, but considerable propagation outwards can jeopardize bone structures of the spine and soft paravertebral tissues as well.

Several types of primary malignant lymphoma, such as: reticular and *adventitial* cell sarcoma, plasmacytoma, *Hodgkin's disease* and *hystiocytosis*, could be found as extradural expansion. Extradural compression of the spinal cord could be induced by a malignant tumor, such as: lung cancer, breast cancer, carcinoma of prostate and kidney.

Teratoma, epidermoid, neurinoma, lipomatosis, etc. are rarely seen as extradural expansive process. Tumors associated with leukemia or thyroid cancer are exceptionally seen.

Radicular symptoms, such as pain and paresthesia, can suggest a level of extradural expansive lesion. Later symptoms caused by compression of corresponding level of spinal cord: progressive weakness, disturbed sensibility below the compression site, etc., depend on the direction of tumor propagation.

Classic native radiographs can show destruction of vertebral bones.

Myelography could prove extradural lesion indirectly.

Extradural tumor is fairly shown by CT scan, especially its relationship to the vertebral bones.

MR imaging is complementary to CT, in order to provide for multiplanar display of extradural tumors (10, 11, 13, 14).

c-1 Plasmocytoma

Plasmocytoma is a diffuse malignant disease that involves bone marrow and contains plasma cells. It is rarely seen as a solitary lesion, with spine being a site of predilection. Apart from bones, plasmacytoma can affect lymph nodes, liver, digestive tract, etc. Pathologic fracture of spine with subsequent paraplegia is usual clinical manifestation. Diagnosis is supported by finding *Bence-Jones* proteins in urine and typical plasma cells by a bone marrow biopsy.

Plasmocytoma was diagnosed on MR tomographs in patient Z.Z. Sagittal and axial images are sufficient for spatial visualization of extradural expansions (Fig. 298).

c-2 Morbus Hodgkin

Morbus Hodgkin (Lymphogranulomatosis) is a systemic disease of the bone marrow and lymph nodes. Lymphogranulomatous tissue is made of reticular mononuclears (Sternberg cells) and eosinophyl leukocytes. Tumor structure resembles granulation tissue. After lymph node capsule rupture, the disease tends to infiltrate surrounding organs *per continuitatem* and give lymphogenous and hematogenous metastases. Spinal vertebra are frequently involved and osteolytic defects are seen.

Extradural invasive *Morbus Hodgkin* from the right thoracic aperture (mediastinal lymphogranulomatosis with direct invasion of lungs) invading spinal canal in cervico-thoracic spinal segment. Advantage of multiplanar MR image of the thoracic apertures is obvious as compared to CT scan. Tumor mass is ideally displayed in coronal MR tomograph (Fig. 299).

c-3 Non-Hodgkin lymphoma

In non-Hodgkin lymphoma, extradural tumefact compromising medulla spinalis can be perfectly visualized by MR examination. Tumor was suspected upon native radiograph of the cervical spine, where vertebral arch and processus spinosus destruction was seen. Non-Hodgkin lymphoma extending from C7 to Th2 compresses medulla spinalis dorsally and reduces its AP diameter, in 24-year old patient (Fig. 300).

c-4 Neurinoma

Radicular neurinoma in a patient D.M. aged 34, is an example of benign, extradural, paravertebral tumor. Huge neurinoma causes a lesion of the arch and body of cervical vertebra (Fig. 301). Further propagation of the tumor can compromise soft tissues in the spinal canal.

Therapy of extradural tumors consist of a complex procedure for systemic diseases (for example M. Hodgkin) combined with local treatment. Tumor is usually surgically removed, but in certain diseases surgery could be combined with radiotherapy.

d) Primary vertebral tumors

Primary tumors of the spinal bones are: myeloma, Ewings sarcoma, osteosarcoma, chondrosarcoma, chordoma, chondroma, osteoblastoma, aneurysmal bone cyst, angioma, etc.

Primary vertebral tumors can compress or infiltrate soft tissues in the spinal canal, especially nerve roots and medulla spinalis. Primary tumors frequently cause bone destruction or pathologic fractures of vertebrae.

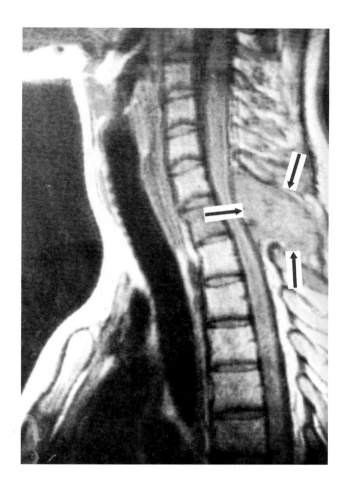

Figure 300. Cervico-thoracic spine. Sagittal image (SE 500/15). Solid portion of the tumor tissue outside and in a spinal canal with unevenly higher signal intensities, extending cranio-caudally and compressing and partly reduces AP diameter of the cervical medulla spinalis - arrows.

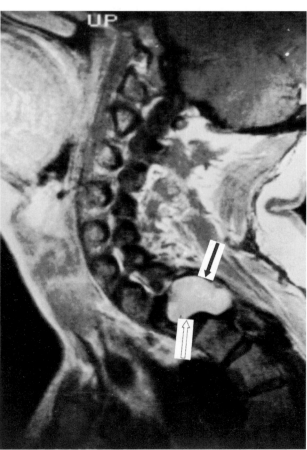

Figure 301. Cervico-thoracic spine. Sagittal image (SE 500/15) after gadolinium-DTPA administration. Arrows pointing at hyperintensive, well demarcated, paravertebral neurinoma.

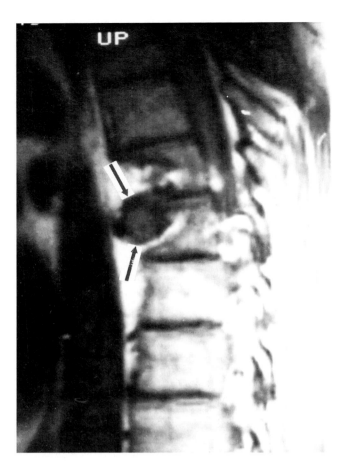

Figure 302. Sagittal image (SE 500/15). Osteoblastoma Th 7-8 - arrows. Osteoblastoma structure is non-homogenous and irregular as compared to the normal vertebral bone structure, with bone destruction of the vertebrae clearly seen.

Pain in the affected vertebra is usually the first symptom. Bony fragments or disc particles are spatiocompressive factors in pathologic fractures, that can cause lesion of spinal nerve roots or medulla spinalis, inducing paraparesis or paraplegia and, if located in the cervical area, quadriparesis or quadriplegia. Spinal shock development is similar to the one seen in spinal trauma.

Classic radiographs and CT examination are neuroradiologic methods of choice for the diagnosis of primary bone tumors. Experienced radiologist can make quick and precise diagnosis of expansive lesions and pathologic fractures.

MR is exceptionally indicated if the multiplanar view of the type and degree of the spinal cord lesion is required (4, 8, 22, 24, 31).

d-1 Osteoblastoma

Osteoblastoma is benign, osteoblastic lesion, usually located in the vertebra. It resembles osteoid osteoma. Osteoblasts, located in abundantly vascularized stroma, produce osteoid and primitive trabeculae. Trabecular mineralization is uneven. The tumor rarely causes bone destruction or rupture of cortex. Differential diagnosis between osteoblastoma and malignant osteosarcoma is of utmost importance.

In patient J.Z., aged 46, MR was needed for the multiplanar display of the relationship of tumor and medulla spinalis. Osteoblastoma Th7 - Th8 in the anterior corpus is ideally shown by MR image in sagittal view. Tumor dose not compress spinal canal or spinal cord (Figg. 302, 303).

d-2 Angioma

Vertebral angioma slightly distends vertebral body, making it porous and scattered in a lattice form. Compressive syndrome is rarely found. Angioma could be associated with A-V malformation of medulla spinalis. Pain is usually present and considerable neurologic deficit follows vertebral fracture.

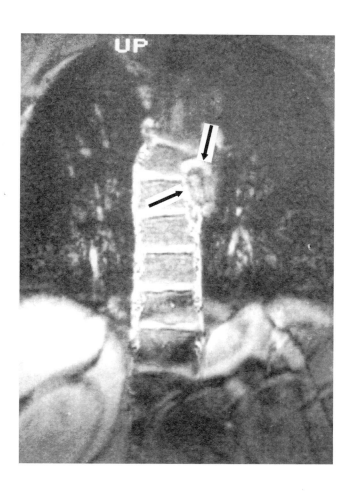

Figure 303. Coronal image (FA 50 TR 189, TE 7). Osteoblastoma Th 7-8 - arrows. Relationship of tumor with normal vertebral bone tissue is clearly seen in FLASH sequence.

Angioma is easily recognized in classic radiographs and CT scan. Complementary MR usually reveals angioma as accidental finding (Fig. 304).

d-3 Aneurysmal bone cyst
According to WHO classification, aneurysmal bone cyst is expansive osteolytic lesion, made of cavities of varying size, filled with blood, with fibrous bands, containing bone trabeculae, osteoid tissue and giant osteoclasts.

Aneurysmal bone cyst is usually seen in the first three decades of life, with spinal vertebra being affected in 15% of cases.

Beside primary, there is also a secondary form, containing predominant compact tissue. Secondary aneurysmal cyst is formed as a reaction to the hemorrhage in benign or malignant bone tumors.

CT and native radiographs are a method of choice for the diagnosis of aneurysmal bone cyst. MR is indicated to display the relationship of tumor and medulla spinalis, i.e. to evaluate type and severity of the medullar lesion.

Indication for MR examination should be decided by a team of radiologist, neurologist and neurosurgeon. MR evaluation deserves wider acceptance (31).

Aneurysmal bone cyst of vertebrae C-7 and Th-1 (bodies, arches and processus spinosus) is shown in MR tomographs in patient M.G., aged 24 (Fig. 305). Pathologic fracture causing compression of the ventral medulla by its fragments, as well as dorsal medullar compression by a cystic tumor mass, is seen. Filiform stenosis of the A-P diameter in cervico-thoracic segment of medulla spinalis is found. Higher signal intensities, corresponding to myelopathy, are seen in a stenosed portion of medulla spinalis. Complete inferior paraplegia is found by neurologic examination.

d-4 Chondroma
These tumors, along with osteochondroma and chondrosarcoma, are hard to differentiate from osteoblastoma sometimes. They are seen in younger patients.

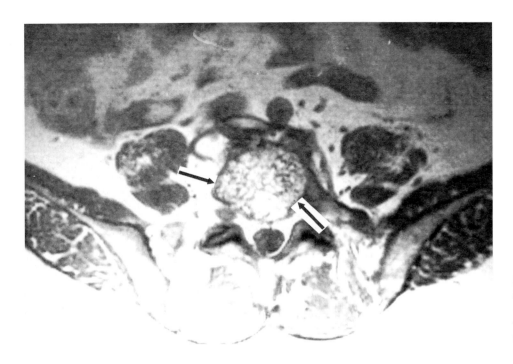

Figure 304. Lumbar spine. Sagittal image (FA 50, TR 190, TE 7). Angioma of the vertebral body of L-4 shown in FLASH sequence - arrows.

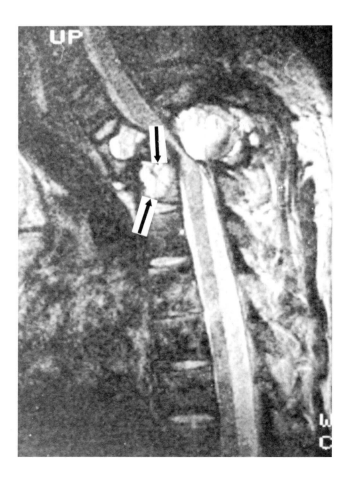

Figure 305. Cervico- thoracic spine. Sagittal image (SE 2000/90). Aneurysmal bone cyst - arrows.

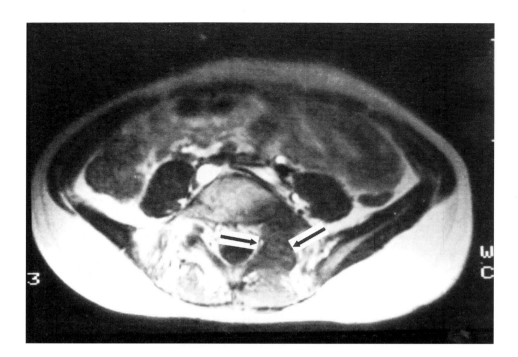

Figure 306. Lumbar spine. Axial image (SE 2500/15). Chondroma - arrows.

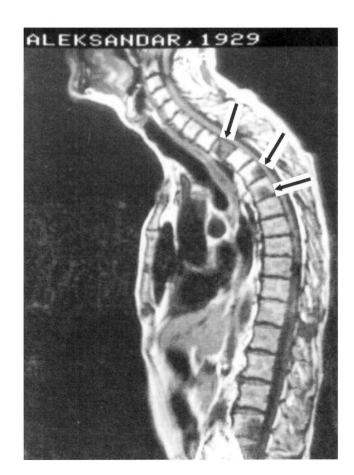

Figure 307. Cervical, thoracic and lumbar spine - Scout scan. Sagittal image (SE 400/15). Arrows pointing at multiple secondary deposits inside vertebral bodies.

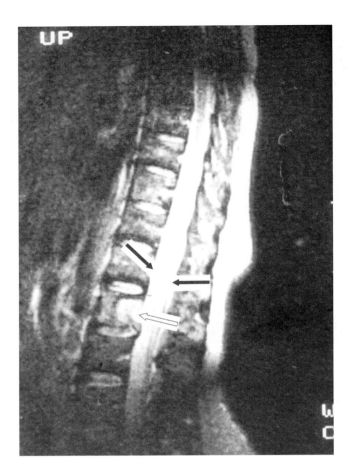

Figure 308. Thoracic and lumbar spine. Sagittal image (SE 2000/15). Metastatic deposit in the terminal medulla spinalis is shown by uneven high signal intensities - black arrows. Metastasis of the dorsal portion of the L-1 body is shown in higher signal intensities - white arrow.

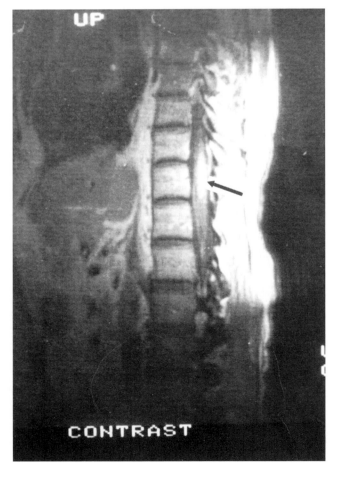

Figure 309. Thoracic spine and spinal cord. Sagittal image (SE 500/15) after gadolinium-DTPA administration. Metastatic malignant melanoma - arrow.

Tumors are usually located in the vertebral column.

Chondroma of the left arch of L-5, without spinal canal compromising, is seen in a 14-year old patient (Fig. 306).

Surgery is a therapy of choice for the primary spinal tumors, whereas adjuvant radiotherapy could be administered in malignancies, based on the features of the neoplasm.

e) Secondary spinal tumors

Secondary tumors of spinal canal are usually seen in middle aged and elderly patients. Solitary or multiple deposits are usually of breast, prostate, thyroid, kidney, bronchus, female genitals cancer or malignant melanoma origin.

Secondary spinal tumors could be located either in the vertebral bodies or in the spinal canal. Metastases usually affect thoracic region, but any spinal segment could be involved. Multiple deposits are frequently seen. Compression could be caused by a tumor itself, or by a collapsed vertebra, or the combination of both.

Classic radiography, tomography and CT, along with other methods of examination (skeletal scintigraphy, laboratory findings), can reach the diagnosis of spinal metastases in a high percentage of patients.

Pain is an usual sign of secondary tumors. Neurologic findings could be negative. Pathologic fracture can cause spatio-compressive syndrome, with spinal nerve roots and medulla spinalis impairment, causing neurologic sequels.

Clinical appearance of secondary spinal tumors is similar to the pathologic lesions induced by a primary spinal tumors. Metastatic tumor frequently invades spinal canal and compromises medulla spinalis. Paravertebral propagation compromises adequate structures, making clinical course even more complicated.

There is no indication for MR in diagnosis of the secondary spinal deposits. (2, 15, 27) MR can reveal solitary or multiple asymptomatic deposits accidentally during the examination for other reasons (Fig. 307).

MR is extremely selective for the early detection of smallest secondary deposits. MR can prove the metastases in vertebrae and medulla spinalis in a patient with positive neurologic finding and negative results obtained by other radiological examinations (20).

Patient with secondary deposits of terminal medulla spinalis and L-1 vertebral body is shown (Fig. 308). Primary tumor is unknown.

Secondary deposit of malignant melanoma in 61-year old patient A.R. is shown inside medulla spinalis in a lower thoracic spine (Fig. 309).

Multiple secondary deposits in cervical spine C-4, C-5, C-6 and C-7, involving bodies, arches and processus spinosus, invading spinal canal and compromising medulla spinalis, are seen in a patient A.R, aged 71, treated for the carcinoma of the prostate (Fig. 310).

Treatment for the secondary spinal deposits is a part of the complex treatment for malignant disease. Radiotherapy and chemotherapy are usually applied, with surgery used for the removal of the tumor portion that have caused the compression of spinal cord and nerve roots. Primary objective of the treatment is to provide for a comfortable life of a patient, with minimal neurologic sequels.

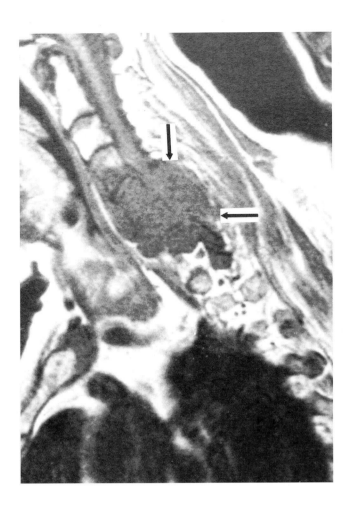

Figure 310. Cervical spine and spinal cord. Sagittal image (SE 380/15). Secondary deposit of the carcinoma of the prostate - arrows.

REFERENCES

1. Aisen AM., et al.: MRI and CT evaluation of primary bone and soft-tissue tumors. AJR, 146: 749-766, 1987.
2. Avrahami E., et al.: Early MR demonstration of spinal metastases in patients with normal radiographs and CT and radionuclide bone scans. J. Comput. Assist. Tomogr., 13: 598-607, 1989.
3. Berger PE., et al.: High-resolution surface coil magnetic resonance imaging of the spine: normal and pathologic anatomy. Radiographics, 6: 573-588, 1986.
4. Brady TJ., et al.: NMR imaging of forearms in healthy volunteers and patients with giant-cell tumor of bone. Radiology, 144: 549-555, 1982.
5. Bydder GM., et al.: Enhancement of cervical intraspinal tumors with intravenous gadolinium-DTPA. J. Comput. Assist. Tomogr., 9: 847-857, 1985.
6. Chi-Zing Z., et al.: MR imaging in the diagnosis of spinal schwannomas and neurofibromas. Radiology, 157 (P): 149-155, 1985.
7. Claussen C., et al.: MR imaging and CT of intraspinal tumors. Radiology, 161 (P): 33-48, 1986.
8. Han JS., Benson JE., Yoon YS.: Magnetic resonance imaging in the spinal column and craniovertebral junction. Radiol. Clin. North Am., 22: 805-814, 1984.
9. Han JS., et al.: NMR imaging of the spine. AJR, 141: 1137-1149, 1983.
10. Holtas SL., Kido DK., Simon JH.: MR imaging of spinal lymphoma. J. Comput. Assist. Tomogr., 10: 111-117, 1986.
11. Kendall B., Russell J.: Haemangioblastomas of the spinal cord. Br. J. Radiol., 39: 817-823, 1986.
12. Keyes WD., et al.: Intradural spinal arachnoid cysts: MR, CT, and myelographic imaging pitfalls. Radiology, 161 (P) 150-155, 1986.
13. Komiyama M., et al.: Magnetic resonance imaging lumbosacral lipoma. Surg. Neurol., 28: 259-272, 1987.
14. Kortman KE., et al.: MR imaging of epidermoid tumors. Radiology, 157: 71-77, 1985.
15. Krol G., et al.: MR imaging of primary or metastatic tumors of the spine: contribution of T1 and T2 weighting and multiple echo sequences. Radiology, 161 (P): 220-233, 1986.
16. Krol G., Sze G., Malkin M., Walker R.: MR of cranial and spinal meningeal carcinomatosis: comparison with CT and myelography. Am. J. Neuroradiol., 9: 709-718, 1988.
17. Levy WJ., Bay J., Dohn D.: Spinal cord meningiomas. J. Neurosurg., 57: 804-815, 1982.
18. Lewis TT., Kingsley DP.: Magnetic resonance imaging of multiple spinal neurofibromata-neurofibromatosis. Neuroradiology, 29: 562-571, 1987.
19. Modic M., et al.: Nuclear magnetic resonance of the spine. Radiology, 148: 757-768, 1983.
20. Parize PM., et al.: Gd-DTPA-enhanced MR imaging of spinal tumors. AJNR, 10: 249-258, 1989.
21. Pomeranz SJ.: Magnetic resonance imaging of the spine. NMR: Update Series, 10: 1-17, 1985.
22. Rosenthal DI., et al.: Sacrococcygeal chordoma: magnetic resonance imaging and computed tomography. AJR, 145: 143-148, 1985.
23. Scotti G., et al.: MR imaging of intradural-extramedullary tumors of the cervical spine. J. Comput. Assist. Tomogr., 9: 1037-1055, 1985.
24. Smoker WRK., et al.: Intradural spinal teratoma: case report and review of the literature. AJNR, 7: 905-917, 1986.
25. Sze G., Drol G., Zimmerman RG., Deck MDF.: Malignant extramedural spinal tumors: MR imaging with Gadolinium DTPA. Radiology, 167: 217-228, 1988.
26. Sze G.: MR of the spine: contrast agents. Radiol. Clin. North Am., 26: 1009-1019, 1988.
27. Utz J., et al.: MR imaging of vertebral metastases. Radiology, 161 (P): 278-286, 1986.
28. Valk J.: Gadolinium-DTPA in MR of spinal lesions. AJNR, 9: 345-352, 1988.
29. Williams AL., et al.: Differentiation of intramedullary neoplasms and cysts by MR. AJR, 149: 159-167, 1987.
30. Wood BP., et al.: Intradural spinal lipoma of the cervical cord. AJR, 145: 174-181, 1985.
31. Zimmer WD., et al.: Magnetic resonance imaging of aneurysmal bone. Mayo Clin. Proc., 59: 633-650, 1984.

VII. DEGENERATIVE DISEASES OF THE SPINE

Miroslav Samardzić, Lukas Rasulić, Gradimir Dragutinović, Ljiljana Djordjić

DISK HERNIATION

a) Introduction

Disk herniation is a protrusion or prolapse of the intervertebral disc into a spinal canal, usually arising in the most flexible segments of cervical or lumbar spine. Very few discus hernia arise in a thoracic portion of the spine.

Clinical symptoms and neurologic signs correlate to a degree of the injury of *annulus fibrosus* and posterior longitudinal ligament, as well as the propagation direction (dorsal, dorsolateral or lateral hernia).

Etiology of discus hernia vary with age: in patients under 30 it is caused by a weak supportive or connective tissue; in patients from 30 years on it is caused by degenerative process; all age groups are affected by repeated trauma of spine, i.e. *annulus fibrosus* and *ligamentum longitudinale posterior*, combination of all mentioned factors.

Nucleus pulposus has jelly structure and compress the injured part of the fibrous ring during the movement of the spine, dependent on the static and dynamic forces, ventrally, and most important laterally towards nerve roots and dorsally towards spinal canal, i.e. medulla spinalis in the dural sac (L-S segment). Dorso-lateral protrusion and prolapse can cause the lesion of the medulla spinalis and nerve roots.

Bulging of the distended or ruptured fibrous annulus with pulpous mass of the intervertebral disc is elongated, like a protrusion, or invades, in a form of prolapse, posterior longitudinal ligament causing the impairment of the spinal nerve roots or medulla spinalis in the corresponding intravertebral space.

Polydiscopathia is a disease of several disks. Subjective symptomatology, clinical appearance and neurologic finding in polydiscopathy is composite and requires a number of complicated diagnostic procedures.

a-1 Cervical disk herniation

Symptomatology disk herniation depends on the affected level. Cervical disk herniation is rare. Site of predilection is C5-C6 and C6-C7, with proximal locations being quite rare.

Disk herniation typical manifestation in patient with acute cervical discus hernia is a pain in the neck and arm, tilt of the head and neurologic symptoms of the cervical nerve root compression (6).

The pain usually arises in the cervical region irradiating towards prescapular area and shoulder, down wards in the arm, resembling brachial neuralgia. Pain in the neck usually ceases with occasional increasing pain in the arm. Pain is deep, lancinating and disabling for the patient. Pain is distributed in segment distribution of skeleton and muscles, rather than in dermatomes.

Sensibility impairment is frequently seen, especially numbness and paresthesia in the involved dermatomes. Sensibility impairment is useful for the detection of the level of the root compression, rather than the pain distribution: thumb (occasionally index finger) for C6, middle finger (occasionally index finger) for C7, small and fourth finger for C8, arm weakness can be noticed in case of C7 lesions, especially extension of the forearm, innervated neglectably by other roots (C8).

The disease has a chronic course in elderly patients, with gradual degeneration of the disc and surrounding structures, followed by recurrent episodes of the pain in the neck and arm. This type of chronic disease is called cervical spondylosis. Degeneration in cervical spondylosis causes disc bulging and development of bony crests, called osteofits, especially on uncinate processes nearby neural foramina and hypertrophy of facet joints with subsequent foramen stenosis.

Sudden onset and intensive pain make a difference between acute and chronic disc disease.

Myelopathy, along with radiculopathy seen in medullar compression, is second important clinical syndrome in cervical disc disease. Acute form is seen in massive central herniation of intervertebral disc. Pain in the neck is not always seen, but gait disorder, instability, arm weakness and urinary bladder impairment can follow. Dorsomedial discus hernia can compress medulla spinalis and cause quadri-

impairment can follow. Dorsomedial discus hernia can compress medulla spinalis and cause quadriparesis. Prompt diagnosis and emergency surgery are required.

Chronic cervical myelopathy is usually caused by cervical spondylosis, by osteofits in chronic degenerative disease. Numbness and arm weakness are seen in the beginning, but leg weakness with hypertonus, spastic gait on a wide basis and hyperreflexion below the spondylotic crest, can follow. Abdominal reflexes are reduced, but sphincter function is usually preserved, unlike in spinal cord tumors.

a-2 Thoracic disk herniation

Thoracic disk herniation is not frequently seen in clinical praxis. It affects males between 30 and 55 years of age, usually below Th-8. Thoracic spinal canal is narrow, so that there is a little space between the disc and spinal cord.

Prolapse of a thoracic disc is usually caused by a disc degeneration.

Persistent pain in the back is the usual symptom, caused by disc degeneration and the painful elongation of the posterior longitudinal ligament. Radicular pain is frequently found. Onset of neurologic manifestation can be either acute or slow (1).

a-3 L-S discus herniae

Discus hernia usually affects the lumbar portion of the spine and that could be easily explained, because it is the portion with maximal exposure to movement and stress.

Of all flexion and extension movements, 75% are located in the lumbo-sacral joint, 20% in the L4-L5 level and the rest 5% in all other lumbar levels, therefore the lumbar discus hernia is usually located in the lowest two levels, particularly in L5-S1 (5).

Pathoanatomically the lesions could be sorted as follows:

- *disc protrusion* (annulus fibrosus retains its continuity, but it is thinned and bulged toward the canal);
- *extrusion* (ruptured annulus with partial disc protrusion, but the protruded part is continuous with the rest of intervertebral disc);
- *sequestration* (completely separate part of pulpous nucleus in the canal).

The prolapse of the disc could be either in a form of hernia of the pulpous nucleus with elongation of the intact annulus fibrosus (protrusion), or annulus rupture with subsequent sequestration of the free fragments underneath posterior longitudinal ligament or through it to the extradural space (extrusion). Disc prolapse is usually postero-lateral, because of the posterior longitudinal ligament which prevents direct posterior herniation, or, exceptionally, lateral with nerve compression in the neural canal.

Prolapsed intervertebral disc causes the compression of the root running along the posterior surface of the disc downwards beneath the pedicle of the next vertebra. Therefore prolapsed L4-L5 disc will compress L5 root, running caudally over the disc and entering intervertebral foramen beneath the L5 pedicle. Likewise, L5-S1 disc will compress S1 root. Exceptional lateral discus hernia will cause compression of the root at a level beyond the expected one, so that in L4-L5 disc the L4 root will be compressed. Massive discus hernia could cause compression of several roots.

Syndrome of cauda equina compression is produced by massive herniation with posterior longitudinal ligament rupture, direct posterior central herniation and compression of cauda with correspondent clinical manifestation.

Clinical presentation of LS disk herniation is recurrent lumbar pain (lumbago) usually following effort and certain movements. In discus hernia pain is located in the lumbar region, irradiating to the hip, sheen and to the toes. Pain is exacerbated by a movement and effort. Hypersensitivity of the processus spinosus nearby herniated disc and painful points along ischiatic nerve. Tests of elongation of the ischiatic nerve, including Lasseque (Lazarević) test, are positive.

Paresthesia or hypoesthesia of the toe suggest L5 lesion and L4-L5 disk herniation. If the outer part of the foot and the smallest toe are affected, the S1 lesion and L5-S1 disk herniation are suspected. Achilles reflex is usually absent.

Motor signs are present in a form of the spasm of paravertebral muscles at the level of the damaged disc and subsequent marked scoliosis. Flexibility of the lumbar spine is limited and gluteal hypotonia, or sometimes in the entire leg, could be observed. Motor root impairment could cause insufficiency of the plantar or dorsal flexion of the toes and foot.

Intervertebral disk herniation between L3 and L4 or L2 and L3 can cause decreased patellar reflex and motor force, hypotonia and hypotrophy of the quadriceps muscle.

Medial discus hernia at this level can cause syndrome of cauda equina, perianogenital hyposensibility, as well along the medial and posterior side of the thigh, like riding. Paresthesia, pain and hypoesthesia can affect lumbar area and leg. Motor root compression causes weakness of the leg muscles and muscular areflexia. Sphincter function can be disturbed as well.

Typical (but not obligatory) clinical manifestation for respective disk herniation level are:

L3-L4 disk herniation:
- pain along anterior thigh,
- hypotrophy of the quadriceps muscle,
- weakness of the quadriceps function and dorsiflexion of the foot,
- hyposensibility of the anterior thigh and medial sheen,
- decreased patellar reflex.

L4-L5 discus hernia:
- pain along the posterior or posterolateral side of the thigh with irradiation to the dorsum of the foot and toe,
- insufficiency of the dorsiflexion of the foot and toe,
- occasional reflex impairment.

L5-S1 discus hernia:
- pain along the posterior surface of the leg irradiation to the plantar portion of the foot,
- plantar flexion insufficiency,
- hyposensibility of the outer foot,
- absent Achilles reflex.

Electromyography (EMG) is neurophysiologic diagnostic method for evaluation of the electrical potentials in muscles, i.e. detection of the motor neuron lesions. Decreased conduction velocity in peripheral nerves is typical for neuropathies. This method of the examination of the nerve conduction velocity, along with neuroradiological visualization of the discus hernia can define morphology and degree of the nerve damage precisely.

b) Neuroradiological examination

Neuroradiologic examination, along with clinical and EMG findings, can reveal the level of discus hernia and degree of the radicular or medullar impairment. They tend to assess morphology of the pathologic lesions of vertebral bony structures and disc, elongation or rupture of the longitudinal posterior ligament and relationship of discus hernia and intrathecal liquor space, medulla spinalis or spinal nerve roots. Neuroradiologic imaging should determine adequate conservative or surgical treatment.

Neuroradiologic examinations for discus hernia consists of classic radiographs, myelography and CT scan.

Classic radiographs (AP, LL, semioblique, special and polytomography) enable visualization of the spinal vertebrae damaged by degeneration and trauma, as well as abnormal position of the vertebrae (solitary or in segments). Change of physiologic curves due to spasm of paravertebral muscles is of utmost importance.

Myelography is an indirect method of visualization of the defects in subdural spinal space filled with hydrosoluble iodine contrast. Neurologic diagnosis of discus hernia could be supported by an indirectly shown defect in intrathecal contrast propagation, thus inducing conservative or surgical treatment according to the features of lesion. Myelographic display of the nerve roots (radiculography) can determine the degree of radicular compression upon the appearance of perineural space filled with iodine contrast, in a form of dislocation, spinal root amputation, etc.

Myelography provides for sufficient information on discus hernia in the cervical, thoracic and lumbosacral spine. Lesions of the cervico-thoracic junction and thoracic segment in obese patients are poorly displayed because of summation effect and artifacts of the massive bones and soft tissues.

Disadvantage of the myelography is its invasiveness and painful puncture, inability to get the contrast in all desired segments and perineural space of all spinal nerve roots and inability to display disc, *ligamentum longitudinale posterior* and tissue qualities of the compromised medulla spinalis.

CT scan is an outstanding method (an ideal combination is **myelo scan**) for direct visualization of bone structures of spinal vertebrae and discs, their relationship with medulla spinalis, dural sac of L-S segment and spinal nerve roots. Computerized tomography perfectly displays calcified fragments of discus hernia, as well as degenerative changes of the vertebrae (osteofits, etc). CT examination is complementary to the neurologic and functional EMG examination for the diagnosis of discus hernia, and it is usually sufficient for definitive diagnosis.

Disadvantages of CT examination are numerous artifacts caused by X-ray examination and overlapping of the vertebral bones, ribs, sternum, clavicles, etc. in the cervico-thoracic and thoracic spinal segments. Postcompressive and posttraumatic myelopathies and myelomalacia of medulla spinalis caused by a compression affect of discus hernia are poorly displayed.

c) Magnetic Resonance Imaging

c-1 General remarks

MR is the most precise and most expensive method for the diagnosis of disk herniation. In the University Clinical Center in Belgrade it is indicated for undefined and uncertain diagnosis of disks herniation or if myelopathy/myelomalacia is suspected.

MR examination is a superb method for the diagnosis of disk herniation of the cervico-thoracic junction, thoracic segment in obese patients to avoid artifacts and for differential diagnosis of the spatio-compressive processes of different etiology. Superior contrast resolution and multiplanar view are additional advantage of MR over CT.

MR should be indicated for the diagnosis of discus hernia only after X-ray plane, myelography or CT scan have been done.

c-2 Examination technique and sequences

Technique of MR examination for all spinal segments is basically the same and use of additional planes and special sequences can make a difference. **Helmholz** coil is ideal for the cervical spine examination, whereas oval spinal coils are used to improve resolution in thoracic and LS segments. If examination of the whole spine is requested, **"body"** coil should be used. Recent models of ARRAY coils could encompass practically the whole spine at once (2).

Spin Echo 500/15 and Spin Echo (SE 2000/90/15) are used. Special rapid sequences TSE, FLASH and FISP are used to display the disc tissue, calcifications (spondylotic lesions), blood, etc. Myelo MR sequences are used as well (14).

Slice thickness is 2,3 up to 4 mm. Slice distance is 0.1 - 0.2 Sagittal, coronal and axial views are used. Paraxial planes are used depending on the physiologic and pathologic curves of the spine.

Paramagnetic contrast is rarely used, because it does not enhance signal in disk herniation, so that it is only needed for the differential diagnosis.

Discus hernia has specific signal intensities in various MR sequences.

c-3 MR of normal anatomy structures

In patients under 20 *nucleus pulposus* contains 85-90% of water, but it is reduced to 70% with aging. *Annulus fibrosus* has 78% water contents, which is reduced to 70% in elder. It is difficult to define *annulus fibrosus* from *nucleus pulposus* in MR image.

The normal disc has medium signal intensity in SE 500/15 sequence. Low signal intensity (stripe form) surrounding discus is caused by a *corticalis* of vertebral bodies, partly by *annulus fibrosus* and "chemical shift" artifact. Joint mass of *nucleus pulposus* and *annulus fibrosus* has average signal intensities in SE 500/15 (3).

In SE 2000/90 sequence *nucleus pulposus* has higher signal intensities, whereas *annulus fibrosus* in peripheral zone has low signal intensities. MR tomographs in sagittal view shows a stripe of low signal intensity in the middle of the disc, corresponding to normal invagination of *annulus fibrosus* into the *nucleus pulposus*. Behind the disc there is *ligamentum longitudinale posterior* with low signal intensity. Liquor in the spinal canal has the same signal intensity as in the ventricular system of brain.

High signal intensity of anterior epidural vein caused by **"flow effect"** should be recognized in SE 500/15 sequence. Epidural fat, dorsal to the vertebral bodies, has high signal intensities in all sequences.

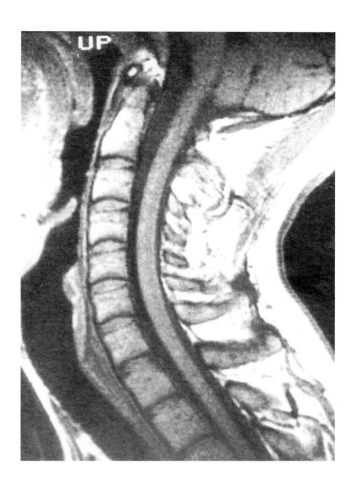

Figure 311. Cervical spine and spinal cord. Sagittal image (SE 500/15). Normal image.

Nerve roots have low signal intensities in axial MR tomographs in SE 2000/90 sequence. Perineural space, filled with liquor, has high signal intensities (11).

It is important to display spinal nerve roots in case of dorsolateral and lateral discus herniae (Figg. 311-316).

c-4 MRI of disk herniation

MR diagnosis of disk herniation should determine whether there is a protrusion (usually reversible) or prolapse with complete rupture of the *annulus fibrosus* and *ligamentum longitudinale posterior* (irreversible process).

In disc protrusion dorsal bulging of *annulus fibrosus* and *nucleus pulposus* with ligament deviation (low signal intensity) towards intrathecal cerebrospinal fluid (high signal intensity) is seen in SE 2000/90 sequence (8). Liquor, medulla spinalis and nerve roots are well demarcated in this sequence in axial and sagittal views (10). Morphology details of the disc, medulla spinalis and vertebral bony structures are best seen in SE 500/15 sequence (Figg. 317, 318).

Relationship of discus hernia and dural sac is best displayed in MR tomographs in SE 2000/90/15 (Fig. 319).

Nerve roots and their relationship with discus hernia, in case of a lateral discus hernia, are shown in axial view in SE 500/15, and especially in SE 2000/90 sequence.

Acute disk herniation has signal intensities like the "rest" of the disc, whereas the chronic one has reduced signal intensities in all applied sequences, due to the reduction of the water contents and degenerative changes. Calcifications have extremely low signal intensities.

Disc prolapse (higher signal intensities), with intact posterior longitudinal ligament (low signal intensity), is demarcated in SE 2000/90 sequence and clearly defined from the liquor space (high signal intensity), medulla spinalis (medium signal intensities) and spinal nerve roots (medium to low signal

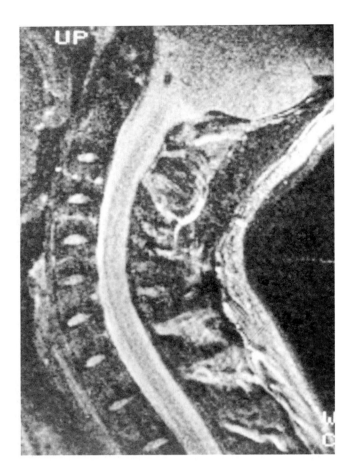

Figure 312. Cervical spine and spinal cord. Sagittal image (SE 2000/90). Normal image.

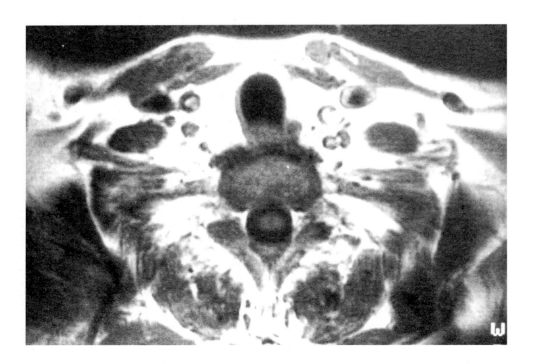

Figure 313. Cervical spine and spinal cord. Axial image (SE 500/15). Normal image.

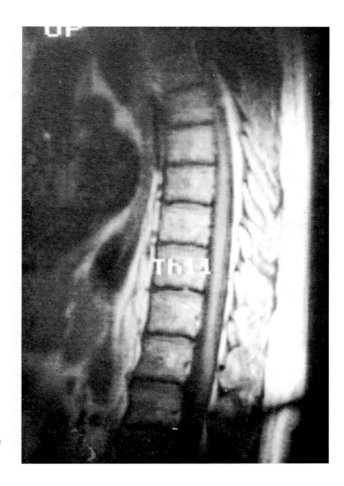

Figure 314. Thoracic spine and spinal cord. Sagittal image (SE 500/15). Normal image.

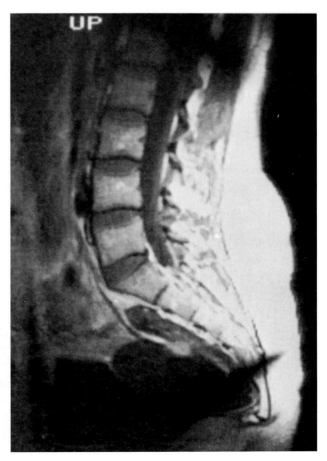

Figure 315. Lumbar spine. Sagittal image (SE 500/15). Normal image.

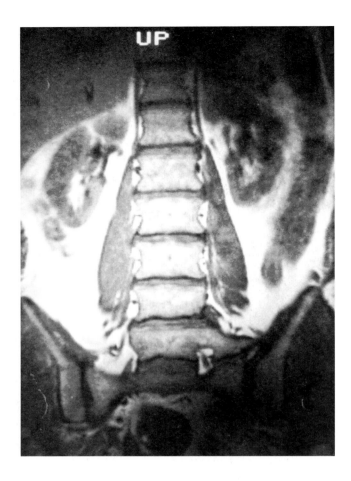

Figure 316. Lumbar spine. Sagittal image (SE 500/15). Normal image.

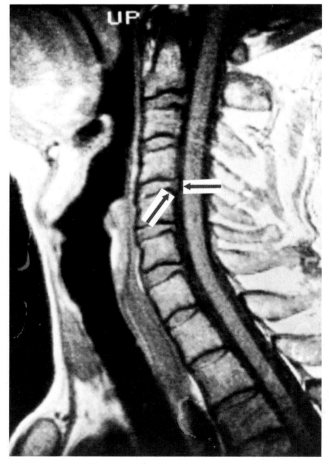

Figure 317. Cervical spine and spinal cord. Sagittal image (SE 500/15). Discus hernia C4-C5 - protrusion - arrows.

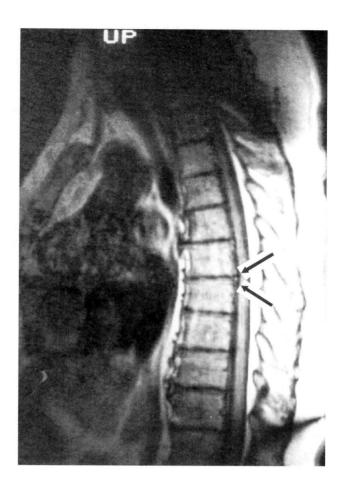

Figure 318. Thoracic spine and spinal cord. Sagittal image (SE 500/15). Discus hernia Th6-Th7 - protrusion - arrows.

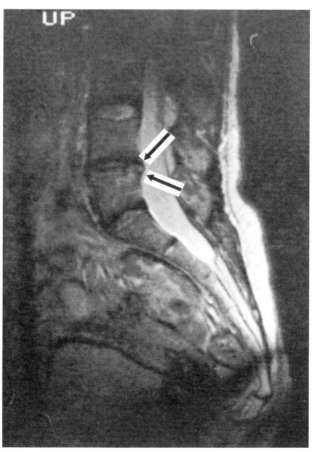

Figure 319. Lumbar spine. Sagittal image (SE 2000/90). Discus hernia - protrusion - arrows.

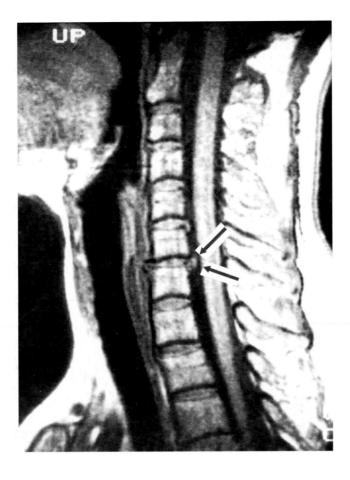

Figure 320. Cervical spine and spinal cord. Sagittal image (SE 500/15). Discus hernia C6-C7 - prolapse - arrows. Discus hernia C5-C6 - protrusion.

intensities, surrounded by perineural space filled with hyperintensive liquor).

Magnetic resonance imaging in disc prolapse with ruptured posterior longitudinal ligament shows disc particles within spinal canal in epidural space (9).

Spondylotic calcification and calcified portions of the disc, in a form of prolapse, are hard to confirm by MRI and special sequences should be used (13). Additional results obtained by classic radiography, myelography or CT examination contribute to the precise interpretation of the complex lesions of bone and soft tissues of the spinal structures (Figg. 320-323).

Compressive effect of the prolapsed discus hernia can cause myelomalacia, shown in SE 2000/90 by higher signal intensities (Fig. 324).

Decision on indications for surgical treatment of cervical discus hernia is specially delicate because of the risk of further neurologic deterioration (4).

Anterior or anterolateral approach is indicated for medial and mediolateral prolapse, because of the reduced risk of the neurologic damage. Surgery, through the anterior cervical approach, should remove the damaged disc and replace it with a bone graft.

Posterior access is successful in treatment of the lateral disc prolapse. Posterior access is exclusively used for the decompression (laminectomy and foraminectomy) in treatment of polydiscopathy with marked degenerative changes.

Apart from the other diagnostic methods clinical appearance and neurologic finding are still the basic parameters for the surgical indications in lumbar discus hernia. Absolute indication for the surgery, based on the clinical course, are:

Massive prolapse with cauda equina syndrome (motor weakness, sensory impairment, sphincter disorders). Surgery should be done immediately, preferably in the first 24 hours of the syndrome onset.

In case of isolated neurologic deficit - muscle weakness in LS innervation area (peroneus) or S1 (tibialis) with radiographically proven discus hernia, emergency surgery is indicated as well.

In younger patients without degenerative changes or motor deficit, if the severe pain is present, surgery should be done, whereas in other cases conservative treatment should be attempted.

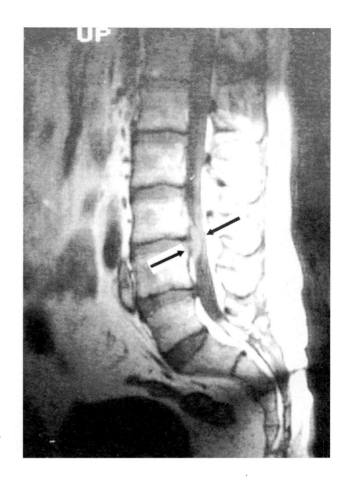

Figure 321. Lumbar spine. Sagittal image (SE 500/15). Discus hernia L3-L4 - prolapse - arrows. Discus hernia L4-L5 - protrusion.

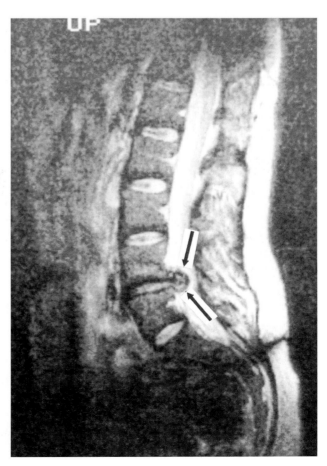

Figure 322. Lumbar spine. Sagittal image (SE 2000/90). Discus hernia L4-L5 - prolapse - arrows.

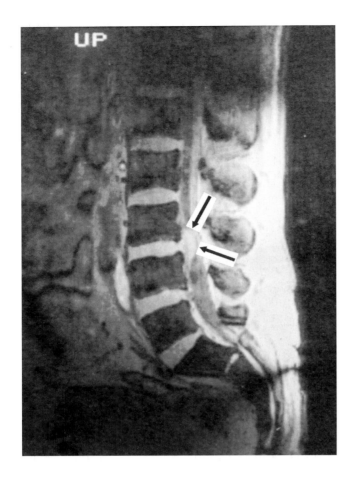

Figure 323. Lumbar spine. Sagittal image (FA 50, TR 19, TE 7). Discus hernia L4-L5 - prolapse - arrows.

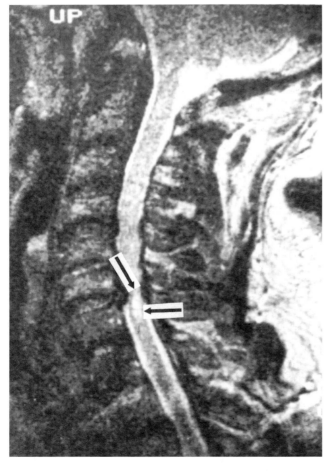

Figure 324. Cervical spine and spinal cord. Sagittal image (SE 2000/90). Discus hernia C6-C7 dorsomedialis cum myelopathy - arrows.

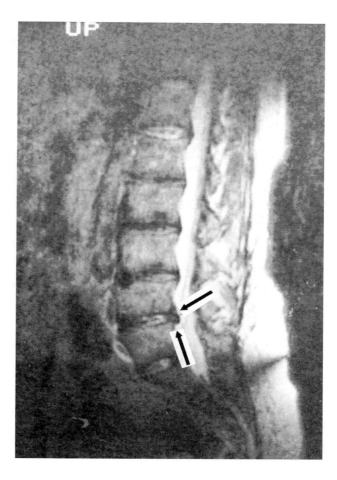

Figure 325. Lumbar spine. Sagittal image (SE 2000/90). Residual/recurrent discus hernia L4-L5 - arrows.

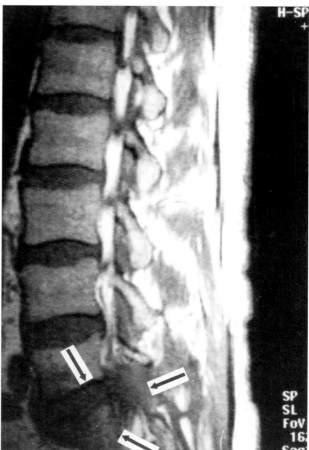

Figure 326. Lumbar spine. Sagittal image (TSE 600/12). Discitis post operationem reg. L5-S1 - arrows.

Nowadays, there are four basic operations for the treatment of lumbar discus hernia:

Classic laminectomy or its modification, partial unilateral, so called interhemilaminectomy, is still the most frequent operation. In younger patients removal of the ligamentum flavum without removal of any bone is usually sufficient. Once the prolapsed disc is removed, foraminotomy should be done to decompress respective nerve root in the bone canal.

Microsurgery, based on the same principles, enables better visualization and minimal bone removal.

Percutaneous discectomy, through posterolateral or lateral approach, is a closed method, using special instruments and pertaining increased risk of the damage. It is usually used for the disc protrusion.

Chemonucleolysis is a chemical method of disc destruction with certain enzymes (chymopapain, chymodiactin).

c-5 MRI controls

MR controls are seldom indicated during conservative treatment, because functional methods (EMG) and neurologic findings are crucial indicators of the therapy effects and cure.

MR is indicated in surgically treated discus hernia, if a recurrence is suspected upon the objective deterioration of patients condition, residual or progressive neurologic sequels or marked subjective symptoms or to evaluate working capacity of a patient. Beside neurologic finding, clinical finding and functional analyses, preoperative MR image and detailed description of the surgery are of utmost importance. Control classic radiographs and CT examination are obligatory.

MR control could be done at least 6 weeks following surgery. It takes 6 weeks to heal the wound, resorb the blood collection, reduce edema, etc. (7, 12).

Technique of the MR control is identical to the initial examination, but additional views could be used depending on the surgical technique and complete condition of the tissue in the operated area (Fig. 325).

Discitis in the operated area is one of the postoperative complications. Severe pain, gait inability and neurologic deficit are the indication for MR control (Fig. 326).

REFERENCES

1. Awad EE., Martin DS., Swith KRJ., Baker BK.: Asymptomatic versus symptomatic herniated thoracic disk. Frequency and characteristics as detected by computed tomography after myelography. Neurosurgery, 28: 180-186, 1991.
2. Berger PE., et al.: High resolution surface coil magnetic resonance imaging of the spine: normal and pathologic anatomy. Radiographics, 6: 573-588, 1986.
3. Chafetz N., Genant HK., Moon KC.: Recognition of lumbar disc herniation with NMR. AJR, 141: 153-166, 1986.
4. Han JS., Enson JE., Yoon YS.: Magnetic resonance imaging in the spinal column and craniovertebral junction. Radiol. Clin. North Am., 22: 805-822, 1986.
5. Hardy RW., Ir.: Lumbar Disk disease. Raven Press. New York. 1982.
6. Houser OW., et al.: Cervical disk prolapse Mayo Clin. Proc., 70: 939-945, 1995.
7. Hueftle MG., et al.: Lumbar spine: postoperative MR imaging with Gd-DTPA. Radiology, 167: 817-823, 1988.
8. Modic MT., et al.: Nuclear magnetic resonance imaging of the spine. Radiology, 148: 757-766, 1983.
9. Modic MT, et al.: Lumbar herniated disc disease and canal stenosis: prospective evaluation by surface coil MR, CT and myelography. AJNR, 7: 709-722, 1986.
10. Modic MT., et al.: Magnetic resonance imaging of intervertebral disk disease. Radiology, 152: 103-118, 1984.
11. Reicher MA., et al.: MR imaging of the lumbar spine: anatomic correlations and the effects of technical variations. AJNR, 147: 891-907, 1986.
12. Ross JS., et al.: Lumbar spine: postoperative assessment with surface-coil MR imaging. Radiology, 164: 851-862, 1987.
13. Takahashi M., Yamashita Y., Sakamoto Y., Kojima R.: Chronic cervical cord compression: clinical significance of increased signal intensity on MR images. Radiology, 173: 219-229, 1989.
14. Van Dyk C., et al.: Gradient echo MR imaging of the cervical spine: evaluation of extradural degenerative disease. AJNR, 10: 627-633, 1989.

VIII. MR ANGIOGRAPHY OF THE SPINE

Gradimir Dragutinović, Vaso Antunović, Miodrag Rakić

MR angiography of the spinal blood vessels is rarely done. Special sequences (FLASH and FISP, etc) enable visualization of AVM. Successful diagnosis depends on location and size of the pathologic lesions. MR angiography, using 3D and MIP localization of AVM, is still limited by artifacts (1-4).

If the vascular pathology in the spinal canal is suspected, MRA is done, but if it is negative, classic angiography should be performed (Fig. 327).

Future development of MRA software should provide for safer diagnosis and precise information of smaller spinal blood vessels (5).

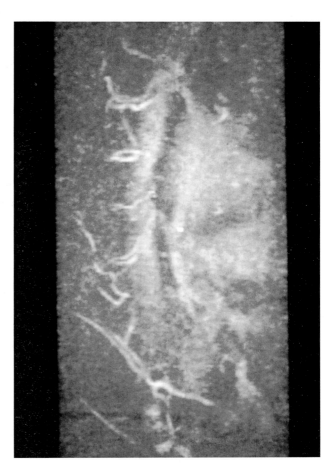

Figure 327. Thoracic spine - MR angiography.

REFERENCES

1. Dumoulin CL., et al.: Three-dimensional phase contrast angiography. Magn. Reson. Med., 9: 139-152, 1989.
2. Keller PJ., et al.: MR angiography with twodimensional acquisition and three-dimensional display. Radiology, 173: 527-536, 1989.
3. Marchal G., et al.: Intracranial vascular lesions: optimization and clinical evaluation of the 3D time of flight MR angiography. Radiology, 175: 443-452, 1990.
4. Masaryk TJ., et al.: Intracranial circulation: prelimanary clinical results with three-dimensional (volume) MR angiography. Radiology, 171: 793-802, 1989.
5. Spetzler RF., et al.: A proposed grading system for arteriovenous malformations. J. Neurosurg., 65: 476-483, 1986.

IX. POSTOPERATIVE CHANGES AND CONTROLS

Miodrag Rakić, Gradimir Dragutinović, Branislav Nestorović

Magnetic resonance control examinations are used for the assessment of the various lesions, during and after conservative, surgical or radiotherapy. Indications for MR controls should be restricted and made with utmost selectivity, because of the high cost and limited capacity of MR machine.

Clinical appearance depends on the type, location and other features of the pathologic lesion, but deterioration of neurologic deficit following surgery or radiotherapy should be considered always. Interdisciplinary consultation of neuroradiologist, neurosurgeon, neurologist and oncologist is indispensable for optimal timing of MR controls.

Initial MR examination of spinal lesion is important for recognition of the lesion qualities. If the control MR examination is the first one, it is difficult to interpret the results. Complete neuroradiologic file is requested for such cases.

Before commencing MR examination, neuroradiologist should become familiar with images and written description of radiography, myelopgraphy and CT scan. Radiologist, performing MR examination, should be fully trained to perform and interpret all of neuroradiologic examinations. Thus he would be able to make his own diagnosis, re-evaluate possible wrong assessment and rule out false positive or false negative results of previous neuroradiologic examinations.

If there is no improvement after the medical therapy, regarding neurologic and clinical findings, MR control is indicated.

MR control should be done using identical sequences, views and slice thickness and distance, with eventual use of the i.v. paramagnetic contrast (5, 6). Additional administration of the paramagnetic contrast, that has not been used during the first examination, could be required upon the clinical and neurologic findings and pathoanatomy of the lesion.

Number of MR controls should be limited and indications based on the knowledge and on the nature of the disease and effects of therapy. MR control should not be done if the multiplication of the known lesion have occurred, because the treatment will remain unchanged.

MR diagnostic is needed to reach the diagnosis and determine effective and properly timed treatment (1).

Postoperative and postirradiation MR controls are seldom indicated. MR imaging in neurosurgically treated patient should be done if the neurologic sequels are beyond expectations, in case of postoperative complications or partial reduction of the expansive lesions in order to assess further expansion of the tumor, etc. (2, 3, 4).

Indication and justification for MR controls are shown in following examples of postoperatively observed patients.

MR control following surgery have revealed big recurrent meningioma, in patient P.K, aged 46, with complete removal of the meningioma in the dural sac, at L2-L3 level, several months ago. Meningioma involving entire dural sac and big cystic postoperative defect, filled with liquor, are seen in the sagittal view (SE 500/15) with i.v administration of paramagnetic contrast and slice thickness of 3mm.

MR control have confirmed the necessity of the reapportion, i.e. removal of the benign residual-recurrent meningioma (Fig. 328).

Patient V.O., aged 66, operated for paraganglioma of *cauda equina* have developed deterioration of the clinical course with *paraparesis flaccida* and *incontinentio alvi et urinae* three months following surgery.

MR control in sagittal view (SE 500/15) after gadolinium-DTPA administration have ruled out residual or recurrent tumor. However, multiple cystic formations, with the biggest one communicating with dural sac and being filled with liquor, are found in the projection of the operative field. Two of subcutaneous cystic formations have expansive nature and cause the bulging of the skin in the lumbar area (Fig. 329).

Complete MR image determines the future treatment of the operated patient.

Neurologic deterioration was observed in a patient T.M., aged 50, five months after complete removal

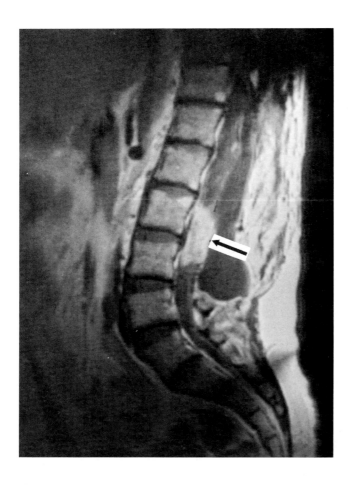

Figure 328. Lumbar spine. Sagittal image (SE 500/15) after gadolinium-DTPA administration. Residual-recurrent meningioma - arrow.

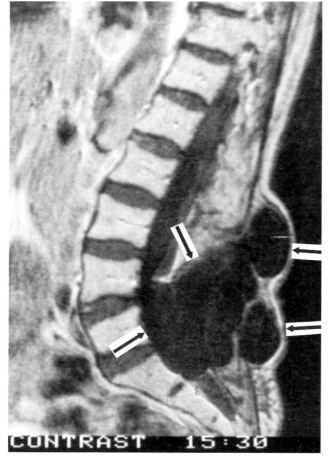

Figure 329. Lumbar spine. Sagittal image (SE 500/15) after gadolinium-DTPA administration. Postoperative cysts - arrows.

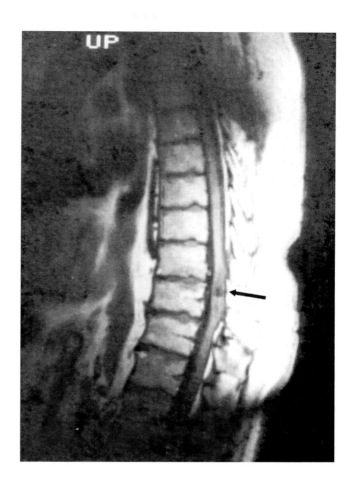

Figure 330. Thoracic spine. Sagittal image (SE 500/15). Myelomalacia postoperative - Cystis intramedullaris reg. thoracalis - arrow.

of the extradural neurinoma with caseous mass, located at Th 10- Th 11. Paraparesis spastica inferior have developed thus making indication for MR control.

Patient did not have preoperative MR examination, so that we had no idea on the preoperative appearance of the tumor or its compressive effect to the medulla spinalis.

MR control in sagittal view (SE 500/15) have ruled out residual or recurrent extradural spatio-compressive process. Cystic cavity is found inside medulla spinalis at Th10-Th11 level, surrounded by hypointensive zone of myelopathy/myelomalacia (Fig. 330).

Etiology of the cyst and surrounding myelopathy/myelomalacia, causing neurologic deficit in a form of inferior spastic paraparesis, could be explained either by previous preoperative compression effect of extradural neurinoma or by intraoperative trauma of respective segment of medulla spinalis.

MR controls in radiotherapy are indicated either for the evaluation of the therapy effect or to correct the radiation field if needed. In patients with clinical deterioration and progressive neurologic deficit, MR is indicated to detect possible irradiation lesions.

Generally speaking, MR controls during or following conservative, radiation or surgical treatment, should be done twice or eventually three times per year.

REFERENCES

1. Heindel W., et al.: Artifacts in MR imaging after surgical intervention. J. Comput. Assist. Tomogr., 10: 596-607, 1986.
2. Hueftle MG., et al.: Lumbar spine: postoperative MR imaging with Gd-DTPA. Radiology, 167: 817-828, 1988.
3. Maas R., et al.: Value of MR imaging with Gd-DTPA for differentiation of scar and reprolapse after lumbar disc operations. Radiology, 161: 309-321, 1986.
4. Ramsey RG., Zachrias CE.: MR imaging of the spine after radiation therapy: easily recognizable effects. AJNR, 6: 247-255, 1985.
5. Ross JS., et al.: Lumbar spine: postoperative assessment with surface-coil MR imaging. Radiology, 164: 851-866, 1987.
6. Ross JS., et al.: MR imaging of the postoperative lumbar spine: assessment with Gd-DTPA. AJNR, 11: 771-786, 1990.

INDEX

Typesetting and printed by Arti Grafiche Italo Cernia - Casoria (Na-Italy)

September 2001